Disease Ecology

'The microbe is nothing; the terrain everything.'
Pasteur, on his death-bed

'Marriages, Babies dead, Broken lives, Men gone mad,
Labour and crime, All treated in bulk, with the tears
wiped off.'
Helen Wilson

'I recall a particularly lovely evening in early summer when I climbed alone to the top of one of our noble hills . . . And as I watched the evening train creeping up the valley with pauses at our three stations, I had this strange thought, that there was hardly a man woman or child in all those villages of whom I did not know even the Christian name and with whom I was not on terms of friendship. My wife and I say we know nearly all the dogs and indeed many of the cats. Now, does not this intimate knowledge of this flock put the country doctor in a superior strategic position for the study of such a topic as epidemic disease?'
Dr William Pickles of Wensleydale, 1948, an exemplar

Disease Ecology

An Introduction

Andrew Learmonth

Basil Blackwell

First published 1988

Basil Blackwell Ltd
108 Cowley Road, Oxford, OX4 1JF, UK

Basil Blackwell Inc.
432 Park Avenue South, Suite 1503
New York, NY 10016, USA

British Library Cataloguing in Publication Data

Learmonth, Andrew
  Disease ecology: an introduction
  1. Epidemiology
  I. Title
  614.4   RA651

  ISBN 0–631–14855–8
  ISBN 0–631–15799–9 Pbk

Library of Congress Cataloging in Publication Data
Learmonth, A. T. A. (Andrew Thomas Amos), 1916–
  Disease ecology.

  Includes index.
  1. Medical geography.   2. Environment induced
diseases. I. Title. [DNLM: 1. Ecology. 2. Epidemiology.
3. Geography. WB 700 L438d]
RA792.L4   614.4′2   87–11768
ISBN 0–631–14855–8
ISBN 0–631–15799–9 Pbk

Typeset in 10 on 12 point Plantin
by Photo·Graphics, Honiton, Devon, England
Printed in Great Britain by T.J. Press Ltd, Padstow, Cornwall, England

Contents

Preface

For a geographer to write under the title *Disease ecology: an introduction* may call for explanation, especially in view of Barrett's 1986 statement, forthright and authoritative, that 'disease ecology is a branch of ecology and not geography.' This book flows from almost forty years of commitment to this borderland study, and it is the ecological viewpoint that I would most like to see young medical geographers taking seriously while still applying geographical techniques of analysis and synthesis. One aim, then, is to introduce them to the huge biomedical literature bearing on this most interdisciplinary of fields. If other readers, from for example epidemiology, community medicine and the caring professions, find interest in geography's contribution, I shall feel particularly rewarded.

Some undergraduate geographers will be studying medical geography as an option chosen from the range of courses available to them, while others may be curious about the impact of health and disease on the quality of life as an aspect of population geography, social geography, welfare geography or – less probably but by no means inappropriately – political geography. In language and concepts the main 'story-line' should be available to interested young people in the later years of school and in technical colleges. The list of references at the end is long, and even so is inevitably selective and in this field one can never be up-to-date; my anxiety has been to stress that workers in more than a few sister disciplines are writing on themes that bear on disease ecology, their contributions far outnumbering those from the still comparatively few medical geographers. My aim has been to provide at least entry points into the literature across a broad spectrum, for students of geography and perhaps other social sciences too. Entry points have not specifically been provided on the philosophy and epistemology of disease ecology or medical geography, though readers interested in these important themes will find at least some in works cited for other reasons. There are glimpses of the post-war history of the field, but for earlier periods interested readers should refer to the continuing series of papers by Barrett, starting with his intriguingly titled 'Medical geography as a foster child' (1980);

and there are valuable countrywise accounts in the pages of *Geographia Medica*.

The bulk of the present book was written between January 1985 and October 1986, with selective updating to July 1987. Many people have helped me in writing it, including the librarians of the Open University and the University of Liverpool, the Liverpool School of Tropical Medicine and the London School of Hygiene and Tropical Medicine. *Dorland's Illustrated Medical Dictionary* and *the Penguin Medical Encyclopedia* (Wingate 1972) have been constant companions, as have the *Tropical Diseases Bulletin and Abstracts on Hygiene*. I owe a particular debt to John Davey and other staff of Basil Blackwell and their medical referee.

Many authors and publishers have been most generous in allowing me to use their material, particularly maps and diagrams. I am heavily in their debt and extremely grateful. There are too many to list here, but the figure captions and quotations include references to the works concerned, full details of which are given in the References at the end of the book. The quotation from Currey on pp. 284–5 is copyright © 1984 by D. Reidel Publishing Company, Durdrecht, Holland. Figure 15.6 is reproduced by permission of the author and publishers, copyright © Harwood Academic Publishers GmBh. Figures 8.1, 8.2, 10.3 and 14.3 are reproduced by permission of the Open University. Most of the cartography is by John Hunt of the Open University. Mrs June Matthews of Penmachno has typed from a manuscript that ranged from the difficult to the impossible; help and facilities were provided by Gwawr Dafydd of Bys a Bawd, Gwasanaeth Swyddfa, Llanrwst. My wife Nancy has helped in time of need even though it is a field of geography that she dislikes, and has also forgone much of my company these many months.

1 Introduction: One World or Three to a Pathogen?

A Geography of Disease?

Even before answering the question in the chapter title, it may be as well to ask 'Is there a geography of health and disease?' And if there is, can professional geographers contribute to its study, as individuals or as members of a research team? The answer to the second question is the theme of this book as a whole, but the first perhaps requires an answer right at the outset, and an example may serve better than abstract argument.

The *Treponema*: Yaws and Syphilis

Figure 1.1 is from one of two complementary world atlases of disease (May 1950–55; Rodenwaldt and Jusatz 1952–61); it deals with the world pattern of a group of related skin infections, caused by bacteria, spiral in shape and so grouped with the spirochaetes by biologists; the genus causing these infections has been given the name *Treponema* (from the Greek 'turning thread'). It will suit this introductory argument to concentrate for the moment on yaws. This is a serious skin disease involving disfiguring, often crippling lesions especially of the limbs (for recent work on yaws in Ghana, for instance, see Osei 1981, *WER* 1982a). For many geographers, a main task is to study and correlate areal distribution patterns, and to identify both comparable tracts where common causes may be at work, and unique areas with a particular complex of charactcristics or problems; granting this, there does seem to be a geography of yaws. There is a marked concentration in the humid tropics, but especially in Africa. While hot and humid climates favour the organism, its spread from person to person is made easier if people's clothing pattern leaves much bare skin and if the limbs are exposed to

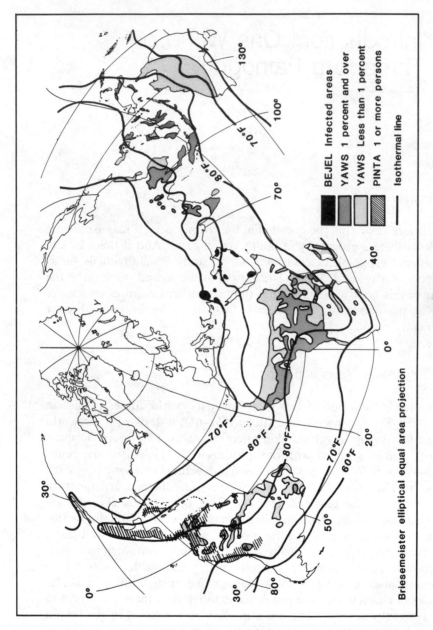

Briesemeister elliptical equal area projection

Figure 1.1 World map of some non-venereal treponemal infections (yaws, bejel and pinta)
Source: May (1950–55)

cutting and jagging vegetation while walking or working. (Viral hepatitis B has been similarly transmitted between fell-runners in Scandinavia – Vellar 1964.) Climate, vegetation and patterns of human work and movement are all involved with the adaptation of a particular organism, in this case the species of *Treponema* known as *T. pertenue*. (*Note*: Where it is readily seen which genus is being discussed the biologists' convention will be used, as here, contracting the generic name to an initial and adding the species or specific name.) Comparable but differing ecological complexes apply to the other diseases mapped in figure 1.1. However, there are other species in the same genus: some occupy ecological niches in the human mouth, and some of these are apparently commensal – that is, living with the host (literally sharing the same table), deriving and sometimes giving benefit but causing no harm; in contrast at least one of these mouth 'germs' is a suspected pathogen, possibly causing gum disease. It may give perspective to consider that the new-born baby builds up a load of bacterial flora, normally of course commensal, some acquired via the umbilical cord but much from the environment starting within hours of birth and very varied within a week according to Rotimi and Duerden (1981). Other species of *Treponema* live on the human skin, including the pudenda, without causing harm. Yet the closely related *T. pallidum*, difficult to distinguish from *T. pertenue* except by its behaviour, is the organism that causes syphilis, one of the classical venereal or sexually transmitted diseases – STD in many modern references to this group of infections.

However, non-venereal syphilis, attributed to *T. pallidum* rather than *T. pertenue*, is also a serious public health problem, usually contracted in childhood and in arid areas, in contrast with the humid tropical environments of yaws; under the name of *bejel*, for instance, it is an active and current problem in oil-rich Saudi Arabia (Pace 1983).

Dr May did not include venereal syphilis on his map, no doubt because it is now a universal disease, closely corresponding to the distribution of population in general pattern. It is easy to think of syphilis and the other STDs as concentrated in seaports and large cities, but in many countries it travels far and wide into rural towns, villages and farms; a map of diffusion of a particular wave of syphilis might be interesting enough, but a map of its static pattern much less so. (For a world survey of the *Treponema*, see WHO 1982 TRS 674.)

Ideas on the Evolution of Syphilis

Syphilis became known in the Old World as a specific disease in the sixteenth century. It was long believed, and many still believe, that the organism came to Europe carried by sailors with Columbus and other early navigators, who had become infected through sexual intercourse with indigenous Carib women, themselves largely or totally immune to its effects. The sailors, and later their sexual partners in Europe, Asia and Africa would have lacked immunity, hence the epidemic syphilis that travelled along lines of communication, affecting people of all social strata, from the time of Henry VIII onwards. A generation ago another theory was proposed (Cockburn 1963): that during the Renaissance more or less communal sleeping and bathing arrangements became much less common and also socially unacceptable, while a little later came more frequent washing of underclothes with the spread of cotton garments. On this argument, *Treponema* that had been able to survive very well as skin infections moving freely from person to person, evolved a specific preference for the sexual organs and for spread by sexual intercourse, causing much more harm to the human host than they had done as skin dwellers. While this theory must remain speculative, as must so much thinking about past changes in the geography of disease, it is very suggestive in accounting for the coexistence of yaws, non-venereal syphilis and venereal syphilis even within one country, as in Australia. Obviously enough historical epidemiology like this must always be speculative and controversial: a recent paper, for instance, notes that historical references to *morbus gallicus* (the disease of Gaul or France) were traditionally regarded as syphilis but may have included both endemic syphilis from North Africa and venereal syphilis from North America (Morton 1985. See also Maleville (1976), viewing endemic treponematoses as bacterial reserves; G. J. Hackett in Hart (1983) and Brothwell (1981) for the archaeologist's view of these infections). *WER* (1981a) and Perine et al. (1984) review the endemic treponematoses, and Willcox (1980) reviews the relations between them in the Pacific islands and Papua New Guinea.

It is perhaps easier for the modern reader, even of newspaper coverage of current changes in disease patterns including the diffusion across the world of 'new' STDs, to give credence to Cockburn's hypothesis, than it was when he wrote: certainly analogies suggest themselves. Twenty years ago not many people, even venereologists, would have predicted the emergence as important STDs, though arguably less serious than syphilis and gonorrhoea, of genital and anal infections by the cold sore or herpes virus, or *Chlamydia trachomatis* (discussed in chapter 9 as an eye infection). These organisms must always have been in the environment, and it seems clear that it is largely changes in sexual mores that has caused the change, offering a close analogy to Cockburn's hypothesis. On the other hand the spread of the acquired immune deficiency syndrome (AIDS), or of the causal virus known as HIV I, appears at present to resemble actual worldwide diffusion of a 'new' disease (see also chapter 2).

Malaria: Map Interpretation and Ecology

Figures 1.2 and 1.3 make the point that there is a geography of disease in a different way (Bentley 1916). Figure 1.2 is a 'contour map' of malaria in (undivided) Bengal about 1911, showing generally high rates in West Bengal and on the whole low rates in East Bengal (now Bangladesh). This was ascribed at the time to the flushing of water-channels in the east by the powerful sheet-floods from the combined waters of Ganga (Ganges) and Brahmaputra during the monsoon rains, but much later the role became clear of a breeding preference of the main local vector mosquito *Anopheles philippinensis* for still water for egg-laying and larval production, not heavily polluted, with rather a low water-table and a moderate (but not light-excluding) growth of aquatic plants. Figure 1.2 shows population increase 1901–11, high in the less malarious area in the east, low – or even decreasing – in the malarious west. The malaria and the population trends were causally linked by the early workers, on visual comparison of the maps. On the population side, too, later knowledge added to understanding that the low population increases in the west were at least broadly related to an increase in spontaneous abortions caused by malaria (indeed some other infections have similar effects) (Learmonth 1957). A geography has, I think, been demonstrated; its far-reaching social and economic effects hardly need demonstration, and a start has been made at showing the complex interactions that underlie apparently simple spatial correlations, a procedure itself carrying some statistical dangers (see chapter 4 on spatial autocorrelation).

Disease Complexes and Human Behaviour

This book links geography with disease ecology. The author was much influenced in this direction, as a young man, by May, a French medical man steeped in the medical ecology of Indo-China and then turned medical geographer with the American Geographical Society (May 1950); it might equally well have been Rodenwaldt and Jusatz in Germany (Rodenwaldt 1956; Rodenwaldt and Jusatz 1956), Shoshin (1962), in the USSR, or Audy, an English medical man whose deep ecological insights were sparked off by the problem of scrub typhus and its complex ecology, during the Burma campaign of 1943–5 (Audy 1949, 1968; see discussion in chapter 9).

The malaria reference just given will suffice meantime as an example of May's major contribution in stimulating professional geographers to

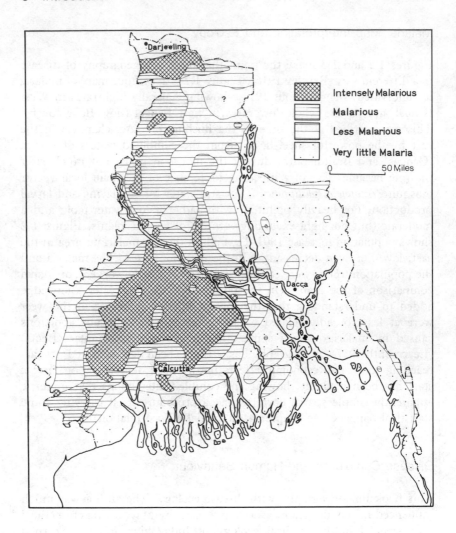

Figure 1.2   Malaria distribution in Bengal (after Bentley (1916)). Bentley used surveys of proportions of enlarged spleen in sample populations, a method suggested by Sir Ronald Ross. He then generalized these as contour maps. There are two sources of error – the statistical 'sampling error' (however careful the sample survey), and possible confusion with kala-azar which also causes enlarged spleens, but as pioneering mapping it is remarkable in itself and in Bentley's cartographic correlation with figure 1.3. *Source*: Learmonth (1957)

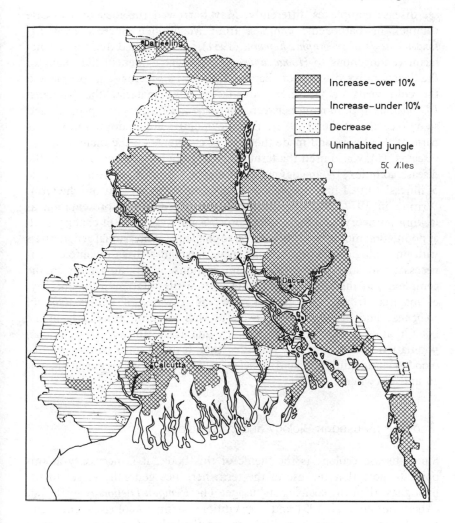

Figure 1.3 Population change in Bengal, 1901–11 (after Bentley (1916)). Bentley was able to compare his malaria map with this map of population increase (and locally decrease – almost unthinkable in modern West Bengal or Bangladesh); the Census of India has long been map-minded!
Source: Learmonth (1957)

see disease complexes differently. May borrowed the idea of a disease complex or pathogenic complex from Maximilien Sorre's great *Les fondements de la géographie humaine* (1951), and classified diseases as one-factor (endogenous to *Homo sapiens*, on present evidence, like many of the degenerative diseases of chapters 2 to 7), two-factor (e.g. people and the cold virus or viruses!), three-factor (like malaria, the pathogen *Plasmodium* spp. moving between *Anopheles* mosquitoes and people), and so on (see also Picheral 1983). This viewpoint will be adopted in various parts of this book, and made the basis of chapter 9 on the main 'tropical' diseases. (May also used the term 'geogen' for geographical factors in the disease complex, by analogy with 'pathogen' – from the Greek for 'cause of illness' – but I find the analogy faulty and try to avoid using the term. Writing in 1977, Melinda Meade has criticized May's presentation as lacking in theory, and therefore in process and neglectful of change, such as population mobility.) May went on to challenge professional geographers with an ecological viewpoint: that to understand a disease complex it is necessary to study the ecological interactions of all the factors in the complex, and therefore to be able to look at the total environment, say, of malaria, from the points of view, as it were, of *Plasmodium*, of *Anopheles* and of people. It may be as well to admit thus early in the book that of these the most complex and least studied is the human population and its myriad activities that bring it into contact with a blood-seeking adult female *Anopheles* – a theme that will recur in chapter 10 and elsewhere.

'Ecology' as used in Biology and in Sociology

Since disease ecology is the theme of this book, it is necessary at this point to note that the use of the term here lies generally closer to the biologists' than the sociologists' usage. The *Penguin Dictionary of Biology* (Abercrombie et al. 1951 and later editions) defines ecology as the study of relations of animals and plants, particularly of animal and plant communities, to their surroundings, animate and inanimate. Given that *Homo sapiens* is an animal species, disease ecology on this definition would be a facet of the total ecology that is the only correct usage to many modern biologists. The sociologists' use of the term is related to biology in that Burgess (1925), for example, described concentric zones of different socioeconomic characteristics within Chicago – and by extension as a model of the western city; he interpreted these zones using biological analogies like invasion, succession, dominance and co-dominance, and so on. Much subsequent analysis of social areas has been done using data from census enumeration districts, city wards, and other administrative units, and when a relationship between, say, an ethnic minority and high infant mortality is implicitly or explicitly inferred from such statistics, the inference is often impugned as subject to the 'ecological fallacy'. This unfortunate but now ineradicable term is a warning that grouped data probably of heterogeneous individuals may not properly be used to draw inferences about individuals within the population. (Neither, of course, is a statistical relation necessarily causal – in that example the ethnicity as such is not necessarily the cause of the high infant mortality. It is worth noting that Susser (1973) avoids the term 'ecological fallacy', preferring the much more precise 'aggregative fallacy'.)

One World or Three?

Figure 1.1 and the controversial piece of historical epidemiology of syphilis are placed at the beginning of the book for a particular reason. Much recent writing on health and disease, and about economic development too, stresses and arguably overstresses the extent to which problems differ in what is rather optimistically called the Developed World and the near-pejoratively termed Third World. The argument about the treponemal infections offers a strong, if to some bizarre, example of the fact that we do live in One World. The American statesman Wendell Wilkie spoke of One World soon after the end of the 1939–45 war, before the idea had been taken up by the ecology movement, the Limits to Growth school, or the thinkers about the North–South relations after the Brandt report. But it is also the title of a book by a distinguished physiologist and physician of tropical disease (Maegraith 1973). One strand of Maegraith's thinking concerns the speed of modern travel in relation to the import of 'exotic diseases', often unfamiliar to general practitioners, to developed countries (Maegraith 1965, 1971). This concern is now widely shared (Diesfeld 1980, 1982; Strong et al. 1982; Pène et al. 1982; Kratochvil 1983) and for a very telling survey of Scots returning from package holidays – 21 per cent had been ill, half with intestinal and half with respiratory troubles – see Cossar et al. (1983). To the venereologist it is the scale as well as the speed of modern tourist movement that is impressive (Willcox 1977).

Later chapters will bring out the greater relative importance of infectious and parasitic diseases, often carried by arthropod, including insect, vectors in the Third World, and in contrast the greater relative importance of the degenerative diseases in the Developed World. So it is all the more important to stress here the One-Worldness of the relations of humankind in health and disease to the whole environment of our globe. Universal diseases like influenza, pneumonia and measles are important in all parts of the world, though it is overwhelmingly in the Third World that they remain among the main killing diseases. As such they are as important as the diseases like malaria, yellow fever or cholera that we are apt to think of as tropical diseases even though many of them, including the three just mentioned, have been epidemic and killing diseases in the past in temperate countries, as we shall see later in the book. Moreover it has recently become clear that the 'western diseases' like heart disease, stroke and certain cancers are tending to increase sharply in Third World minority groups adopting a western life style (Trowell and Burkitt 1981). And infections remain important in developed countries, mainly as causes of morbidity rather than mortality, with some changes of 'new' infections for old to an extent (see, for instance, Velimirovic 1984).

If the two main strands in the chapter so far are interwoven – that yaws in an African rainforest community and syphilis in a Sydney suburb may have evolved from the same skin organism, and that the universal infectious diseases are just that, while the 'western diseases' are becoming much more universal, can one achieve a new world-model or world-view stressing the One-World aspect? Possibly. For one thing we may see ourselves, wherever we live, as seeking some kind of *modus vivendi*, some sort of balance, some ecological equilibrium, for as long a lifetime as is attainable and reasonable, in our own particular environment, physical and social (including life style). Perhaps we can achieve a sort of satellite view, but taking account of the distribution and movement of organisms and people, and of ideas and communication too, that escape even the miracles of modern remote sensing equipment. (For a very broad view of the relations between disease and human behaviour, in evolution and change even today, see Stanley and Joske 1980.)

A World-view: from Rocks to Ideas?

One approach to a world-view is to start from the rocks and the water, the lithosphere and the hydrosphere, then add the biosphere, the living things on land, sea and in the air (the atmosphere), from viruses, algae and bacteria to the larger plants and animals in all their variety including *Homo sapiens* – so-called, for humankind constitutes the most creative and the most destructive species of all? But we must add, too, the world of ideas, of the exchange of ideas, of communication and diffusion of ideas, that has been called the noösphere or sphere of the mind from the Greek noös (Teilhard de Chardin 1960). Clearly the geography of health involves mainly the biosphere since people are animals, in interaction with plants and with many other animal species in an ecological web –

complex even in relatively self-sufficient self-contained and immobile societies, and much more so in the modern world of long-distance trade and rapid travel. There are many relations too with the hydrosphere, both as regards the chemical content of drinking water and the many wholly or partly aquatic forms of life. But the noösphere has a part to play too. People's perception of disease varies in different societies as well as in individuals, though surely the extremes or limiting cases of health and disease must be universally perceived – birth, death, a severe fever, a crippling arthritis and so on. Human culture embraces medicine in a broad sense, covering a wide spectrum of ways of viewing and treating disease. Sociologists point out that illness implies a number of different roles in both patient and professional (doctor, witch-doctor, nurse, midwife, wise woman and so on). Health and disease are to some extent social constructs, varying in different societies and cultures – subcultures too. Many illnesses are relative to some perceived norm of what constitutes normal or what is good health. Again the extremes or limiting cases must approach the absolute – violent paroxysms in cerebral malaria or in rabies, the severe dehydration of cholera, a crippling stroke or massive heart attack can scarcely be regarded as merely mental images or social constructs (though some are arguably inevitable products of ageing). Yet the interpretation of these may vary from the very narrow search for a causal organism and a wonder drug to kill it, to an attribution to witchcraft or previous sin – or to poverty linked with the post-imperial (or neo-colonial) world economy.

All these relativities carry methodological difficulties – to be borne in mind in reading the later, more empirical and substantive chapters! Much research involves the deliberate donning of blinkers in the hope of making progress on some narrow front: thus my own studies of the spatial diffusion of malaria across India in 1965–76 are largely mechanistic though taking account of some variables from human geography, and do not cover the perception of hyperendemic malaria among tribal people in jungle tracts. A research exercise completed, it is important to recognize that one sees in part and prophesies in part!

Changing Viewpoints over Time

This relativity of health and disease has affected their study in relation to differing social and biophysical environments across the globe and over time – between historical periods as well as between cultures at some particular time period. To take only the last 150 years or so, Pasteur's penetrating intuitions and brilliant discoveries ushered in 50 or more years, perhaps almost a century in which the 'germ theory' of disease causation profoundly affected thinking even about disease *not* involving specific infection, at least on present knowledge. (For instance, *must* all mental deviation from some culture-related norm be due to a specific disease, and therefore fall within the competence of the psychiatrist?) This approach is often referred to as 'reductionist', a special sort of over-simplification that consists of offering only a single-variable explanation for a phenomenon without taking account of its complex or multi-variable causation. In the present context a reductionist approach involves the assumption that any illness must have a specific and ultimately traceable physical cause; this is justified in a research project, but not justifiable if one neglects altogether the wider societal view of the relativities, subjectivities and cultural aspects already noted. It would nowadays be almost unthinkable in a cholera campaign to include only action against the bacillus, *Vibrio cholerae*, without taking account of poor housing, personal hygiene or water supplies – and ultimately of their socioeconomic context, usually poverty.

The phase of over-dominance of the germ theory very much affected the study of the geography of disease. By the mid-nineteenth century the growth of scientific thinking had brought a strong stream of what was then called medical topography. It was most unfortunate that the great achievements of the germ theory carried with them an almost complete neglect of spatial and environmental analysis, with too little integration with ecology even though that science was growing at about the same time; too seldom were the pathogenic organisms seen in their environmental context beyond the immediate desiderata for their spread. Thus it was that after the 1939–45 war there was in a sense a fresh beginning in the field with the atlases of disease of Rodenwaldt and Jusatz, and of May, already noted, and a great expansion of applied medical geography in the USSR also. However, it is worth noting that in the Third World in the late nineteenth and early twentieth century the then colonial and tropical territories saw a continuous stream of environmental, ecological and geographical writing about disease, though seldom by geographers: there the post-Pasteur thinking was much better integrated into a broader view of disease incidence and distribution, and it seems that the intervention of arthropod or insect vectors or infections was at least one very strong underlying factor in this difference.

In both temperate and tropical countries, however, 'western' and scientific medicine became increasingly professional; in time not only doctors but also nurses, physiotherapists, radiographers, laboratory technicians, hospital and health service administrators and, more recently health educationists, became increasingly – and perhaps inevitably and rightly – subject to professional training and professional bodies with their own, doubtless legitimate, vested interests. With this tendency came a rejection of traditional medicine, and only recently in the Third World has there been some reaction to this, with moves, sometimes by governments, to combine the use of traditional healers with some scientific training. In India there are two or three main streams of traditional medicine, each with a long history and a considerable literature, and esteemed and recognized by governments since the end of colonial rule. In some countries this trend merges with the increasing use of 'barefoot doctors' following their very successful use in China since the Communist revolution there; in part this movement springs from the impossibility of meeting the demand for health care by western-trained health workers. It is worth noting that even in the USSR the universal health service provision makes considerable use of paramedical workers known as *feldshers*, and that in some western countries there is a move towards the employment of 'nurse practitioners'. In some later chapters traditional medicine will be included as an essential part of the picture of health and disease.

What *is* Health?

If illness and disease are to some extent relative matters and to an extent social constructs as the sociologists say, then health is very much more so. The International Geographical Union for many years had a Commission on Medical Geography as one of a dozen or so similar groups set up to encourage work in different fields within the discipline as a whole; it was mooted at the first post-war International Congress at Lisbon in 1949, and formally constituted at the next Congress at Washington in 1952. Dr J.M. May, then of the American Geographical Society's atlas project already cited, was very influential in its formation and was chairman of the Commission until 1964. There were several moves to change its title to Commission on the Geography of Health, consistently resisted by Dr May on the ground that health could not be defined. Yet the World Health Organization uses the term, and moreover adopted 'Health for All by the year 2000' as an objective for WHO and for its member countries at a conference at Alma Ata in Soviet Asia in 1978. It was perhaps under the influence of this strain of international thinking that the International Geographical Union abolished the Commission on Medical Geography at the Moscow Congress in 1976, preferring to set up a Working Group on the Geography of Health; however it had been clear at the Montreal Congress in 1972 that a strong current of geographical research had developed, particularly in North America, concerned with the locational analysis of health services. It is probably easier for workers on that side of our study to regard themselves as geographers of health than as medical geographers – itself a term used in English largely because nosogeography (Greek *nosos* disease) somehow sounds bizarre as an English word though common in several other languages.

There are issues apart from the mere niceties of nomenclature. The Alma Ata declaration and subsequent literature alike stress that by 'health for all by 2000' is meant not merely the availability of health services, but 'a personal state of well-being – a state of health that enables a person to lead a socially and economically productive life' (Mahler 1981). That international agreement was attained is remarkable, a matter for praise and even wonder. It is equally clamant that the difficulties of definition remain formidable.

The late Ralph Audy, already cited for his ecology of scrub typhus, suggested that it would be possible to quantify – to graph and measure – health defined as adaptability in a special sense, namely 'the individual's ability to rally from insults, whether chemical, physical, infectious, psychological or social' (Audy 1971). Apart from its immediate contribution, this paper gives a valuable summary of some ideas on health in the second century AD onwards from Galen, often with the idea of balance at their core, as also in millennial Indian and Chinese thought. Balint (1957) is quoted thus in Abbott (1982): 'health is a state in which a person is unaware of the function of his own body' – unfortunately a state destroyed if one asks questions in search of quantification of the proportion healthy in a population! For a similarly broad, indeed evolutionary approach to the other side of the coin, disease, see McKeown (1985).

Within immediate grasp, then, are there any useful or potentially useful tools of measurement and definition, and in particular any geographical approaches to the problem?

Physiology seems an obvious sister science to invoke if one is interested in the health of the whole man, whole woman or whole child; only some work in physiological climatology has come to my notice – much of it done by or for the armed forces in various countries interested in climate and appropriate clothing in relation to military efficiency in foreign operations. So far as I know broader links with normal living and working remain to be explored though I shall be happy to be proved wrong. Sports medicine too seems a promising link with physiology, but apart from some work on mountain populations little geographical research has been done. Recruits to the armed forces are a possible source of information on the health of young adults; if there is a very high rate of rejection on health grounds, as in early twentieth-century Britain, a spur to improved diet, exercise, etc. may result, but I know of little if any geographical work on this topic. Medical examinations for insurance purposes might offer information about a wider set of age groups than data from recruiting offices, but in most countries they would be subject to bias in socioeconomic groups taking out insurance, and this applies also to the tempting idea that general health screening data may prove useful. As long ago as 1972 an attempt was made to use such data from Hawaii (Brownlea 1972b), but apart from problems of confidentiality and access to data, there have been many doubts expressed in the last decade about the usefulness of *general* health screening in preventing disease or in maintaining 'a personal state of well-being' (*World Health Forum* 1980). (Specific health screening, for instance against cervical cancer, is another matter – see the wide review in the *British Journal of Hospital Medicine* (1982).) Medical sociologists, again, have produced some very interesting results from various kinds of survey about how individuals perceive their health: often personal well-being is equated with cheerfulness in British surveys, and the findings seem to be related very closely to the cultural matrix of the society – or sub-culture within it – and to become less subjective and easier to analyse only as inquiry moves in the direction of use of health services or of satisfaction with these, and correspondingly farther from the elusive concept of health as such. So the late Dr May was perhaps justified in his reluctance to adopt the term 'the geography of health' for the international Commission. With the best will in the world to reach out towards geography's potential contribution to 'health for all by 2000', this book will contain much more about disease than about health: even indirect indications of the general health status of a population such as infant or child mortality, or average or general nutrition for a whole population or for a stratum within it, will often concern the negative and unsatisfactory rather than positive health.

Conclusion and Prospect

This book is one man's approach to ecological medical geography – or nosogeography! – or to the geomedicine of the Heidelberg school (see for instance Jusatz 1984). Inevitably there will be much overlap with epidemiology, the branch of medicine concerned with disease in populations rather than in individuals, and with geographical pathology which focuses on spatial patterns of disease usually on the evidence of hard laboratory findings. Students of geography should appreciate the overlapping field of epidemiology – see Susser (1973) and Barker (1982). Ecological medical geography suggests an attempt to approach a borderland study from the methodologies of ecology and geography (physical, biogeographical and human), and to keep in touch with the changing concepts and techniques of these parent disciplines. Sub-disciplines that fail to keep in touch with changes in parent fields inevitably run the risk of becoming fossilised in their methods. Ideally of course this and many other problems of interdisciplinary fields of study would be solved by team work, and this does occur, but too seldom. Very few trained geographers are able to face the long period of medical training, though one or two are qualified in public health; just occasionally a medical doctor undergoes training as a geographer, and both directions of movement are to be welcomed. However, team work seems the likelier to yield results within a few years, and it is hoped that this book will encourage this.

Within geographical studies of health and disease there is a strong stream of research concerned with health services and growing in vigour and importance over the last 15 years or so. Recent surveys of the field will be referred to in a later chapter, in the hope that even within geography closer integration may be achieved in the near future between ecological medical geography, studies of need, and research on optimal location and health provision in a socioeconomic context. There is a need for intradisciplinary teamwork as well as interdisciplinary teamwork! Health education, or health promotion as it is increasingly termed, may also have a geographical dimension, as yet comparatively little explored, and this will be discussed in the conclusion to the book.

So the broad shape of the book is that this introductory chapter 1 is followed by Part I comprising several chapters on health and disease in developed countries, one of which is historical. Part II includes several chapters on health and disease in Third World countries, and one on the geography of hunger, both in the history of what are now developed countries and in recent years in the Third World. Part III includes a chapter on disease patterns and health care in both developed and developing countries. The concluding chapter is an attempt to draw together from the whole book the main threads that bear on the two main pleas of this introduction – a One-World view, and the marriage of disease ecology with geographical studies.

Part I   Western Diseases?

2 Introductory: Health in Industrial and Post-industrial Countries

'Universal' and 'Western' Diseases?

Chapter 1 referred briefly to the importance throughout the world of the universal diseases like measles, influenza and pneumonia, as against the 'western' ones like heart diseases, stroke and certain cancers, important in developed countries whether socialist or with mixed economies, and in contrast too with the so-called 'tropical' diseases, mainly vector-borne and parasitic illnesses, that remain relatively more important in the Third World (Burkitt 1973; Trowell and Burkitt 1981; Hutt and Burkitt 1986). This chapter introduces studies focused mainly on the developed countries. Probably most readers of this book will be more familiar with western Europe or North America, but it is important to retain the One-World perspective put forward in chapter 1. One way to reinforce this perspective is perhaps to remind ourselves that in developed countries one important reason why heart disease, stroke and the cancers are common in middle and later years is that, unlike most people in the Third World, citizens of developed countries have an expectation of life long enough for these to be important causes of death. As noted earlier, they are of increasing importance as public health problems in the Third World among the comparatively small elites with western-type life-styles. Moreover, infections like measles and influenza in developed countries normally figure as causes of 'morbidity' (the technical term for illness) rather than of mortality. In contrast, in the Third World such diseases, along with the vector-borne and parasitic diseases, are important killers as well as causing much illness, of profound social as well as economic importance. This change in relative importance from infections to degenerative diseases has been termed the epidemiological transition (Omran 1971) and is discussed more fully later in this chapter. Migrant populations and rapidly 'modernizing' groups offer a kind of laboratory of the epidemiological transition in progress; see for instance Crews and MacKeen (1982). Burkitt, already cited, has for many years urged the importance of adequate dietary fibre in western diets and in urban elites in the Third World adopting western-type eating habits.

General death rates for developed countries tend to have a group of leading causes of mortality, the order perhaps differing from country to country or from time to time – the heart diseases, strokes and certain cancers already mentioned, along with accidents on the road, at work and not least in the home. Some figures will be given of these causes of death presently, but first it may help some readers to look a little more closely at these 'western diseases'.

Heart Diseases

These diseases include the various conditions affecting the coronary (Latin, crown-like) arteries supplying blood to the heart muscle or myocardium (Greek, mys, muscle). The commonest of these diseases is the deposition of atheroma (Greek, gruel + swelling), a fatty material, in the artery linings, producing narrowings of these blood vessels. This is the usual cause of what is known as ischaemic heart disease (Greek, ischein, to suppress, haima, blood); here the reference is to insufficiency of blood supply to the heart muscle, which in turn causes the pain of angina (Latin but from the Greek for 'choking'). Angina can also be causes by anaemia, or by replacement of some of the oxygen in the blood by carbon monoxide because of smoking. Tobacco may also cause deterioration in the arteries including the coronary arteries. The other major result of coronary artery atheroma, or narrowing of the coronary arteries, is that of myocardial infarction (Latin, 'stuffing in', referring to the coagulation that may cause necrosis or death of muscle tissue), otherwise known as coronary thrombosis or heart attack.

Strokes

The strokes of popular usage are part of the cerebrovascular group of diseases (Latin cerebrum, the brain). Stroke or apoplexy covers three conditions (Greek apoplektikos, applied to the illness with the sense of 'strike completely'): cerebral haemorrhage – bleeding into the brain from a weakened artery; cerebral embolism – sudden blockage of an artery by material from a diseased artery of the heart or occasionally from other parts of the body; and cerebral thrombosis (Greek, curdling) – a more gradual blockage of a cerebral artery by blood-clotting within it. The brain cannot function without continuous supplies of glucose and oxygen, hence the well-known symptoms of paralysis, often of one side of the body, in severe strokes – slight ones may cause little or no disability. Like much heart disease, strokes are associated with atheroma (Greek, gruel + swelling), the deposition of greasy material in artery linings, mainly cholesterol (Greek, solid bile!); atherosclerosis is also common (Greek, hard gruel), a consequential hardening of artery walls. Hypertension or high blood pressure is associated in a general way with strokes, and with a possible additive effect along with atheroma, but it is difficult to define because of individual and ethnic variations in apparently well people. It is also associated with particular diseases, notably of the kidney. Some 80–90 per cent of hypertension is thought by some workers to exist in its own right as an individual idiosyncrasy – the so-called essential hypertension. Again there are probably links with diet, for instance with cholesterol, as we are reminded in much advertising of margarine etc., and possibly with another phenomenon very hard to define and especially to measure – stress. (On alcohol and stress, see McQueen and Celentano (1982); and on 'type A' or simply very tense behaviour, Radley (1982, 1984). For geographical gropings on the topic see Foster (1979) and Dean (1979).)

Soft water has been found to relate to cardiovascular disease in the Federal Republic of Germany, but with discrepancies in some towns of Lower Saxony (Keil 1979); similar studies in Ohio proved negative (Bain 1979), but in Quebec there was a positive correlation accompanied, however, by socioeconomic influences (Thouez 1978). Nitrates in high concentration in drinking water (a suspected but not proven cause of some cancers also) have been related to early onset of hypertension in Colorado (Malberg et al. 1978).

A comparative study of blood-pressure levels and cerebrovascular mortality in Australia and the USA confirms higher blood pressures and mortality in Australia: in men of 40–69 strokes are 49–55 per cent higher and cause some 4200 deaths per annum. This is thought not to relate strongly to alcohol consumption (MacMahon and Leeder 1984).

The Cardiovascular Diseases as a Whole

A broader international comparative study by the WHO focuses on trends of cardiovascular diseases in 27 countries, bringing out the sharp contrasts already noted, along with a general slight decline, but increases in Bulgaria, Czechoslovakia, Denmark, Hungary, Poland, Yugoslavia and (for males only) Northern Ireland (Pisa and Uemura 1982).

On heart disease in black Africans in the Republic of South Africa, see Walker (1980) and, from the geographer's viewpoint, McGlashan (1983). Hazra (1984b) writes on the – probably partial – data on heart disease in West Bengal, India; while the South Asian population in Britain seems to have rather higher rates not accounted for by diet or smoking and in which racial tension is therefore suspected (Russel 1986). Complementary to such surveys are first reports of preventive campaigns: examples include the very impressive Karelia project in Finland (see, for instance, Notkola et al. 1985) and campaigns in the UK and in Belgium. On prevention, a WHO report states the position as known in 1982 (WHO TRS 678): the association of coronary heart disease with the saturated fat and cholesterol content of diets in many western societies is sufficiently strong, in the view of the panel of experts, to justify moderate shifts in dietary habits; also justified are modification of overweight and moderate reduction in dietary salt. The link with smoking is also such as to add weight to the campaigns against the habit activated by concern about the epidemic of lung cancer – even though the link is less clear for the cardiovascular diseases. (See also *Preventive Medicine* 1983.) An extremely temperate and authoritative view of preventive measures against coronary heart disease in Britain covers smoking, hypertension, exercise and diet (*Lancet* 1982), and for a conspectus on survey methods see Rose et al. (1982). For a sceptical, sometimes iconoclastic view, of many such proposed measures, see the controversial exchanges in *World Health Forum* (1984) in its Round Table item on coronary risk factors initiated by Professor Michael Oliver of Edinburgh. (When doctors disagree. . . !)

The Cancers

Cancer (Latin, crab) is a disorder in which cell growth is no longer coordinated with the body's normal needs for new cells, generating a colony of generally relatively undifferentiated cells, drawing on the body's nutrient supplies but contributing nothing and in time outnumbering healthy cells in their neighbourhood within the body. If unchecked by natural or therapeutic processes, the growth may cause much pain and ultimately death by stopping vital organs from functioning, depending on the cancer site. The common features of cancers have stimulated the search for universal causes, such as stimuli to cell mutations of the type indicated (mutagens), including ionising radiation (also used in some treatments), carcinogens (Greek *karkinos*, cancer + *genesis*, origin) such as tars in tobacco smoke, and possibly certain virus infections (Milne

1984). However, a cautionary note by Weatherall (1982) stresses that laboratory demonstration of mutagenicity of a substance as affecting bacteria need not imply that it is mutagenic in the human body, simply because of our inbuilt defence systems. See also Anderson (1982) on monitoring mutagens. For a concise account of carcinogens and the balancing of risks, see Badger (1981); some possibly carcinogenic chemicals are listed in IARC (1982) – dental use of fluoride has been cleared, so far at least. And see Wyke (1981) on oncogenic viruses.

On the fundamental question of the origin and growth of tumours, a series of papers locates the topic on the borders of genetics and immunosuppression (de Carvalho 1977). On the other hand many studies have concerned particular types of cancer and specific sites in the body. The main types are: carcinoma (Greek, crab *and* the disease) in which epithelial cells tend both to infiltrate adjacent tissues and to spread to distant tissues, causing secondary growths known as metastases. (Epithelium, Greek, lierally 'upon the nipple' – cells containing cementing material to form both the external skin and internal surfaces in the body including the mucous membrane; and metastasis is Greek, literally 'standing beyond' and implying change or transfer). In contrast are the sarcomas (Greek, flesh-growth) in which the abnormal cells form tumours within connective tissue rather than in epithelium; some are tumours of undifferentiated cells, while some are differentiated and named according to their distinctive characteristics, e.g. fibrosarcoma, osteosarcoma. The leukaemias are sometimes grouped with the cancers: leukaemia is a cancer-like disease but seems not to start from single cells like most cancers, but to be a widespread malfunctioning of the bone marrow so that it produces, instead of normal white blood cells, abnormal cells lacking the power of combating infections.

Not all cancer sites are of major importance as public health problems in developed countries, while some, as we shall see later, are of great importance in Third World countries. Since cancers of particular sites in the body thus have a macro-geography – and some have a geography for smaller areas – analysis by site seems justified, though without closing one's mind to the holistic view of cancers as a group. As with other 'western diseases', however, one should note that some of the developed-country cancers are tending to become important in the Third World: this is true, for instance, of lung cancer, by now almost a byword as a main – and largely preventable – cause of *premature* death in developed countries, associated with much personal, social and economic loss. Other important cancers of developed countries are breast, uterus and stomach in some – though tending to decrease. Among cancers relatively less important *as public health problems* are liver and oesophagus cancers, important in the Third World (see chapter 13).

Trends over Time

Is anything to be learned from variations over time in the relative importance of these main causes of death in developed countries? (For a world survey, see United Nations 1982.) National campaigns against road accident deaths, against lung, breast and uterus cancers, and in some against stomach cancer, even against heart disease, can be important in avoiding *premature* death and the personal and societal losses noted earlier. Table 2.1 on this topic of loss of productive and enjoyable years of life from different causes in Canada is very thought-provoking: many developed countries with broadly similar life-styles must present a similar picture. See also Catford et al. (1984) on the unfavourable picture in the UK in cardiovascular disease compared with other countries in Europe. A recent report on the health of New Zealand, long a pioneer in concern for the national health, cites a 66 per cent increase in road accidents in 20 years, continued importance of hepatitis A and of sexually transmitted disease (with an increase in syphilis and non-specific urethritis), a doubling of lung cancer and smaller increases in other cancers, and a 50 per cent increase in bronchitis. As in the US and Australia there was a decrease in coronary heart disease and in strokes that the authorities found difficult to attribute to particular changes in life-style etc. (*World Health Forum* 1981b). The Canadian table will be referred to again later in a comparison with data from Ghana as a Third World country for which broadly comparable information is available.

Table 2.1 Years of life lost by Canadian males of 1–70 years, with causes

Cause of death	Percentage of total years of life lost
accidents	38.9
diseases of circulatory system	24.3
cancer	15.7
diseases of nervous system	5.2
respiratory diseases	4.2
diseases of digestive system	3.8
allergic, endocrine and blood diseases	1.8
infectious diseases	1.3
diseases of genito-urinary system	1.1
all other causes	3.7
all causes	100.00

(data from Romeder and McWhinnie, 1977, tables 2 and 4)
Source: Open University, 1985, III, p. 17

The Epidemiological Transition

The opening sentence of this chapter referred to the importance of the 'universal' diseases like measles, influenza and pneumonia in developed and developing countries: however, in developed countries their import- ance is mainly as a cause of morbidity rather than of mortality and premature death. However, there are exceptions. It is easy to overstate the extent to which the problem of intestinal infections is a Third World problem. Waddington (1983) suggests that in Europe, particularly Mediterranean countries, deaths in the years 1973–7 ranged from 140 000 to 680 000, with higher figures in the later years – and six countries had cholera outbreaks in 1980. And for a bench-mark survey of infectious disease in developed countries, see Murdoch and Gray (1973). At times, for instance, an epidemic of influenza gives an opening for several kinds of bacteria and viruses to cause pneumonia and in such circumstances there may indeed be many premature deaths in developed countries. It is perhaps one legacy of the long period of dominance of the germ theory of disease that most laymen do not need explanations and definitions of at least the commoner infections in the same way as seems useful for say heart disease or stroke. (Or is it perhaps that one tends to shy away from confrontation with details about leading causes of death from degenerative diseases in a culture that has lost the habit of looking death in the face?) However, there are so many organisms which cause – or may in particular circumstances cause – infectious or parasitic disease, some vector-borne, that in this book it has seemed best to include definitions and brief descriptions of them as they arise.

The epidemiological transition idea was referred to early in this chapter – the idea that there is a sequence linked with socioeconomic development in which the burden of disease shifts from the infectious to the broadly degenerative ones (Omran 1971, 1977). A world view of lessening mortality trends over the last century is in Preston (1977). A Japanese climatologist and medical geographer has argued that a good index of such changes may be found in decreasing seasonal variations in mortality as diet, clothing and domestic heating insulate people from adverse effects of the seasons (Sakamoto-Momiyama 1977, 1978). On seasonality and infant deaths in England and Wales, see Hare et al. (1981), and on possible links with the cot deaths syndrome in Tasmania, McGlashan and Grice (1983). A group of workers in the USSR make a point by considering separately the age-dependent causes of death as a whole, as compared with those unrelated to age that may occur at any time, for example during epidemics. They note that the reduction in mortality in developed countries has largely been in the non-age-dependent group, but also that, while age-dependent mortality has remained relatively stable, the causes of death recorded on death certificates have tended to change (Gavrilov et al. 1985). The issue invites both present speculation and future research? On the overlapping concept of disease competition, see Greenberg (1985). The epidemiological transmission idea runs parallel to the demographic transition model of Chung (1970): that in demographic trends over time, low-technology societies tend to have high birth rates and high death rates (usually with fluctuations but maintaining some sort of ecological equilibrium in the long term); with economic development there tends to be a phase of continuing high birth rates but much lower death rates – and so of rapid population growth – related to curative and especially preventive medicine, improved hygiene, nutrition and housing; and that this is followed by a phase of renewed population stability or slow increase, linked with low birth rates *and* low death rates (and probably with increased proportions of old people). The health economics of this are discussed in Gori and Richter (1978).) It is argued that several western countries have undergone changes along these general lines, though with differences stemming from individual social, economic and cultural differences and, indeed, some evidence that seems not to fit well with the theory (Preston 1976; Madsen 1973). McKeown (1976) has opened up a large area of debate about the modest influence, as he sees it, of medicine in these changes in nineteenth-century England, as compared with the major role of the public health movement, but for some critical comment on certain key aspects of his findings see Wrigley and Schofield (1981, p. 484, note 60).

Development and Health

In the Third World today socioeconomic development is often assumed to be more important than health services in lowering mortality (see, for instance, Sembajwe (1983) on Tanzania). Pendleton and Yang (1985) find evidence that health services are important early in the demographic transition, declining as the society moves towards 'maturity'. The role of specific health measures in the control of tuberculosis, as against economic development and improved living standards, has been much disputed: Collins (1982) finds that the environment in New Zealand was such that medical measures had little effect, but that particular age cohorts in England and Wales, and in Italy, were benefited. It is accepted that the developing countries of today may not follow the model very closely assuming progress in socioeconomic development, but there is some evidence that at comparatively modest levels of improved living standards (and interest in consumer goods?) the small family may become a widely accepted norm (see, for instance, Learmonth 1971). It is not difficult to link the two transition models, the high death rates with the high burden of infections, the falling death rates with immunization programmes etc. Ultimately (though still uncertain and controversial) the greater confidence of survival of children along with greater prosperity and interest in consumer items, better housing etc., may lead to a small family ethic, an ageing population and a dominance of the degenerative diseases like heart disease, strokes and the cancers common in developed countries. McGlashan (1982a,b) uses cluster analysis to demonstrate a spectrum in the epidemiological transition in the English-speaking West Indies from underdeveloped St Vincent to affluent Trinidad and Tobago.

Some Recent Trends in Developed Countries

The USA has in fact experienced two recent periods of decline in mortality rates, one when antibiotics reduced deaths from infections, and in the last few years a reduction in cardiovascular disease (Crimmins 1981). Perhaps the best explanation for the reduction in mortality from heart disease in the USA is from the long-term observation of an age-cohort in Framingham near Boston. The reduction seems to be a combination of some improvements in medical treatment and perhaps especially surveillance of people at high risk, and more general changes in diet along the lines noted in chapter 14; and changes in life-style with more emphasis on exercise and relaxation to control stress. The second generation, still young at the beginning of the 1980s, show signs of reduced blood-pressures and blood cholesterol (McQuade 1980, Gordon and Kannel 1983). The topic remains controversial: large scale experiment on human populations is of course ruled out on ethical grounds and, moreover, results from survey of large groups of people subject to intensive health education campaigns, as compared with control groups (in the USA and in North Karelia-Kuopo in Finland), have been to some extent confounded by the fact that the control groups have also shown a decline in heart disease. This may well be because of the influence of human ideas and communication systems – part of de Chardin's noösphere mentioned in chapter 1 ? – influencing the control group almost as much as the campaign population. (The Round Table in *World Health Forum* for 1984, already noted, reflects the controversy: Professor M. Oliver, a cardiologist in the University of Edinburgh, deprecated, even debunked, attempts at mass control, apart from anti-smoking campaigns and urged the policy of concentrating detailed guidance and treatment on high-risk groups, provoking on the whole adverse comments from an international panel of authorities. A little later J.T. Hart, a general practitioner from

South Wales noted for his trenchant views, urged that mass hypertension control, while of doubtful benefit for coronary prevention, could reduce strokes.) For a brief account of views and action from the USSR, see Oganov et al. (1985).

It is worth noting that even within infectious diseases, developed countries have seen a further epidemiological transition within the last forty to fifty years. Diphtheria, scarlet fever, poliomyelitis, measles, bacillary dysentery, viral hepatitis and pulmonary tuberculosis are generally on the wane in modern Britain, for example, while 'new' diseases – largely in fact newly identifiable through improved laboratory methods or new identifications of existing pathogens – are still being reported in increasing numbers. Thus for the now well-known Legion-naires' disease, it was not the infection that was diffused across the world, but knowledge of the bacterium now named *Legionella pneumophila*, once the enormous resources of the US Centre for Disease Control at Atlanta were deployed following the outbreak among delegates at the American Legion (veterans') Convention at Philadelphia in 1976. Other examples include enteric bacteria like *Campylobacter* (Greek *campylos*, curved), and several enteric viruses; viral haemorrhagic fever; and the 'toxic shock syndrome' occurring mainly in women and at first linked with the use of tampons in menstruation but now established as generally due to *Staphylococcus* (Greek, 'bunch of berries'), familiar as a cause of boils. (For a retrospect on the toxic shock syndrome ten years after it became widely known, see Dowler 1982.)

In the USSR death rates for males rather unexpectedly began to rise in 1956, and for females in 1970 especially in some age-groups; in part this is attributed to increasing infant mortality (see Jones and Grupp 1983); but in men it seems that there may be quite a marked rise in coronary heart disease (Cooper 1981, 1982). Somewhat comparable trends are reported from Poland (Cooper et al. 1984).

Sexually Transmitted Diseases (STDs)

In the United Kingdom in recent years the sexually transmitted diseases (STDs) have been the leading infections in morbidity calling for medical treatment (Communicable Disease Surveillance Centre UK 1985). The treponemal infections including venereal syphilis have been discussed in chapter 1. While the two leading 'classical' venereal diseases, syphilis and gonorrhoea, have tended to decline slightly, there has been an almost world-wide development of resistance to penicillin by the gonorrhoea organism *Neisseria gonorrhoea* (from Dr A.L.S. Neisser and Greek, seed-flow), see OPCS (1983). Anal infection in homosexual males, and in some women, is proportionately more important than in recent years (Willcox 1981a,b). Venereal diseases have long been known as a cause of illness in many Third World countries, with a tendency to spread back to rural areas with returning male migrants after temporary work in the cities (see Piot and Meheus 1983). A disquieting paper from Zaria in Nigeria gives evidence of gonorrhoea in children from some form of sexual contact including at least some sexual abuse (Mathur et al. 1985).

The change in terminology from venereal diseases (VD) to the modern STD seems to be at least largely a response to the rise in 'pelvic inflammatory disease', and other diseases such as sexual transmission of the protean organism *Chlamydia trachomatis* and the cold sore *Herpes simplex* (though usually of a different strain from that causing facial cold sores; the attempt to reduce the stigma of the older term is because these 'new' infections occur far more widely among non-promiscuous couples than did the classic VDs (Dunlop 1983). This change appears to be connected with changes in sex mores during recent decades, including more adventurous approaches to intercourse and an acceptance of several changes in partner, perhaps in early maturity, with the availability of the contraceptive pill. Conclusive evidence is of course difficult to gather, and there is some dialectic exchange in the literature. At risk of over-simplifying complex arguments, there is a school broadly advocating single sexual partners and the avoidance of oral and anal intercourse, while this smacks of 'victim-blaming' to defenders of the change in sex mores (see, for example, Willcox 1981a,b; Order of Christian Unity 1985). The suggestion that cervical cancer may be in a sense sexually transmitted (see chapter 3) adds a further dimension to the debate.

Acquired Immunodeficiency Syndrome (AIDS)

The newest STD at the time of writing, the acquired immunodeficiency syndrome (AIDS), is the subject of widespread public concern in many western countries. Several other diseases, and probably severe stress also, compromise the immune system, complicating attacks of malaria, tuberculosis, influenza and measles. But the immune system recovers in surviving patients. With AIDS the immune deficiency is permanent. Already several books on AIDS have been published, such as the racy human-interest one entitled *The Plague Years* (Black 1986) subject to occasional scientific solecisms, and the more scientific one by Daniels (1985). It was first reported from the USA in 1981, though one or two reports from elsewhere have proved to concern the same disease; initial reports linking the disease with male homosexuals and with immigrants to the USA from the Caribbean brought widespread stigmatizing, especially when it became clear that the disease had been spread through blood transfusion to haemophiliacs and others – a route of transmission now effectively blocked. Transmission between drug addicts sharing needles to inject themselves is an important mode of transmission causing concern in cities as different as New York and Edinburgh. (For Europe see WER 1985a). The virus does cause illness directly, often slight and resembling mononucleosis or glandular fever caused by the Epstein-Barr virus, but sometimes including acute neurological symptoms, including seizures and temporary paralysis. However, the deficiency in the immune system, referred to in the name AIDS, makes patients very vulnerable to many 'opportunistic' diseases affecting different body systems, but two soon came to be widely known: a rapidly malignant form of a skin cancer previously known as a milder and more slowly developing lymphadenoma (cancer spreading through the lymphatic system) Kaposi's sarcoma; and a pneumonia caused by organisms not commonly causing severe illness, including *Pneumocystis carinii* and *Legionella pneumophila*. Numbers with the full-blown disease are still comparatively low, about 1500 in the USA, half of whom are dead, and about the same in Europe. There are reports from most western countries, but almost none from the Soviet bloc countries or from China, and, in contrast say with the knowledge diffusion in Legionnaires' disease, this does seem an instance of disease diffusion on a world scale in an age of rapid travel and, some would add, of sexual permissiveness. It is now possible to lend some perspective to a view of AIDS (see, for instance, *Guardian* 1985, or *Population Reports* 1986, and on the Third World, PANOS Dossier 1986).

The root cause is a retrovirus with an incubation period now thought to vary from four months to six years or even more, so that the people infected, many of whom will develop the disease proper, outnumber the overt cases. The virus was first identified by Montaignier and his team at the Pasteur Institute in Paris, and named lymphadenopathy-associated virus (LAV) from its links with lymphadenoma as already noted. Meanwhile, workers in the USA had been working on analogues in several animal leukaemias which share the AIDS characteristics of damaged immune mechanisms and involvement of the lymphatic system. In 1983–4 they identified several human T-cell leukaemia viruses (HTLV), of which HTLV–III appeared to be identical with the LAV virus. HTLV–III has been the common term in English language journals, and LAV in French, but to acknowledge the first discovery one could call it LAV/HTLV–III. However, in May 1986 the International Committee on the Taxonomy of Viruses recommended that the virus be known as human immunodeficiency virus or HIV, and this term is widely though not yet universally used.

After this section on AIDS was first drafted, a report in *Nature* from Montaignier and the Institut Pasteur in Paris claimed the discovery of a second AIDS virus, found in two West African heterosexuals and named LAV–II; it appears to be very similar in form and effects to HIV–I/but to have genetic coding 30 per cent different, and different antibodies (possibly affecting the efficiency of screening say of blood for transfusion purposes) (Teddera and O'Connor 1987).

The logic of LAV has already been noted; that of HTLV may call for slight elaboration. The body's immune defence system includes two types of cell: the B-cells (from Latin *bursa*, a wine-skin, because they were originally studied in birds, in which these cells originated from the 'bursa of Fabricius', an organ not found in man; but also in English an easy mnemonic for their origin in *bone*-marrow), able to produce antibodies to control invading 'foreign' or 'non-self' organisms, and the T-cells thought to originate in the thymus, a small gland between the lungs now regarded as part of the lymphatic system. T-cells include the white blood cells termed T-4; most of these are 'helper' cells, inducing or helping other T-4s, the 'killer' cells, to fight invading organisms whilst some T-cells *reduce* antibody production when the invading cells are under control. The LAV/HTLV–III virus has a 'recognition site' that precisely fits a 'receptor site' on T-4 cells. Once there, the RNA (ribonucleic acid) strand of the virus is 'transcribed' into DNA (deoxyribonucleic acid); it then 'takes over' the T-4 cells' DNA, using it to replicate the viral DNA and generate new viruses. The virus may lie dormant within T-cells, possibly for years (hence one possible explanation of the 'slow-virus' element, and also a complication in evolving safe vaccines). Moreover, the white cells in the blood are left with an excessive proportion of 'suppressor' cells; their function in a normally balanced immune system is to damp down the 'killer' cells once invading cells have been controlled, thus restoring homeostasis or balance. Given the excessive proportion of 'suppressor' cells in AIDS, the immune system is simply suppressed. Thus it is a blood disease, transmissible as noted earlier by blood transfusion or by shared syringes of drug addicts. (For a report from a locally concentrated haemophiliac population in the area of Newcastle-upon-Tyne, UK, see Jones et al. (1985).) The virus is transmitted in semen, and it has been thought that anal intercourse involving thin epithelium with blood vessels near the surface involves high risks of transmission direct from semen into the blood stream – as compared with the thicker muscle involved in vaginal intercourse. However, there is some evidence that mucous membrane in the vagina can also receive infection, and thus that a woman can be infected by a man carrying LAV/HTLV–III, though less likely to transmit the virus to other sexual partners simply because she does not emit semen during intercourse. For detailed reports of limiting cases of transmission – by a single episode of anal intercourse, and by semen artificial insemination by donor (before relevant regulations were changed), see Reiss et al. (1985) and Stewart et al. (1986). The virus is also transmitted during the process of birth from infected mothers, in the milk of infected mothers, and possibly in saliva. Early in 1987 AIDS-related deaths were reported as the leading cause of deaths in young women in New York.

AIDS has been thought to be endemic in central Africa, where it seems to be equally common in both sexes in at least many groups, and where there is thought to be little association with homosexual or bisexual intercourse, but rather with promiscuity, and it is associated mainly with comparatively mild and slowly developing Kaposi's sarcoma. Reports speak of epidemic rather than endemic conditions, however, with thousands of deaths from 'the slim disease' as it is called in Uganda. It is conceivable that the virus has only recently come to affect humans and may be primarily an infection (possible not even a disease) of monkeys and possibly cats – a zoonosis like plague or yellow fever. The African Green monkey often carries a very similar virus or antibodies to it, and seems to suffer little or no illness (*Annals Internal Medicine* 1985, but see doubts in Zuckerman 1986a). As to means of transmission, one author has argued for blood-sucking insects such as *Cimex* bed-bugs (Cook 1985). Mosquitoes are thought to be ruled out because they often bite children in preference to adults, and this is an adult disease (Zuckerman 1986b) – though there is the analogy with Burkitt's lymphoma which may be caused by a mosquito-borne virus (see Tran Ba Loc (1976) for an animal experiment in this field). The Caribbean may also have endemic areas, and it seems that migration to the USA and homosexual permissiveness must be involved in the high incidence in cities like San Francisco, drug addiction and, for a time, blood transfusion playing a part. The world total of infected people was thought to be two to three million, prior to alarming reports from Central Africa. There may be 1.75 million infected in the USA (not all ill, and many may never be so), mainly in Los Angeles, San Francisco, New York and Miami; Europe and Latin America are thought to have about 800 000. Central Africa may perhaps have millions *of both sexes* and perhaps tens of thousands dying if – as some observers believe – the disease is present in epidemic form there (*Population Reports* 1986). In a small country like Britain it is thought that there may be between 12 000 and 20 000 infected, of whom 2000 may develop the overt disease in the years to about 1990. A full-scale programme of health education in the newspapers has been launched and if this is effective in changing practices in sexual intercourse this disease may be controllable. Meantime an effective vaccine may be evolved, though there are many problems (World Health Forum 1985, 30–4; *Guardian* 1985, 1986; and for a bench-mark bibliographical review, Peterman et al. 1985). A report from the USA indicates marked behavioural change in homosexual men since AIDS became widely known – so human behaviour can be changed! – but sombrely indicates that much greater changes towards single-partner stable relations would be needed to halt the epidemic (*MMWR* 1985).

Geography and STDs?

Geographical aspects of this discussion of STDs have mainly been on the macro-scale. There seem to be rather few geographical studies for smaller areas. One study of gonorrhoea in 'upstate' New York using a static geographical framework demonstrates distance decay round main urban centres, with concentric circles of diminishing incidence round these, and a 'tendency towards geographic clustering' on contact tracing (Rothenberg 1983). Girt's (1978) paper on linear programming as an approach to areas of high and low risk in disease diffusion processes uses gonorrhoea in Ontario as a worked example. A paper on the mountainous Trentino area of Italy shows distance decay away from the provincial capital, Trento City, but with rates concentrated along main valley routes and tailing off into inaccessible mountain tracts, while the detailed map of the city shows distinct clustering in both inner city and some suburban areas (Staluppi 1983). A study of clinic attenders reviews demographic and social factors, personality disorders (not found important except to a limited extent for gonorrhoea), sexual activity (forms of which may affect transmission, as indeed noted above), and of course the differential risks associated with the different individual diseases (Fulford et al. 1983). A population dynamics model for a heterogeneous population is used to compare the effectiveness of six alternative combinations of population screening and contact tracing, concluding in favour of selective contact tracing rather than general population screening (Hethcote et al. 1982). Finally, the concept of social networks, which may of course have spatial implications, is used to study on the micro-scale the transmission of AIDS, using diagrams covering 40 cases in Los Angeles, San Francisco and New York (Klovdahl 1985).

Road Accidents

Road accidents may well rank as one of the western diseases, and one that, like others, is tending to spread to Third World countries – Selya

(1980) even suggests that the move from seventh to third place as a cause of death between 1960 and 1977 of road accidents in Taiwan is one measure of economic development! (See also Levy (1980).) Oil-rich Kuwait is perhaps an extreme example, with road accidents among the leading causes of death (Bayoumi 1981). A broader survey of 'non-war violence' including road accidents ranks the countries for which comparable data were available in four groups (Day 1984): (1) Chile, USA (non-white), Finland, Norway, Austria; (2) Northern Ireland, Japan, the Republic of Ireland, New Zealand, USA (white); (3) Australia, Switzerland, Scotland, Sweden, France; (4) England and Wales, Denmark, The Netherlands. In the USA it took from 1900 to 1952 for cars to kill their first million people, but only from 1953 to 1975 for the second million. On current trends the third million will be killed in the 16 years 1976 to 1991 (Sondel 1983). The USA is by no means the worst country in the world when considering its vehicle density in relation to population, and it has high casualty rates in rural areas – 55 per cent of travel is on city streets but two-thirds of deaths are on rural roads (Australia has a similar problem). In the USA 42 per cent of all deaths in men of 15–19 and 35 per cent in the 20–24 age group are from road accidents, and the picture in Britain and most developed countries is similar. In Britain urban accidents predominate in number and in causing deaths, though less severe in damage and cost; a slight reduction in total deaths, from 5934 in 1982 to 5445 in 1983, was accompanied by disquieting increases in accidents involving children or pedal cyclists (For broad reviews, see Adams (1985), and it may be worthwhile to look back at older sources like Ministry of Transport (UK) 1967, and Norman 1962). Whitelegg (1985), pointing out these trends, goes on to make a plea for greater geographical participation in the interdisciplinary field of accident research, on various scales from the beneficial effects on accident rates of subsidized public transport on the national or metropolitan scale, to systems-analytic approaches to time–space clustering; monitoring the changing surface of city-centre pedestrian precincts and consequential changes in traffic flow; or modification of suburban design in the interests of all road users including cyclists and pedestrians, especially children. Interestingly enough an analysis concentrating on the age-group 15–19 for males found rural areas to present higher risks than urban (in contrast with the overall figures noted earlier), and that distance from hospital accident and emergency facilities is a factor in higher mortality, and one in course of being exacerbated by current policies of centralization of hospital facilities in areas like East Anglia from where the study emanates (Bentham 1985). From the USA again, Brodsky (1984) argues that the higher rural risks, because of inevitable delays in calling emergency services and their travel time, demand much more preparedness on the part of bystanders. (Given American litigiousness, it may be, however, that 'Is there a doctor present?' might not be answered.)

Alcohol

Alcohol is, of course, a cause of many road and possibly industrial and home accidents, while later chapters will include many references to alcohol and tobacco as causes of disease; there is a case for considering them both as addictions and diseases in their own right. The alcohol problem has a very large literature. An overview of Europe, bedevilled by lack of comparability of data, is in Davies and Walsh (1983). The important 'Rand Report' in the USA is drawn on in Armor (1978) and this aspect of the long-term Framingham study in Gordon and Kannel (1983). C.J. Smith's intriguingly titled 'The wrath of grapes. . .' (1985) records persistently low rates of alcohol consumption in Mormon and traditionally fundamentalist areas, but with sufficient convergence of regional rates to make the author suggest that prosperity has its dangers, with little action available except to tax the prosperous, addicted or not, to help pay for this particular consequence of the consumer society. On alcohol in the Third World, a WHO workshop in Manila exemplified the concern, and see also Smith (1982). Chambwe (1982) compares drinking patterns in young people in Zimbabwe and in the UK, and a survey method potentially useful in both types of society is suggested in Smart et al. (1980). On vitamin deficiencies in alcoholics, see WHO (1980, TRS 650), and for a specific example of beri-beri in beer drinkers Whyte et al. (1982). A review of treatment policies is in Orford and Edwards (1977). McGlashan (1980) reports on the social correlates of alcohol-related mortality in Tasmania (for cancer of the oesophagus, country of birth; for cirrhosis, masculinity and marital status; for road accidents, young maleness). Ritson (1973) gives a good general survey on alcoholism as a reflection of environment, and comments on high rural rates in Scotland. Holtermann and Burchell (1981) analysed the costs of alcohol abuse in England and Wales, but specifically did not try to estimate the benefits of moderate consumption. There is evidence of serious concern about alcoholism in France in a series of major reports, some with substantial geographical input from Professor Henri Picheral and others (Premier Ministre: Haut Comité d'Etude et d'Information sur l'Alcoolisme 1983), and also a paper on alcohol in migrants, including the impact of Islamic prohibitions (Thévenin 1983). Perhaps this quotation from one of the papers by an outstanding medical educationist puts the alcohol problem in perspective:

> . . . if a team of young psychologists were to devise a really effective alcohol education programme for an adolescent and young adult population, this might do more to affect patterns of illness twenty years later than a hundred liver specialists devoting their lives to ameliorating the end results of alcohol excess.
>
> (Maddison 1980)

Tobacco

While alcohol is well-nigh universal, except perhaps in very strictly Islamic countries and groups, there are western patterns of social drinking that spread in urban and professional elites in Third World countries, and lead on to alcoholism in a proportion of people, mainly men, just as in western society. Tobacco is a clearer case of a disease-causing addiction that is spreading – or even being deliberately spread by vested interests, advertising and so on. Milio (1985) notes the fall in cigarette smoking in developed countries, and at faster rates of decline (except notably, even tragically, among young women), and the concurrent increase in developing countries; she suggests an urgent need for targeted information to reach policy makers in the Third World, and probably assistance with planning transitions needed to reduce tobacco consumption. The *Medical Journal of Australia* (1983) outlines recent battles in that country. In a study from Malaysia, a survey of school children at a mean age of 16 years revealed patterns of early smoking comparable with western experience, especially in boys, of whom 33 per cent had smoked (a smaller proportion admitting to current smoking), with mean starting age of just over 13 years (Thambypillai 1985). In Bangladesh over 405 km^2 of land (100 000 acres) that could produce food are used for tobacco, and respiratory diseases including much (and increasing) lung cancer follow. At least equally serious and probably more urgent, smoking only five cigarettes a day in a poor household may result in 8000 calories less a month (33.5 MJ), over 250 calories a day or perhaps 50 per person, a serious deficit in marginal diets (Cohen et al. 1983).

Inequality

One could go on discussing 'western diseases' and their tendency to spread to the Third World. Inequality in health matters is a matter of serious concern in many developed countries, and receives further comment in chapter 16. A continental review of inequality is in *World Health Forum* (1981a) looking forward to the implications for 'Health for

All by 2000'. (See also the *WHO Chronicle* for 1980.) And for a Marxist interpretation of higher mortalities in peripheral parts of the world economy, and in the working-class in more developed areas, see Gregory and Piche (1983). Baird (1973) provides chilling evidence of the effects of deprivation in the slump of the 1930s on female foetuses then in the womb, leading to malformed babies in the 1960s and 1970s. See also Alvarez (1982). A pioneer geography of regional disparities in Britain is in Coates and Rawstron (1971). The 'Black Report' on inequalities in Britain a generation after the National Health Service was formed – named from its chairman – was commissioned by a Labour government but presented to a Conservative one (DHSS 1980a); a short review is in *World Health Forum* (1982a). See also Townsend et al. (1986); Whitehead (1987). On what are identified as slightly greater inequalities in France, see Leclerc et al. (1984), and for a regional view across Europe, van Poppel (1981). A series of papers from Italy present that country as in some ways transitional between western and Third World standards (Bellezza 1983). For the particular case of apartheid, see WHO (1983). Inequality in health can hardly be seen in the same way as say heart disease or certain cancers, likely to spread to developing countries, for such disparities are no stranger to the Third World. Inequality is indeed endemic in much of the Third World – India did after all evolve the stereotypic though by no means the only caste (and out-caste) system – but perhaps western patterns of inequality within prosperous communities can be seen in their limiting case in Third World manufacturing cities. Certainly the following chapters will contain many studies in which inequality is an ultimate cause of the persistence of this or that disease, and others in which it causes important differences in access to health care. So it seems better to leave this theme meantime.

On the specific issue of unemployment in developed countries, see Colledge (1982) on economic cycles and health, Spruit (1982) on the macro-scale of analysis, Brenner and Mooney (1983) on economic change, and Schwefel (1986) on data from German-speaking countries.

Ageing

As the last of the 'western diseases' it is perhaps worth considering ageing or at least the increasing proportion of a developed-country population in the older age-groups; this is not, of course, a disease, but in some circumstances may well be a problem. Examples of the copious literature on ageing are: on the problems of provision of facilities for increasing numbers of the very aged in Denmark, Leeson (1981); on socio-spatial aspects of 'health-seeking behaviour' in an elderly population, Henry

(1981); and on a positive view of health and potential in the elderly, Riley (1982). From generally prosperous Australia Gibson and Rowland (1984) review the severe problems ahead in both community and institutional care for the aged, while Fries (1985) points out the tendency towards a 'compression of morbidity' in the last few years of life in an ageing population. (For a geographical contribution, see Dear (1981).)

Conclusion

The chapter title has a question mark: Western diseases? There are ways in which the burden of disease differs as between the developed world and the Third World, and I have tried to do justice to these without losing sight of the common elements and experiences that link us in One World, yesterday, today and tomorrow.

One more point before moving from descriptive generalities towards the more geographical chapters: geographical presentation of data, and especially serious geographical analysis, seem so far to have been more successful in relation to infectious, including vector-borne, disease than to the degenerative diseases, though this is less true today than it was even ten years ago. Readers may care to check this statement for themselves in the following chapters culling some of the literature in medical geography. As a geographer, the writer has severely limited competence in sister sciences, and this must cause a bias towards work by fellow-geographers, but some of the research described will be by biomedical and biostatistical workers adopting an essentially geographical approach. This cross-discipline view is particularly true of the next chapter dealing mainly with relatively straightforward mapping of disease data – for geographers have no monopoly of cartographic skills – while chapters 5 to 7 on ideas like 'surface' and spatial diffusion patterns, on analytical use of change of scale and so on, will draw mainly on research by professional geographers.

In a sense this chapter has really continued the One World theme of chapter 1: the universal diseases are important in developed countries mainly as morbidity rather than mortality, while the degenerative diseases, along with accidents, dominant causes of death in the developed world, are already important in urban elites in the Third World. Though the chapter is mainly descriptive and scene-setting as background for the geographical discussions that follow, some geographical contributions have been noted that seem to fit better here than in later chapters.

3 Mapping Cancer

The Howe Atlases and Standardized Mortality Ratios (SMRs)

The United Kingdom owes to Professor G.M. Howe, with backing from the Royal Geographical Society, its first modern and comprehensive atlases of disease mortality (Howe 1970). These maps are based on standardized mortality ratios, so that *after* allowing for the age and sex structure of a particular census unit they show if it is 'over-represented' or 'under-represented' for a cause of death, as compared with the national expectation of death from that cause. Thus for a retirement resort with a high proportion of the elderly, it is easy to see that 'crude' death rates would show a very high ratio for a disease common in the elderly, say heart disease, compared with a nearby area with a mainly youthful population; the standardized mortality ratio (SMR) is one commonly used way of allowing for this factor to give a general picture of relative mortality. The direct method of calculating the SMR is more strictly known as the Comparative Mortality Index or CMI; it requires age and sex populations and mortality data for both the local and the national area: death rates for each age group are summed for the nation; then the total is divided into the sum of the death rates derived from applying the local mortality rates to the national population for each age and sex group. The answer is then multiplied by 100. Thus a local rate equal to the national expectation is 100, 'over-represented' areas have ratios over 100, and 'under-represented' areas ratios under 100 (McCracken 1981). The indirect method requires age and sex mortality rates for the national area but only age and sex *populations* for the local area – so it can be used where the data base is less comprehensive: the total number of deaths for the local area is divided by the total 'expected' if one applies the national age-group mortality rates to each local age-group population in turn, summing to yield the 'expected' total deaths; the result is multiplied by 100. Again local areas 'over-represented' in mortality are over 100, 'under-represented' under 100 (Howe 1970). The standardized mortality ratio can miss quite significant differences in mortality in particular age groups (Keig and McAlpine 1980; McCracken 1981; both with Australian examples); for some purposes age-specific mortality data are preferable, for instance where a particular disease is known to attack a particular age group. Thus one might select middle-age data for lung cancer. Other ways of looking at premature deaths in groups of people are mentioned from time to time in this book.

Cancer of the Stomach, England and Wales

Figure 3.1 is the map of cancer of the stomach for males 1954–8, taken from Howe's 1963 atlas. There is a great swathe of high rates running across both rural and urban Wales and the north and north-west of England, the areas long associated with 'traditional' industry based on coalfields; there is an extension of high rates into the Midlands industrial conurbation, and an important outlier in parts of London, mainly in eastern boroughs; there is also a less important outlier running from the fen country in Kesteven south through Northampton and Bedfordshire: could this be linked with brick manufacture? That the map for females (not reproduced here) shows more strikingly high rates illustrates the problems of map interpretation without detailed local studies. High rates elsewhere are mainly urban. The picture from Scotland and for Northern Ireland (not reproduced here) is broadly consistent with these spatial patterns. In contrast is figure 3.2, of the same disease for a later period, 1959–63. This uses a demographic base map – that is, the square or diamond-shaped symbols are drawn in proportion to the population size of the area represented; this is done in order to avoid over-emphasis of areas with high SMRs but low population such as much of North Wales. Howe's maps in this series distinguish areas whose SMR is found to have statistical significance in differences above or below the national expectation (by solid boundary lines to symbols, as compared with pecked lines for non-significant differences). This particular map has a very stylized shape, but apart from this there is a loss of any representation of a continuous surface for England and Wales. Along with the stylized shape, this makes comparison difficult with maps on a conventional projection, say of relief, rainfall, geology and the like. Urban rates can be distinguished from those classed as rural in the then administrative structure. The reader may agree that the *broad* pattern is similar to that in figure 3.1, and the present author believes that in spatial analysis of disease it is generally best to study groups of areas with common shadings, rather than single areas or single symbols, for that may mislead and cause

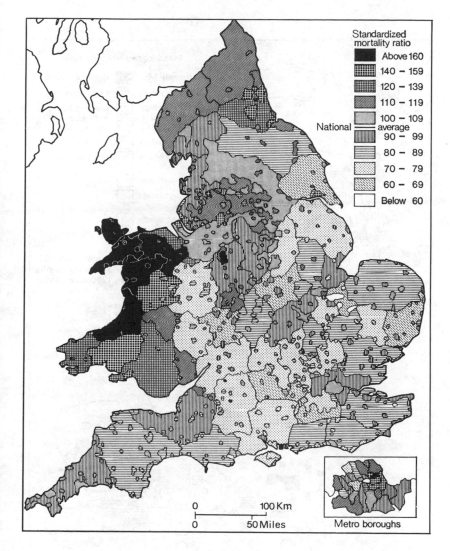

Figure 3.1 Stomach cancer, males, England and Wales, 1954–1958
Source: Howe (1970)

unnecessary alarm, or even unjustified complacency, in areas showing high and low rates. However, there are exceptions, such as areas or even a single town where a disease is associated with a particular occupation such as nasal cancer and woodworking. It is fair to add that often the link may be well known to local health workers before the mapping is

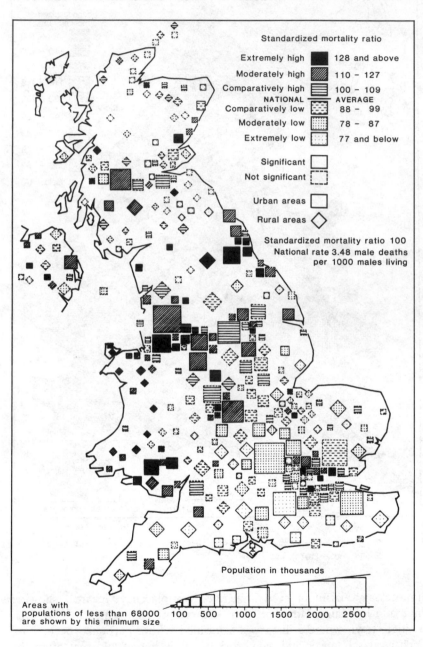

Figure 3.2   Stomach cancer, males, the UK, 1959–1963
*Source:*Howe (1970)

done (Gardner 1984); a study in wood-processing areas in twelve countries points to sanding of hardwoods as a particular risk in nasopharyngeal cancer – see Wills (1982).

Figure 3.3 is one of Howe's more recent published maps, again for stomach cancer in males for 1970–2 (Howe 1979). Here the demographic base map has been put on a conventional map of the land area. The much more familiar shape of the British Isles has been preserved by

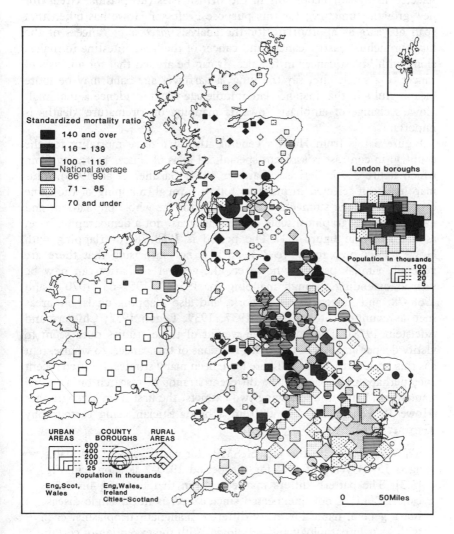

Figure 3.3 Stomach cancer, males, the UK, 1970–1972, 15–64 years
Source: Howe (1979)

using three instead of two symbols – circles for county boroughs, squares for urban districts and diamonds for rural areas. The clean effect of the map has probably sacrificed differentiation of statistically significant differences, the solid and pecked lines of figure 3.2. However, there is one further and important technique introduced: Howe has used SMRs as before, but has selected the age-groups 15–64, the main productive years economically and demographically. This map is from a paper on selected malignant neoplasms in the British Isles (neoplasms, Greek for new growth, tumours): for this purpose Professor Howe has taken that span of years as appropriate for the analysis *together* of cancers of the lung–bronchus, gastric cancer and cancer of the large intestine in males, along with breast cancer in females. It can be argued that for analysis of cancer of a single site, say the lung, a narrower age-band may be more meaningful – in that instance late middle age when incidence is maximal. Howe's change of emphasis towards mapping of 'premature' deaths is important.

Figure 3.1 is from Howe's general atlas of disease mortality for the country; in contrast is a recent specialized atlas of cancer mortality from which figure 3.4 is derived (Gardner 1984; Gardner et al. 1983). This map has been selected in order to follow through mapping of the same cancer, that of the stomach; it uses SMRs for the whole population, and uses normal geographical scale for census areas, not a demographic base, as did Howe in figure 3.1. The period is 1968–78, overlapping with Howe's 1972 map in figure 3.3, so it is not surprising that there are generally similar patterns; however, the general similarity can now be seen as extending through mapping for 1954–8, 1959–63, 1970–2 and 1968–78, and indeed to older work, and also mapping on larger areas such as counties (Stocks 1936, 1937, 1939; Legon 1952; Chilvers and Adelstein 1978). The cumulative weight of these studies does seem to justify deeper analysis of the space-relations of this cancer: to what extent has this been forthcoming? There have been many studies, but two recent ones perhaps pull together the different strands of research on a spatial framework, hence the following two extracts, the first from a geographer (Howe 1979) and the second from a biostatistician using cartography (Gardner 1984).

The distribution in the UK of SMRs for gastric cancer for males, aged 15–64 years of age, for the period 1970–2 is shown in Fig. [3.3]. The pattern differs markedly from that for lung–bronchus cancer. This is not unexpected since cancer is not a single disease but a general name for many different malignant neoplasms, each with its own pathology and aetiology. With the exception of certain of the London boroughs (e.g. Barking, Greenwich, Newham, Southwark), the remainder of southeast Britain enjoys favourable

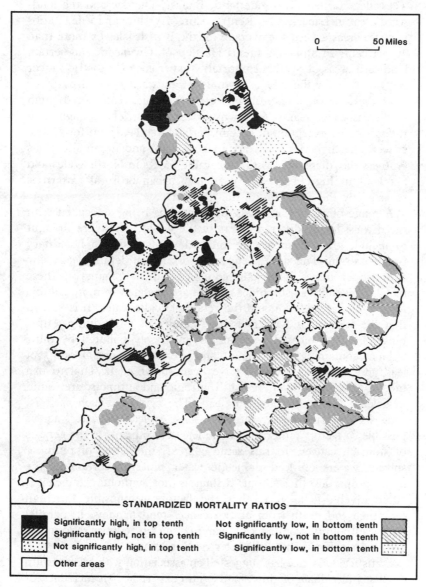

Figure 3.4 Stomach cancer, males, England and Wales, 1968–1978
Source: Gardner (1984)

mortality experience from gastric cancer. Major high risk areas
include southeast London, Gloucester, Newport (Gwent), West
Bromwich, Stoke-on-Trent, and the urban districts of Staffordshire,
Oldham, Salford, Bury, Bolton, Warrington, Bootle, Gwynedd,

Teesside, Hartlepool, Sunderland, Belfast, Dundee and the land-ward areas of Lanarkshire, Renfrewshire, Ayrshire and Fife. Ratios in these areas exceed the average for the British Isles by more than 40 per cent. In Stoke-on-Trent, Hartlepool, Gwynedd, and certain landward areas of Scotland, mortality experience for gastric cancer is twice that for the UK as a whole. [Landward = rural.]

In the case of lung–bronchus cancer, already considered, high risk areas occur mainly in towns or urban districts (though with the intriguing exception of certain parts of Scotland) but for gastric cancer, the high risk areas are in both rural and urban situations (witness the 'diamonds' with high value SMRs in North Wales and Scotland in Fig. [3.3]). No particular urban or rural pattern is revealed by the geographical distributions.

A range of factors has been postulated as being associated with the disease in the different parts of the world. These are thought to include trace elements in soil and water and also hereditary predisposition. The spoil heaps and workings of defunct lead, zinc and copper mines in Britain contain residual amounts of these metals, generally as sulphides. These are changed to more soluble form by aerial oxidation and the action of acidic water. It is known that the streams and rivers in the vicinity of mine dumps (tips, bings) in parts of Wales are almost invariably polluted by mine effluent containing these metals and even very slight amounts of lead and zinc (e.g. 3 ppm) have been shown to be fatal to fish life. . . Selenium, silver, bismuth, arsenic and antimony are found in galena, the main source of lead. The evidence, such as it is, suggests that zinc/copper ratios in soils, or lead in water, act as possible co-factors rather than complete determinants in the genesis of stomach cancer. In this same context, the action of plumbo-solvent waters on lead domestic water pipes in certain of the older properties throughout Britain is not without significance. Alternatively, it may be that the factors responsible for high incidence and death from gastric cancer tend to move in parallel with lead pollution of drinking water or the zinc/copper ratio in the soil, both being themselves not strictly relevant.

Statistical evidence has suggested an association with blood group A, that individuals of this blood group experience an incidence of gastric carcinoma which is greater than individuals of the other ABO blood groups. . . The inherited element does not appear to be responsible for the distribution of mortality from gastric cancer (Fig. [3.3]) since the eastern parts of Britain, known to have the highest proportion of people of blood group A in Britain, have some of the lowest SMRs for gastric cancer. . . This spatial pattern would lend weight to the importance of environmental factors in the aetiology of gastric cancer.

Geographical differences in the incidence of and mortality from gastric cancer which have been observed globally and nationally . . . support the view that gastric cancer (and probably the majority of human cancers) are environmentally induced.

(Howe 1979)

Gardner takes other cancer sites for detailed regional analysis in this particular paper, but his discussion of general environmental factors includes some useful remarks on stomach cancers, along with other cancers that may have factors in common.

An area where the epidemiological evidence is not yet definitive is the possible role of environmental nitrates in human cancer. A study of stomach cancer mortality in an English town with high nitrate concentration in the drinking water suggested high death rates from the disease. However, a recent re-assessment of this town and its surrounding areas indicated that the local population contained a high proportion of coal miners, whose stomach cancer rates are known to be high. Another site of cancer thought to be possibly involved is the oesophagus, and this derives partly from the fact that the major source of nitrate intake into the human body is from food. The main items of dietary nitrate are vegetables, which themselves have been suggested to be protective against gastric cancer. A recent study of salivary nitrate secretion found higher levels in Oxford (low for stomach cancer) than in the north-east of England and north Wales (high for stomach cancer). These salivary nitrate levels reflect green vegetable consumption, but are inversely related to stomach cancer rates. Thus, the evidence from epidemiological studies that nitrate is involved in the aetiology of stomach cancer is very weak (P. Fraser, personal communication).

In the late 1970s, with the publication of a geochemical atlas containing the distribution on a 1 km grid scale of trace elements in soil over England and Wales there was a suggestion that cancer mortality (in particular, cancers of the lung and prostate)—as well as other morbidity and death rates—might be high in the village of Shipham in Somerset. This had been the site of an old zinc mine, and high levels of cadmium had built up in the soil where home-grown vegetables were produced. These high levels were distinctly noticeable in the geochemical atlas, but [later] epidemiological work did not find high cancer rates among Shipham residents. Other uses of the geochemical atlas in relation to human health are discussed by Thornton and Webb.

Other areas with particularly raised death rates which may be related to the local geology or soil composition include North Wales, which has high rates for cancer of the oesophagus, particularly in women, as well as stomach cancer. This was noted many years ago by Stocks, and the excess levels still persist. Cattle feeding on bracken fern, which are also infected by a papilloma virus, have been shown to suffer a high incidence of alimentary tract cancer. This may have relevance to man and a study of the relationship between the geographical distribution of bracken and cancer mortality is underway (C.P. Taylor et al. in preparation). It has been suggested that the recycling of water may be responsible for the high stomach cancer rates on the east side of London. However, a study taking into account the social class composition and the size of the boroughs with excess rates showed no relationship with water re-use.

(Gardner 1984)

Some Possible Factors

Much research has been devoted to the possibility that nitrates in drinking water are transformed into nitrites in the body, possibly with carcinogenic effects. In the UK various inconclusive studies were made (for example, Clough (1983) on Kent), then a large scale survey sampled 253 urban areas, taking into account varied socioeconomic status and size of urban area; results were negative even analysing separately areas with nitrate levels over the EEC guide level (Beresford 1985).

Aalborg in Denmark has been known for decades to have a high nitrate level, but any effect in causing cancer is thought to be weak (Jensen 1982). A study in Piemonte, Italy, suggests some association between nitrates and stomach cancer, and a threshold level of serious risks (Gilli et al. 1984). An ingenious way of using data of moderate quality in Chile brought out aspects of the problem, though the study was of mortality as a whole (Haynes 1983): the nitrate mining area proved comparatively low in cancers with higher rates in the main areas of intensive agriculture and horticulture. From the US Corn Belt the costs and benefits of nitrogen fertilizers have been estimated, allowing for costs of water treatment where levels are regarded as undesirable, cancer being one of the risks (Commoner 1977). In Quebec a broader survey of hard and soft drinking water (the latter *prima facie* a cancer risk) was inconclusive, if only because other factors might be the real causal ones (Thouez et al. 1981a). WHO have published a general survey of the health aspects of nitrates, nitrites and N-nitroso compounds (*WHO Environmental Health*

Criteria 1978). A study from northern France, for instance, showed no relation between cancer and nitrates in drinking water (Vincent et al. 1983); in Britain salivary nitrate and nitrite have been found to vary inversely with stomach cancer, and the risk queried, though monitoring should continue meantime (Forman et al. 1985). The changing age-structure of the population must be a factor, and the different risks to which different age-cohorts are exposed (Osmond et al. 1982).

Stomach Cancer: a World Context

Before going on to consider more briefly some further studies of stomach cancer patterns within individual countries, it may be helpful to place them, and indeed the United Kingdom material just reviewed, in a world context, as in figure 3.5 (Gillis 1977). The rates are crude death rates, not SMRs as in the earlier maps, but they take another line to make the map meaningful by selecting for analysis age-groups at high relative risk from the disease, covering the years 35–64. Gillis notes the suggestion of a gradient from Eastern Europe and Western USSR with very high rates, through a belt with moderate rates in Western Europe including the United Kingdom, and then across the Atlantic to generally low rates in North America (but with high rates in parts of Latin America). Gillis notes that limited surveys using modern technology to make early diagnosis of the cancers in Japan suggest very high rates there. He reviews the wide range of possible factors that have been studied, and notes that there are no important epidemiological associations between gastric cancers and the intake of alcohol and spices, the extent to which food is chewed, and rapidity of eating, or the temperature of the food as eaten. (Other world views of the cancers as a whole are in Parkin et al. 1984; Waterhouse 1985.)

The high rates for Japan just noted occur with marked within-country variations (see figure 3.6); this also shows a marked decrease in age-adjusted mortality between 1960 and 1970, perhaps due at least partly to the high-technology surveys noted by Gillis, and partly to changes in life style in Japan. Climate and river waters (as a surrogate or substitute variable for drinking water) have been investigated without establishing strong relations. Dietary salt in locally esteemed foods is also suspected but not proven as a causal factor, a possible causal factor lying in its postulated effect in raising blood pressure (Takahashi 1978, quoting Sato et al. 1959); the high rate area in northern Honshu is also high in cerebrovascular diseases, where salt is also suspected, but not yet proven, as a causal factor. Figure 3.7 of crude mortality rates (not age-adjusted) for China shows very widespread incidence, least in the tropical south,

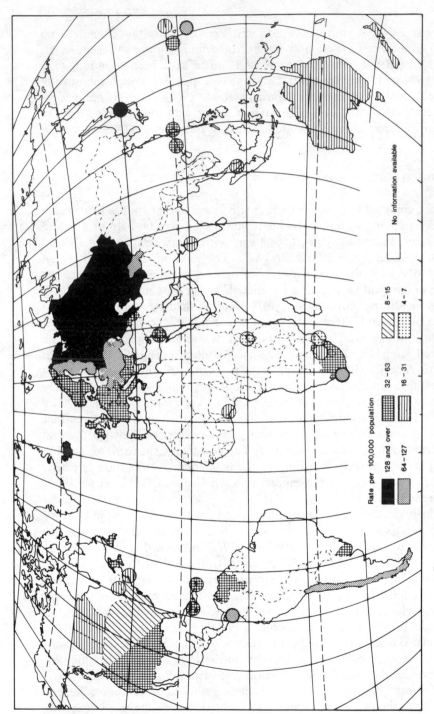

Figure 3.5 World map of stomach cancer, males 35–64 years, probably c.1960
Source: Gillis (1977)

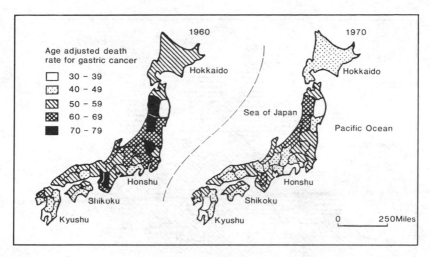

Figure 3.6   Stomach cancer, males, Japan, 1960 and 1970
Source: Takehashi (1978)

with no particular concentration on cities, and a much less focused pattern than that for cancer of the oesophagus (Day 1984). This map will be discussed also in Part II of the book dealing with Third World countries.

In the USA age-adjusted rates of male stomach cancer show a strong predilection for the north and west (figure 3.8, Baker 1980). The author, approaching medical geography from medicine, points out the possibility of confusion in diagnosis between stomach and pancreas cancer because of the close proximity of the two organs in the body, but the corresponding map of cancer of the pancreas (not reproduced here), blurs rather than eliminates the regional pattern. (See also Percy et al. 1981.) He also points out that in a high incidence country like Japan the early detection by high-technology routine surveys may be much more cost-effective than they would be in a country of low and decreasing incidence like the USA. The strongest indication so far is that the disease may be commoner among Finnish Americans. There seems to be a trend towards convergence of urban and rural rates for cancers, and, apart from changes in medical practices and reporting, convergence of life-styles seems to be linked with these changes (Greenberg 1984). The problem of long latency in cancers (specifically stomach cancer in the USA) is tackled in an elegant model including genetic factors and competing causes of mortality in Tolley et al. (1978). (See also Anderson (1984) on north-eastern USA.)

Stomach cancer in Belgium is higher in the Flemish-speaking north (figure 3.9) and there is a statistical association with socioeconomic variables – recent housing, large households, high proportions of labourers,

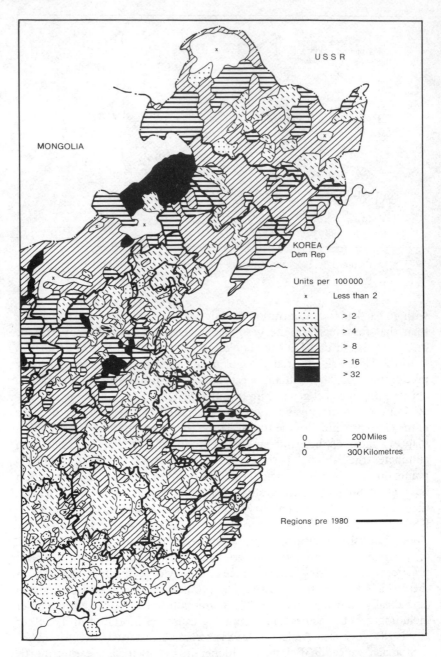

Figure 3.7   Stomach cancer, females, China, *c.*1975. The corresponding map for males shows similar patterns
Source: Day (1984)

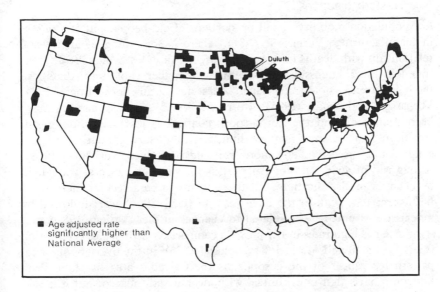

Figure 3.8 Stomach cancer, males, the USA, 1950–1969 – significantly high rates
Source: Baker (1980)

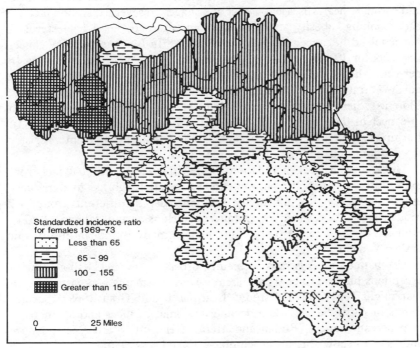

Figure 3.9 Stomach cancer, males, Belgium, 1969–1973
Source: Verhasselt (1981)

low population mobility, small proportions of old people and of workers in manufacturing (Verhasselt 1981). There is something of an inverse relationship with deaths from cerebrovascular diseases, which are concentrated in the French-speaking south (with higher cholesterol diets), so the concurrence noted for Japan does not occur here (Logie 1984; Verhasselt and Logie 1984). In recent years stomach cancers have been decreasing and the north–south contrast is lessened, though still significant; the change may be linked with dietary change, with less smoked and saited food and more fruit and vegetables (Verhasselt 1985). A long run of good data for Antwerp is for stomach cancers, bedevilled by changes in classification, but there seems to be a secular increase in both sexes to a peak in the later years of the 1939–45 war, followed by a decrease assumed to be related to changes in diet (Vrijens 1982).

France has high rates in Brittany – a comparison with Wales is tempting (see figure 3.10 and Mesle 1984; Picheral 1976): in the overlapping areal pattern for cancer of the oesophagus the Calvados area has long been known to have high rates, linked with alcohol and tobacco, but it is said with domestic rather than high-grade commercial production of the cider-based liqueur (Tuyns 1983). On urban cancers, see Picheral (1979). A study in Italy, using international comparisons also, considered cancer and coronary heart disease together and suggested several common factors; age, smoking, obesity and diabetes, but regarded blood cholesterol as not involved in cancer (Menotti et al. 1981). In Italy, respiratory cancer accounts for 19 per cent of cancer deaths, cancer of the stomach for 16 per cent: the Po basin is high for lung, oesophagus and breast cancer; a north-central tract for stomach cancer (Parma, Cremona, Forli, Pesaro, Florence, Siena, Arezzo); the northern and southern extremes are high in cancer of the uterus, and Trieste in bladder cancer (Palagiano 1984). For first cartographic results of high and low total cancers from a registry for Piémont and the Val d'Aosta, see Panero (1976).

The arrival of large populations of Jewish immigrants to Israel from quite different cultural environments a generation ago led to some very interesting surveys of morbidity and mortality in different groups by Modan and others (see, for instance, Tulchinsky and Modan (1967)). Stomach cancers, for instance, were high in many European groups but low in Yemenis.

The pattern in Australia is mainly urban (figure 3.11) though with exceptions like the Cape Yorke area, eastern Tasmania and east of Perth that might repay further study (Learmonth and Grau 1969). Secular trends in Australia include a decline in stomach cancer and an increase in pancreatic cancer (Rohan and McMichael 1981). New Zealand does not seem to show this urban emphasis (Kendrick 1980).

Last of these examples, figure 3.12 (a) and (b) shows a remarkable pattern in South Africa (Bradshaw et al. 1983): the authors can only hint

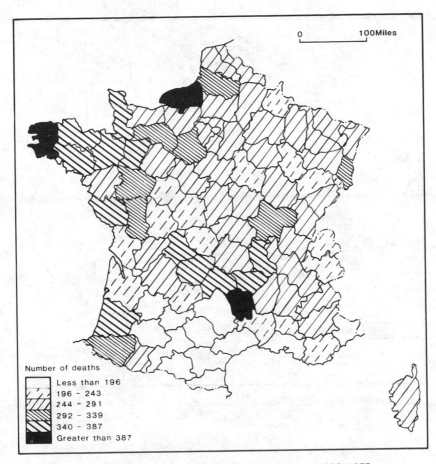

Figure 3.10 Stomach cancer, both sexes, France, 1968–1975
Source: Mesle (1984)

that this remarkably non-urban pattern may in time prove to relate to trace elements in crops and locally derived foods, or possibly in drinking water containing 'derived factors' coming from the catchment.

To sum up, there is a consistency across place and time that regional patterns of stomach cancer seem to exist: it is not distributed across areas merely proportionately to the population. However, so far attempts at causal analysis remain inconclusive and to some extent contradictory, though the apparent contradictions may of course be due to multiple and interacting factors. As so often, the conclusion is that further research seems to be justified: it should preferably be interdisciplinary and it should encompass spatial analysis and studies of individual patients and

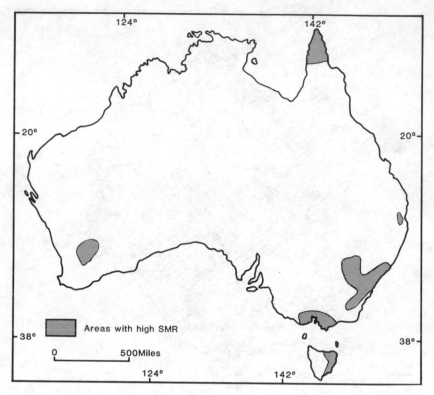

Figure 3.11 Stomach cancer, males, Australia, areas with high rates in both 1959–1963 and 1965–1966
Source: Learmonth and Grau (1969)

local clusters, as well as life-histories and migration patterns. This will be extraordinarily difficult to plan and execute even for one country, and more so if international comparisons are included, as probably they should be, but not impossible given the will.

A good deal of space has been devoted to stomach cancer, since its study shows both the potential of mapping, and that maps and atlases are apt to raise questions rather than answer them, unless their analysis is followed by other research along the lines just suggested. A quite comparable scale of review could be mounted for several other cancers – indeed for other causes of death as in later chapters – but in a short book such a full discussion cannot be justified. In necessarily briefer and much more selective discussion of maps of cancers of some other sites in the body it is tempting to focus on maps showing some dramatic contrast between regions, even if a map for a different period presents a less clear-cut picture; however, an attempt will be made to put each example in context with what is known of other study periods or of trends in that particular cause of mortality. Lung cancer is an obvious starting point since that has been the subject of much public discussion.

Lung Cancer

Figure 3.13 is of lung cancer for males of 15–64 years for 1970–2 in the United Kingdom (Howe 1979). As Howe points out, this map is of particular interest because of the strong link between cigarette smoking and lung cancer, well established a whole generation ago (Doll and Hill 1952) to which must now be added links between smoking and bronchitis and also cardiovascular diseases. Data on present and past smoking show maximum proportions (of smokers to male population over 15 years) in Wales and East Anglia, whereas the highest lung cancer rates are concentrated in the urban north and west of England, in lowland Scotland and in parts of London (and these are less exclusively the East End boroughs than in figures 3.1–3.4 on stomach cancer). Howe suggests that these anomalies may in time be explained by synergistic or additive influences of air pollution, as by chemicals like polycyclic aromatic hydrocarbons, physical materials like asbestos, and in some places by radiation, natural or man-made. Gardner (1984) points to the strong urban bias as linked with heavier cigarette smoking in cities, and the rising female incidence as linked with increased smoking by women. In addition to the factors mentioned by Howe, in fact overlapping with them, are occupational links, but these well illustrate the multiple factors likely to be at work in addition to cigarettes, for occupation is linked with smoking patterns and, over populations, so is social class. So while the campaigns to reduce cigarette smoking are well justified in relation to lung cancer and the other important causes of death mentioned earlier, mapping reveals the need – or strengthens the case – for further research into lung cancer patterns. Not unexpectedly, bronchitis shows considerable overlap in pattern with lung cancer. In France, lung cancer rates are high in the industrial north-east, but also in the Midi and in the Gironde area, a pattern contrasting with the high rates for bronchitis and emphysema in the Massif Central (Perdrizet and Liard 1981). Even excluding nuclear plant disasters and the like, the literature on air pollution is vast: the spectrum is perhaps illustrated by Dockery et al. (1982); Lawther (1982); and Shabad et al. (1982).

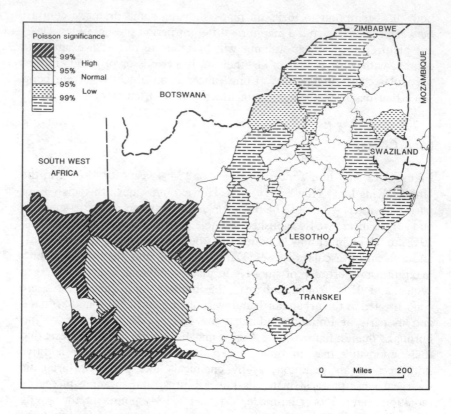

Figure 3.12 (a)   Stomach cancer, males, South Africa, for all three races combined
Source: Bradshaw et al. 1983

Cancer of the Breast and Uterus

The maps of breast cancer and of cancer of the uterus show marked contrast in pattern (figures 3.14 and 3.15). The breast cancer map is for the United Kingdom for 1970–2 in women of 15–64 (Howe 1979), the cancer of the uterus one for 1954–8 for England and Wales, using SMRs for all age groups (Howe 1970). The breast cancer shows no strong regional pattern except perhaps for high rates in rural Scotland that are not confirmed by maps for other periods. Rates for Scotland as a whole, however, are regarded as high and rising slowly, stimulating efforts to improve data (Kemp and Smith 1982). Israeli immigrant data suggest links with higher socioeconomic groups and with western countries of

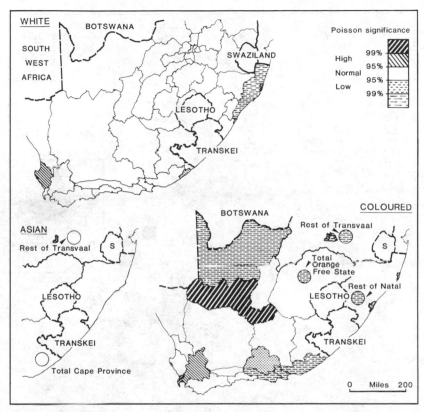

Figure 3.12 (b) Stomach cancer, males, South Africa, for whites, and Asians and coloureds separately. (No data on black population.)
Source: Bradshaw et al. 1983

origin (Bertini et al. 1971). Despite national and regional differences in rates, breast cancer in several countries tended to decrease until about 1900 and then to rise (Stevens et al. 1982). The map for cancer of the uterus shows a massive predilection for the north and west – in this instance including Cornwall; the pattern in London does not have a bias towards the East End. Elsewhere high rates in rural Norfolk, Bedfordshire (rural and urban) and parts of the Isle of Wight are interesting but not confirmed by the map for 1959–63 (not reproduced here).

It is possible that screening programmes may be a factor in rising *reported* incidence of cervical cancer in Britain (Cook and Draper 1984); Roberts (1982) raises a cautionary issue on the effectiveness of screening in that high-risk groups may be the very ones less represented among

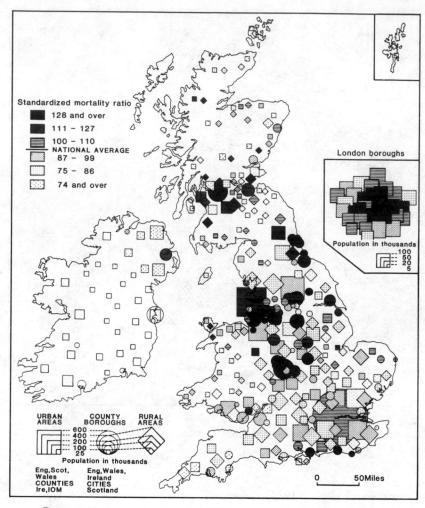

Figure 3.13 Lung cancer, males, 15–64 years, the UK, 1970–1972
Source: Howe (1979)

those coming forward for tests. Cancer of the cervix of the uterus, a large proportion of these cancers, is now confidently linked with the papilloma or wart virus, and specifically with penile warts (e.g. Schwarz et al. 1985). Given this, would one still think of linking the regional pattern with poor housing and bathing facilities, poor health education and poor penile and vaginal hygiene? Increased screening against the disease by means of vaginal smear tests, now with semi-automatic processing, is certainly called for and with regional priorities indicated by mapping.

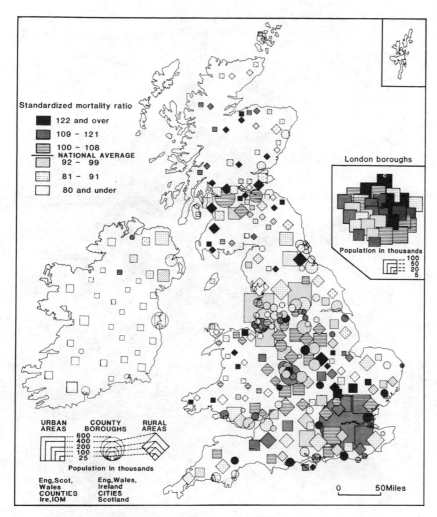

Figure 3.14   Breast cancer, females, 15–64 years, the UK, 1970–1972
Source: Howe (1979)

The unique population recording system in Sweden, combined with high rates of screening, offers some of the most convincing evidence of benefits (Stenkvist et al. 1984). Thus this cancer is now regarded as both preventable and curable given early detection. But beyond the available technologies lie problems of poverty, housing deprivation and health education.

In Japan, breast cancers show no clear areal pattern, but areas high in uterine cancer are concentrated in the southern half of the main island

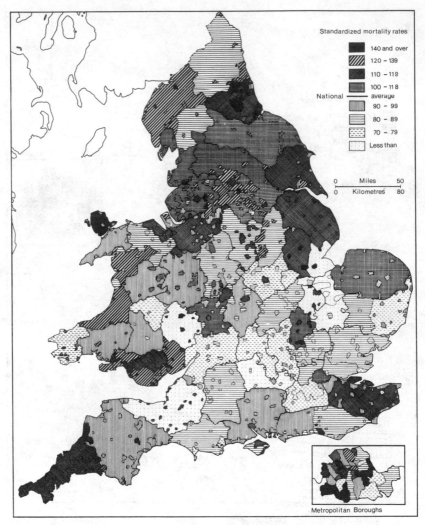

Figure 3.15   Cancer of the uterus, England and Wales, 1954–1958
Source: Howe (1970)

of Honshu (Ohno and Aoki 1981). Fukushima et al. (1985) report that
the papilloma virus, while frequently associated with precursor lesions,
is not consistently found in invasive squamous cell carcinoma. (For
overviews of the role of viruses in cancers see, for instance, Melnick et
al. 1985.)

A valuable source on cancers in the USSR in English has recently
become available (Napalkov et al. 1983). Age-standardized rates have

been declining in both sexes for cancers of the lip, oesophagus and stomach, and for cervix uteri in women; skin cancer in women is stable but rising in men. All other sites analysed in the book show rising rates: trachea, breast and lymphatic and haematopoietic. Cancer of the oesophagus, discussed in chapter 13 has the most striking regional disparities, with very high rates for both sexes in the Turkmen and other Soviet republics bordering Iran, Afghanistan and China, where pharyngeal cancers are also common. In 1969–71 stomach cancer was still the commonest site, but by 1979 it had been overtaken by lung cancer in men; this last cancer is still highest in the north-western republics bordering eastern Europe, and in Estonian men it was already commoner than stomach cancer in 1969–71. Breast cancer rates rose markedly from 1965 to 1980 and are high in the Baltic republics but are among the lowest in the world in Asian republics. Cervical cancer rates are much lower and, in contrast to breast cancers, they are declining. (See also Levin 1980.)

Some Possible Causal Factors

International comparisons are suggestive of some environmental relations of a few cancers. Thus Armstrong and Doll (1975), point to meat eating as probably connected with cancer of the colon and rectum, and fat with cancer of the breast and corpus uteri; and international trends raise questions about the reasons for the widespread decrease in stomach cancer in both sexes and in cancer of the uterus (Hayakawa and Kurihara 1981). This almost concludes the discussion of cancers so far as this chapter is concerned – there will be later discussion of some geographical techniques that have been applied to some cancers in chapters 5 and 13. Two brief points, however, should be made.

There may be a genetic element in cancer. For instance people with blood group A seem, on statistical evidence, to be somewhat more liable to gastric cancers than do people with other ABO blood (for discussion and references see Howe (1979)); however, in that instance as in others it has not so far been shown to explain the spatial pattern – that is, maps of the blood group are not closely similar to maps of high and low rates of the cancer. Up to now blood groups have been the best-studied and best-mapped of the genetic markers because of their importance in blood transfusion (Mourant et al. 1976). More recently, broader studies of genetic markers in France using intensive sample surveys of local populations may point the way forward to deeper studies of genetic factors in cancer and indeed in other disease (Cambon-Thomson et al. 1984).

The genetic element in health and disease receives only occasional mention in this book, on topics where the geography of a suggested link has been explored to some extent. An entry point into 'genetic epidemiology' is in Ward (1980). However, for cancers it is now widely accepted that a large proportion – some claim 80 per cent – is environmental rather than genetic.

Cancers and the Environment

One of the most influential indications of the proportions of cancers due to the environment and largely preventable is in the report to the US Congress by Sir Richard Doll and R. Peto (1981): the largest component is the 30 per cent of cancer deaths due to tobacco, with only some 4 per cent due to occupation as such, industrial carcinogens and the like (as against boring jobs being a factor in addiction to smoking).

There is also a growing literature on possible psychosocial bases of cancer, such as emotional factors that may influence some oncogenic growths, and on factors promoting early or late presentation for diagnosis and treatment (see, for example, Pettingale (1985)). There may well be geographical implications, apparently little explored as yet.

Cancers as a Whole

It is sometimes suggested that despite the widespread and accepted convention of analysing cancers of different sites separately, viewing cancers as a group of diseases and not a single entity, there may be merit in conducting some studies, including geographical ones, of cancers as a whole. The hypothesis here would be that there may be some master variable or set of interacting variables tending to initiate all or at least most cancers; given the presence of such a master variable, individuals or even groups of people, including spatially differentiated populations, might tend to acquire cancer of a particular site – lung, oesophagus, liver, stomach etc. – as a result of some genetic predisposition or environmental factor. So far, it is fair to say, geographical studies have not advanced far in this direction, though this picture may change. However, there may be considerable value in studying and mapping cancers as a whole in health care geography and this point is developed in Pyle (1971).

Cartographic Techniques

Finally, all the cancer maps discussed so far are based directly on administrative or census areas, except for figure 3.11, taken from one of two atlases of disease mortality produced by the author and two research assistants from the Australian National University. Figure 3.16 is yet another map of stomach cancer, one of the two from which figure 3.11 was drawn. It is a contour or isopleth map, representing as it were hills and valleys of cancer mortality. Clearly most researchers, whether from geography or from biostatistics, have preferred the administrative unit or choropleth map (Greek *khora*, land). One reason for my preference is that people in a single administrative unit appearing with high expectation

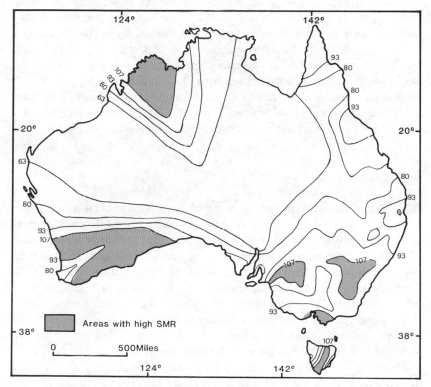

Figure 3.16   Stomach cancer, males, Australia, 1965–1966 using isopleths ('contours')
Source: Learmonth & Grau (1969)

of cancer deaths may receive alarmist rumours. That the single-unit high may be due to occupational disease, or possibly a specific factor like a particular source of drinking water has already been noted. The case for isopleth mapping, not to supplant but to complement choropleth maps, is developed in a wider context in Part II of this book dealing with geographical research techniques applied in ecological medical geography.

Some Useful References

On the world scale, a benchmark bibliographical survey is in Peeters (1980); Tromp (1976) reviews the possible effects of soil, water and meteorological factors, Tran Ba Loc (1981) reviews water pollution as a factor, and a special issue of the *Journal of the Geological Society* (1980) is on geology and health; Verhasselt (1976) illustrates world patterns with maps from her atlas of 1975 and ways in which geographers may approach the many questions raised. A number of papers make methodological points, often cautionary: Magnus (1982) stresses the importance of time trends in incidence and mortality data and the pitfalls in the data. Cleek (1979) suggests that the many problems of scale-related differences in spatial patterns obtained in mapping the same data on different scales may be used positively in hypothesis formulation; Glick (1979a,b) similarly proposes a positive approach to spatial autocorrelation, links theoretical models of carcinogenesis to spatial patterns in incidence and offers a major review of geographical approaches to this field of research.

Conclusion

Examples of various types of mapping of cancers have been represented, some from general atlases of disease mortality, some from atlases of cancers. The accompanying text is descriptive and analytical to the extent of seeking for possible causes, but generally raising rather than answering questions, itself a useful function. So far there is a role in putting the spatial pattern before research workers in case avenues of future research are suggested by them, and before laymen too as a matter of appreciation of the geography of disease – an aspect surprising to many. Pyle's work cited in chapters 5 and 16 shows that there can be a logistic or health-planning function for mapping of forecast needs.

There are two essential works for any student interested to follow up this chapter with further reading and map study: Professor G.M. Howe's splendid edited volume *Global Geocancerology: a world geography of human cancers*, 1986, Edinburgh, Churchill-Livingstone, and the equally important short book on *The Geography of Non-Infectious Disease* by M.S.R. Hutt and D.P. Burkitt, 1986, Oxford University Press, in which the combination of a professor of geographical pathology and a world-famous tropical surgeon compels the attention of geographers.

4 Further Cartographic Studies

Introductory

In this chapter we continue with the main 'western diseases' – heart diseases, strokes and 'accidents' (not of course really a disease) – then turn to just one more atlas-based study of a specific disease, diabetes, before looking briefly at infant mortality, again not a specific disease but a valuable general indicator of the health and welfare status of populations that covers a large number of specific causes of death. As in the latter part of chapter 3, the text is deliberately short and selective, but the resources available in the literature are sufficient for more comprehensive studies to be made by any interested reader with access to a good library.

Cardiovascular (including Cerebrovascular) Diseases

Turning to the cardiovascular (including cerebrovascular) diseases, the definitions and discussion of chapter 2 have established that there are at least some common proven factors and more suspected ones in the heart diseases and the strokes etc., relating to the environment, specifically to life styles – smoking (certainly), lack of exercise (probably), excessive alcohol consumption (certainly), and dietary fat (probably but with controversy still raging around cholesterol, saturated fats, or just the proportion of fats in the total diet). See WHO (1982 TRS 678). Sugar, it seems, is mainly involved through its contribution to excess calorie intake in relation to physical exercise in many people's diet. From USSR comes evidence that suggests that the rural life style encourages cardiovascular disease more than does the urban (Furmenko et al. 1982).

Starting with one of the main types of heart disease, ischaemic heart disease, a world map (not reproduced here) is suggestive of high rates in developed countries and – of course on imperfect data – of low rates in the Third World (Howe et al. (1977), figures 17.2 to 17.5, pp. 436–9 using crude death rates for ages 35–64 for males and for females, 1969–71). For within-country patterns Howe's 1954–8 map for males, covering a wider spectrum of heart deaths, offers a useful starting point of conditions a generation ago (figure 4.1). This is one of many maps in Howe's 1963 and 1970 atlases to show a heavy bias towards high rates in the north and west of England and Wales, and usually covering much of Scotland

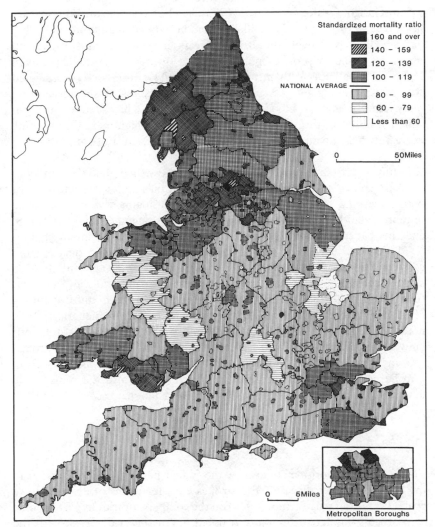

Figure 4.1   Arteriosclerotic heart disease, males, England and Wales, 1954–1958
Source: Howe (1970)

and Northern Ireland also. The map for females is broadly similar, as are the maps for both sexes for 1959–63 (not reproduced here). Outside the north and west there seems to be an urban bias, even away from the great cities. London is mainly above the national expectation of deaths from these diseases, but there is not the concentration of high rates in the East End noted for some of the cancers, while there is perhaps a suggestion of high rates in commuter-land – though East Sussex, for instance, does not show such high rates in the 1959–63 maps. On the within-Glasgow scale, see Howe (1983). A class relationship of coronary heart disease is now well established for the United Kingdom: mortality has steadily risen over the last 40 years in working-class men, but remained stable in professional men: thus the rate is now 26 per cent higher in social class V than in social class I. The difference is associated with more smoking and less exercise in the lower class, to shorter stature, more obesity, higher blood pressure and lower glucose tolerance but which are genuine differential causal factors and which merely co-varying characteristics remain to be proven and even identified (Rose and Marmot, 1981).

Figure 4.2 from Australia shows the areas with high SMRs in both 1959–63 and in 1965–6 with a mainly urban bias and some oddities for both males and females in 'outback' areas. Tasmania was later mapped in more detail by McGlashan and Chick for the same periods (figure 4.3) and this paper is discussed from a complementary viewpoint in chapter 5 (McGlashan and Chick 1974). A substantial decrease in deaths from coronary heart disease in New Zealand has been attributed to a smaller consumption of dairy products, less smoking and more exercise (Beaglehole et al. 1981, cf. Walker (1983) on USA). A thoughtful survey of decline in many but not all developed countries is in Picheral (1981), noting changes of various kinds. Winterstein (1980) notes relations between circulatory and cardiovascular diseases in different Israeli groups and in their countries of origin, with high rates in immigrants from Europe, and low (but rising) rates in Asian Jews – also the remarkably low rates among the Druse (non-Jewish) population.

Strokes, etc.

Figure 4.4 is a world map to give the global perspective as we turn to the cerebrovascular diseases, the strokes etc., for males of 35–64 (Howe et al. (1977), and see Marmot (1984) on the complex topic of hypertension). It is broadly similar to the pattern noted for the heart diseases, with the caveat that data from the Third World may not be comparable. However, Japan here is amongst the highest rates – it is quite low in the heart

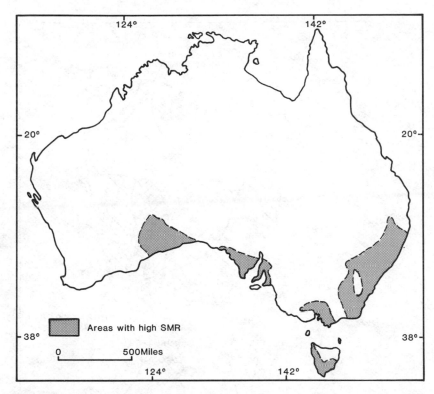

Figure 4.2 Arteriosclerotic and degenerative heart disease, males, Australia, areas with high rates in both 1959–1963 and 1965–1966
Source: Learmonth and Grau (1969)

disease map. Britain as a whole is not quite so high, nor South Africa, Australia or New Zealand, while Portugal, Bulgaria and Argentina have higher rates here. This illustrates the tendency for a small group of main causes of death to be common to developed countries, but to change in order of importance from country to country or from time to time. For a Japanese view of cardiovascular disease in Europe, see Takahashi (1967).

Howe's map of strokes and related diseases for 1954–8 is not reproduced here, though it is well worth study in the original: it shares the heavy bias towards high rates in the north and west of England and Wales, over most of Scotland and considerable parts of Northern Ireland. There are some high rates in eastern England in fen and in brickfield areas, and perhaps in commuter-land round London, though these are lower in the 1959–63 map. The highest London rates are in the north and

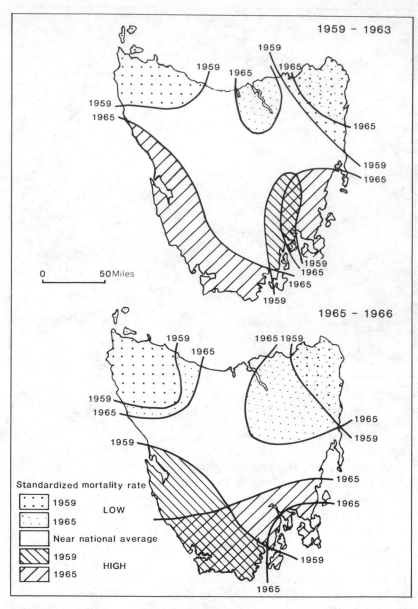

Figure 4.3 Ischaemic heart disease, males, Tasmania, 1959–1963 and 1965–1966
Source: McGlashan and Chick (1974)

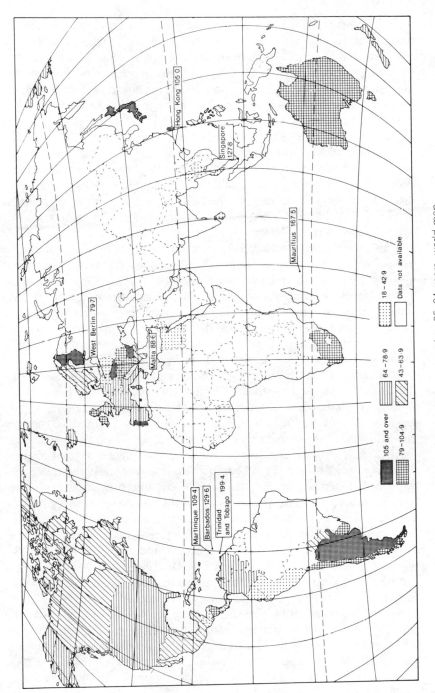

Figure 4.4 Cerebrovascular disease, males, 35–64 years, world map
Source Howe and Burgess (1977)

west. The maps for females are broadly similar, with very high rates in much of the north-east of England, over nearly all Lowland and Border Scotland, and much of Northern Ireland. In England and Wales mortality from strokes is higher in men aged 15–64 in 'lower' socioeconomic groupings, and a survey of blood pressure in the North East shows higher pressures in lower classes, with a maximum at about 30 years (see e.g. Caldwell et al. (1983)). On the contradictory evidence on salt as an influence on hypertension, see, for example, Cummins (1983).

This concordance between the heart disease and the stroke maps stands out as quite a dramatic contrast with Japan, and moreover the regional contrasts within Japan are equally sharp (figure 4.5). Note the very marked concentration of high stroke rates in the north of the main island of Honshu (Takahashi 1981; Omura et al. 1987). This is only one of several maps of related diseases, remarkably consistent with each other and also over time (see also Shigematsu 1978, 1979). This remarkable pattern will be discussed in chapter 5 on geographical methodology, but meantime it is worth pointing out that while Takahashi has analysed a wide number of variables, including for instance the calcium sulphate content of water supplies, the prime suspect to many researchers is high salt content in many esteemed local dishes, though until laboratory proof is forthcoming hardline medical scientists are reluctant to accept the findings. A study of salt intake and strokes (and stomach cancer also) used a coarse areal network of 46 prefectures and 12 regions, and this did not support the hypothesis of salt as a causal factor (Kono et al. 1983). A recent symposium included several papers on this topic, mainly negative in 'hard' findings, but a report from the USA on reduced weight *and* salt intake was encouraging (Tuomilehto and Wolf 1984).

An almost equally dramatic regional contrast comes from Belgium. The map of SMRs for cerebrovascular diseases is almost the inverse of figure 3.9 of stomach cancer: there is a heavy concentration of high rates in the southern, French-speaking part of the country and comparatively low rates in the Flemish north, linked at least suggestively with the consumption of butter in the south and margarine, mainly from vegetable oils, in the north (Logie 1984; Verhasselt and Logie 1984). For the within-Brussels picture see Moens (1984). There is a methodological problem in comparing two distribution maps for likeness or contrast, especially if statistical correlation measures are used: there may well be a 'spatial autocorrelation' effect, that is contiguity as such may be influencing a particular pattern, rather than the proposed causal factor. This has been investigated, for example, in relation to patterns of chronic diseases in Montreal: there was a slight but significant autocorrelation effect, yet other factors such as socioeconomic grouping etc. were probably more important (Bouchard 1976).

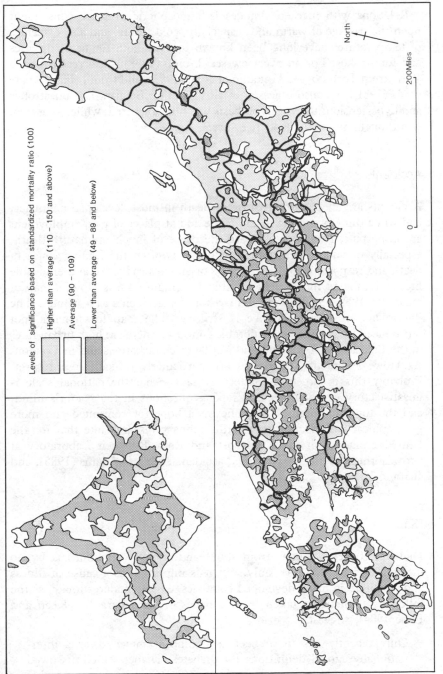

Figure 4.5 Cerebrovascular disease, males, Japan, 1969–1974
Source: Takehashi 1978

Relations with marked changes in atmospheric pressure consequent upon the passage of warm and, especially, cold fronts, and also extremes of temperature, have long been known to exist both for heart diseases and for strokes. For an overview see Tromp (1973); for a recent urban study from Toronto, see Mukammal et al. (1983); and from Dakar, Koate et al. (1981). See also Staessen et al. (1981) on Belgian data on strokes and hypertension: the salt hypothesis was not supported, while potassium was thought to *lower* blood pressure.

Accidents

Accidents are an important cause of death in most developed countries, and while those occurring in the home and at places of paid employment are important, road accidents are the cause of much premature death, especially of young men among whom it is often the leading cause of death and responsible for many years of loss of productive and enjoyable life, as estimated for Canada in table 2.1. Figure 4.6 is Howe's map of males for 1959–63 (the 1954–8 map was for accidents as a whole). The importance of rural residence is striking. The map for females (not reproduced here) shows considerable contrasts: there are high urban rates in the Lancashire, Yorkshire and Midlands conurbations and in London. As Howe comments, the maps are particularly difficult to interpret. Probably this is largely a matter of scale – that the national scale is unsatisfactory except indeed in raising questions in the reader's mind, and the topic so complex that one must hope for continued and more geographical participation in interdisciplinary research like that for the United Kingdom in the Transport and Road Research Laboratory at Crowthorne in Berkshire. On road accidents, see also Adams (1985), and chapter 2 above.

Diabetes

Diabetes (Greek, siphon, from thirst and copious urination) is by no means a 'western disease' only, but it is important as a cause of illness and disability in many developed countries, easy to underestimate, as the following quotations, taken from a paper on its geography (Keen and Ekoe 1984), suggest:

Only recently has there been a significant move towards inter-nationally agreed definitions for diabetes. Diabetes mellitus owed its diagnostic origins to a striking *clinical* syndrome of unassuagable

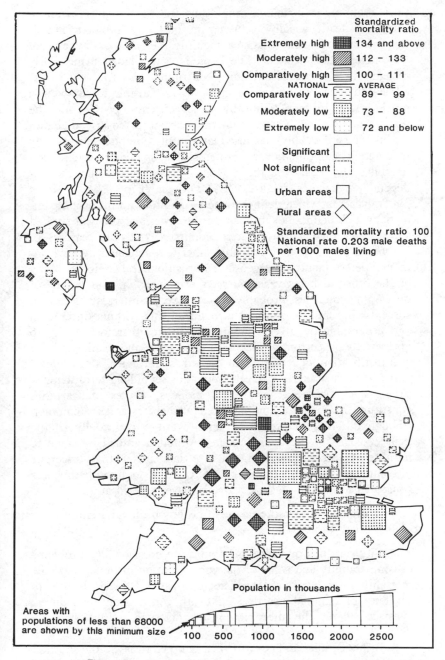

Figure 4.6 Road accidents, males, the UK, 1959–1963
Source: Howe (1970)

thirst, voluminous urination, rapid physical wasting progressing to coma and death, usually occurring in youth or childhood. This is the insulin-dependent diabetes mellitus (IDDM) or Type 1 of the current classification. The copious, sugar-laden urine, early recognized as a constant feature, contributed descriptively to the name and, in more recent history, was responsible for drawing a much larger group of clinically rather different people into the diabetic designation. Though sometimes heavily glycosuric, diabetics of this type are usually diagnosed later in life, are often obese, only moderately symptomatic, free of ketosis and spared the progression to coma and death of the classical case. This is non-insulin-dependent diabetes mellitus (NIDDM or Type 2) ... It is hyperglycaemia which defines diabetes mellitus and the accompaniments which define its subtypes. In the genesis of the well studied subtypes of diabetes in Western countries, the twin features of individual susceptibility, probably inherited, activated by environmental determinants emerge as a major aetiological complex. Many of the other diabetes variants, seen principally in populations of developing countries, probably also involve the interplay of genetic susceptibility and environmental determinants. Ethnic differences and geographically diverse environments are, therefore, likely to give rise to a spectrum of diabetes mechanisms and manifestations.

A justification for retaining the diabetic syndrome as a nosological entity is the characteristic development of a set of long-term sequels. Progressive damage to the eyes, kidneys, nerves and arteries constitute the so-called complications of diabetes and are common (though differing in prevalence and severity) to virtually all the many variants of the diabetic state. Although argued by some to indicate a common underlying cause to the diabetes, this stereotype of complications seems more likely to point to common pathogenic consequences of the diabetic state, however arrived at.

Keen and Ekoe introduce the theme of geographical variation in diabetic mortality thus:

Mortality statistics by causal groupings are notorious for problems of comparability and some of the wide variation in the age-specific mortality rates attributed to diabetes (Table 1 [4.1]) is due to diversity of national practices in death certification procedures. West considered the interpretation of data such as these in some detail.

In Britain, Fuller and co-workers attempted to assess the shortfall in the true contribution of diabetes to mortality by analysing death certificates with any mention of diabetes and noting the frequency of accompanying contributing causes also recorded on the certificate.

Circulatory diseases were disproportionately more frequently associated with mention of diabetes; deaths in such individuals are most commonly classified to cardiovascular cause without mention of diabetes. In a cohort of about 6000 diabetic patients assembled between 1965 and 1969 by the British Diabetic Association, the standardized mortality ratios for vascular disease and ischaemic heart disease were all in excess of 100, especially in women; women aged 15–44 years on entry into the cohort had an 11-fold greater risk of ischaemic heart disease death than comparably aged non-diabetics. In general, cause-specific mortality rates may greatly underestimate the contribution of diabetes to mortality, a conclusion endorsed by Tokuhata et al. and West. The high rates for Malta and Mauritius are notable in Table 1. The health departments of both countries have initiated WHO-sponsored enquiries into national diabetes prevalence and its associations and a study of glucose tolerance, nutrition and diabetic complications on an approximately 1% sample of the Maltese adult population has recently been completed.

Table 4.1, the 'Table I' of the quotation, gives a world perspective of diabetes mortality. While morbidity data would be more useful than

Table 4.1 Diabetes mortality by country or area (rates by age per 100 000 reported between 1973 and 1976)

	Age group				
	35–44	45–54	55–64	65–74	75+
Africa					
Egypt	4.3	15.9	38.9	67.2	67.7
Mauritius	12.6	68.3	158.5	316.9	391.8
America					
El Salvador	3.8	7.9	26.4	58.1	79.4
USA	4.2	10.3	29.3	75.2	174.3
Venezuela	4.8	22.5	72.8	155.6	283.8
Asia					
Hong Kong	1.2	5.6	26.6	56.4	90.5
Japan	2.1	5.5	18.1	54.2	97.0
Singapore	3.5	16.9	64.6	182.7	236.3
Europe					
England and Wales	2.1	3.6	12.0	37.5	93.3
Malta	8.7	28.1	146.4	491.9	1243.9
Norway	2.0	3.6	6.8	23.3	70.3
Sweden	6.1	8.2	17.6	57.8	214.4

Source: Keen and Ekoe (1984), p. 359

mortality data, the table probably reflects the relative position well enough, and the same is true for the within-country picture revealed by figures 4.7 and 4.8, Howe's maps for females for 1954–8 for Scotland and for England and Wales respectively (Howe 1963, 1970). The author must confess that the selection of these maps is because they make the case for within-country analysis of health and disease so dramatically. The maps for males for the same period are only a little less dramatic, and with some very curious differences – high urban rates, for instance, in Lincolnshire and East Anglia (sugar-beet growing, marketing and

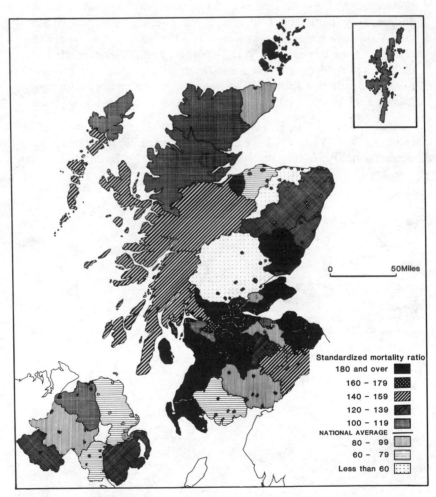

Figure 4.7   Diabetes, females, Scotland, 1954–1958
Source: Howe (1970)

processing? – it is hard to credit). The corresponding maps for 1959–63 are less dramatic, deliberately so to the extent that the demographic base map reduces the visual impact for large areas of low population say in parts of the Scottish high-rate area. The strong bias towards Scotland, parts of Wales and parts of North-East England remains clear, however, surely inviting more detailed studies? The evidence from Howe's atlases

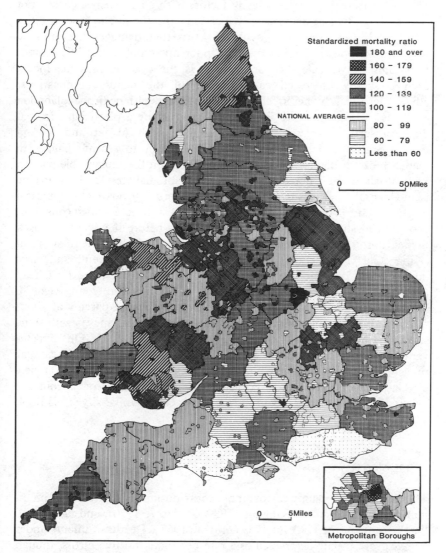

Figure 4.8   Diabetes, females, England and Wales, 1954–1958
Source: Howe (1970)

surely tempts one to hypothesize that regional differences in diet must
be a factor in the regional contrasts, and possibly even in the variations
in the areal patterns for the sexes? A review by Keen (1982) aimed mainly
at preventive measures neatly sums up the risk of diabetes as 'susceptibility
challenged by appropriate environmental triggers'. Noting war-time
privation as *reducing* diabetes, probably mainly the non-insulin-dependent
type, over-nutrition seems a likely factor, with sugar suspected but not
proven. This type of diabetes in 'Caucasians' may be due to susceptibility
triggered by an infection, possibly a virus that damages the immune
response with destruction of B cells. Under-nutrition, on the other hand,
is thought to damage the pancreas, as is the cyanide in some foods,
such as badly processed cassava. One of the many complications,
atherosclerosis, is higher in females than in males, with no firm explanation
available: a possible cause is iatrogenic (caused by a physician), in that
diets prescribed for patients were usually high in fat and low in
carbohydrates, and often high in salt also prior to recent changes in
management of diabetic diets. (This may bear on the remarkable pattern
in Scottish women noted above.) A study of diabetes in three Pacific
island populations assumes three risk factors – overweight, physical
inactivity and urbanization, and although these were found inconsistent
and to need study in specific societal contexts before they could be used
in identifying groups at risk, it is tempting to ask if they apply in Scotland
(King et al. 1983). For a recent review of genetic elements and virus
infections as possible causes of juvenile-onset diabetes, see Craighead
(1981). A possible environmental link for diabetes in young men in
Iceland is the eating of smoked cured mutton by the parents at about
the time of conception and by the mother during pregnancy – with some
support from animal experiment (Helgason et al. 1982). On diabetes
viewed as a social disease in Italy, see Brancato (1983). On the similar
prevalence in both sexes in China, see Zhong (1982). For a sceptical view
of diabetes treatment, see Posner (1977, 1984) and for a rounded
discussion of the orthodox and the sceptical, Open University (1985 Book
1); on relativism in diagnosis see Hunt (1985).

Infant Mortality

The last of these mainly cartographic contributions is figure 4.9 of infant
mortality in the United Kingdom 1959–63 (Howe 1970), and figure 4.10
for the same in the USA for 1959 (Murray 1967). Deaths of infants under
one year are usually expressed as a rate per thousand live births, though
for many Third World communities, tragically, it would be as appropriate
to use a percentage because the rates are so high. Apart from this

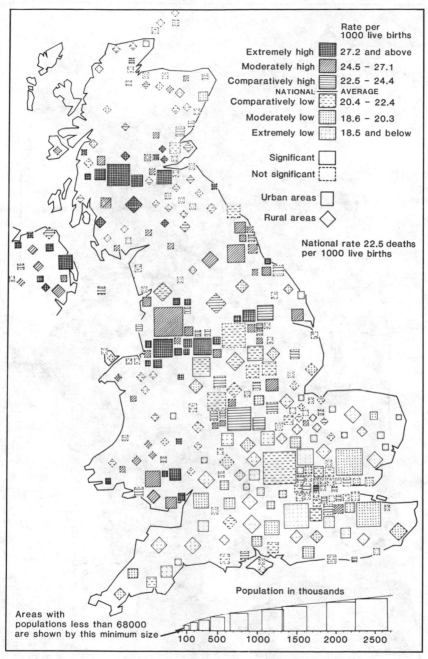

Figure 4.9   Infant mortality, the UK, 1959–1963
Source: Howe (1970)

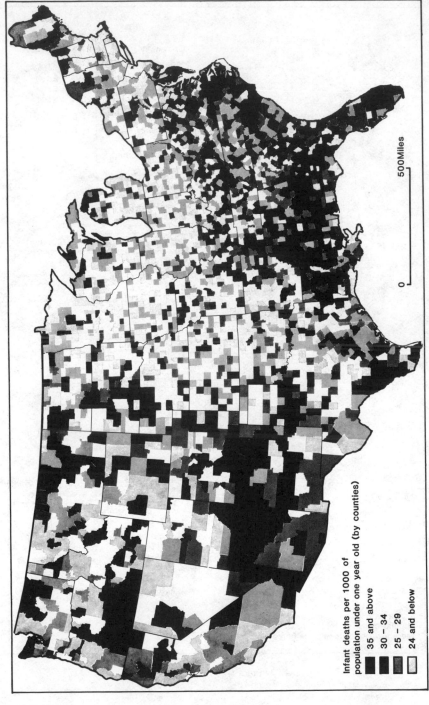

Infant deaths per 1000 of
population under one year old (by counties)

■ 35 and above

■ 30 – 34

■ 25 – 29

□ 24 and below

0   500Miles

Figure 4.10 Infant mortality the USA, 1959

difference from the various maps of death rates or ratios to total population by sex or for selected age groups by sex, these maps differ also in that they cover a wide spectrum of causes of infant deaths. They are included because infant mortality is one of the best widely available indices of general levels of material living and welfare, and one that is available with relative accuracy for less developed countries also, thus offering one of the few fairly reliable bases of comparison between developed and developing countries. For Britain the high rates of South Wales stand out, as also those of many of the older-industry towns and cities of the North of England, lowland Scotland and Northern Ireland. Along with the bias to heavy disease burdens in the north and west noted earlier, these patterns tell their own tale. Murray's paper is a pioneer study which attempts to put health data into the geographer's endeavours to include standards of living in analyses of population density in population geography. It is primarily a comparison of infant mortality mapping compared with maps of total death rates. He prefers the infant mortality map as a measure, or as at least a strong reflection, of standards of living, pointing to the 'more uniform gradation in density from the North-east and Mid-west towards the South . . . the map properly reflects, more accurately, the gradation of level-of-living conditions'. Readers wishing to test this for the United Kingdom will find total mortality maps in Howe (1970).

For developed countries with good vital statistics' recording, data on perinatal mortality are often taken as better indications of standards of living and of health, and also of quality of health care (Waaler and Sterky 1984). In highly developed countries it is suggested that in recent decades the association between socioeconomic factors and infant mortality has been weakened (Markides and McFarland 1982). Newland (1982) again suggests that if infant mortality rises or even fails to fall as income rises – as in Washington DC in recent years – then something is wrong with the health of society (she goes on to compare the lower infant mortality in poor but socially conscious Kerala in south-west India with the higher rates in the much richer Punjab). A specifically geographical contribution is Knox's (1981) paper on regional convergence and divergence in trends over time in infant mortality in the United Kingdom 1949–54 to 1970–2. Most local areas showed no significant change, but the study highlights areas that, with no worse deprivation than others, have fallen behind in the twenty years. Some have experienced sharp deterioration in conditions while other quite prosperous areas seem to have reached an irreducible minimum of infant mortality; among favoured areas, some are rural but apparently progressive areas, while some showing marked improvement are among the notoriously deprived parts of the country. While raising rather than answering questions about underlying causes of change, the paper is one of great challenge. Wilson (1978) found in Sydney links with social disruption rather than poverty as such.

Todson (1980) tested for effects of distance from infant care facilities in Hillsborough County, Florida, but came back to socioeconomic factors – better-off people could overcome the friction of distance! Several Australian studies suggest some association with living standards and life style, not necessarily with poverty as ̀such in 'the lucky country', but perhaps rather social disorganization, with Aboriginal groups as the extreme cases (Wilson 1979). Dube and Youde (1981) note high rates in a 'poverty crescent' within Quebec City, but an Inuit ('Eskimo') group in northern Quebec province have seen rates falling from Third World levels of 330 per thousand live births in 1945 to a moderate though still serious level of 136 in 1970 (Normandeau and Legare 1979).

Conclusion

This chapter is less specialized than is chapter 3 on the cancers, and being selective, raises the obvious point that quite a different selection might have been made. It includes the other two main 'western diseases', heart disease and strokes etc.; accidents as a main cause of premature deaths, or lost years of useful, productive and enjoyable life; diabetes as a main cause of blindness in developed countries, the spatial patterns of which raise questions surprising even to the well-informed; and infant mortality as an indicator of between-country and within-country differences, regional and in terms of social stratification, of major public importance. Again it raises more questions than it answers, but this is often a necessary stage in finding and planning research themes for the future.

Hutt and Burkitt (1986) on *The Geography of Non-Infectious Disease*, already referred to in chapter 3, is a work equally important to any reader wishing to follow up this chapter, as is the second atlas from the Southampton project (Gardner et al. 1984).

5 The Idea of 'Surfaces'

Before Surfaces, Dot Maps!

Figure 5.1 is not, in fact, by a geographer, but by a Medical Officer of Health (Allen-Price 1960); he was following an essentially geographical method using one of the simplest mapping tools – the dot map (like Dr John Snow in the map of cholera in Soho during the London epidemic of 1854, referred to in chapter 6). Both Snow and Allen-Price were working on the micro-scale, that is working on large-scale maps of small areas, and their work shows how effective a simple method can be to a prepared mind. Allen-Price noticed that in the village of Horrabridge in Devon, the area north of the river Walkham had one-third of its deaths due to cancer, compared with one in twelve in adjacent parts of the village regarded as homogeneous in all known aspects of community life except that the source of water supply was different. He was sufficiently convinced that there was a causal relation to campaign successfully for an appropriate change in the water supply. (For a more recent analysis of the effects of different water supplies in a small area, in that instance a city, see the discussion of primary acute pancreatitis in Nottingham after Giggs in chapter 8.) This brief reference to Allen-Price's dot map is really to point up this fact: that though there are various ways of mapping mortality or indeed morbidity data, death and illness are in fact point patterns occurring in an individual at some specific point on the earth's surface. So a dot map is a fundamental way of representing the occurrence, though often some other method of representation on a map is more convenient for a particular kind of illustration or analysis. A choropleth map represents, say, mortality as spread across an administrative area or census unit, in a series of steps or plateaux as it were, whereas isopleth maps represent 'hills and valleys', of, say, cancer mortality – or

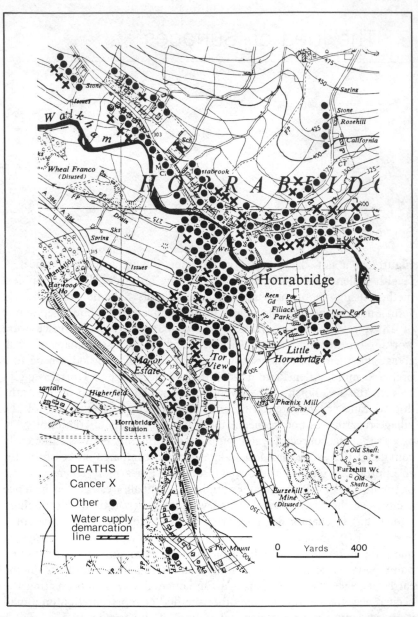

DEATHS

Cancer X

Other ●

Water supply
demarcation
line ┅┅┅

Figure 5.1 Cancer deaths, Horrabridge, Devon: the areas of three different sources of water were separated by the river and the hatched line.
Source: Allen-Price (1960)

to put it more abstractly, in terms of more general gradients or surfaces. It is this concept of surfaces that is now developed a little further. (There are other assumptions in this type of analysis that may in some circumstances invalidate results: one major difficulty is mobility and migration of people so that one really needs a life-history of exposure to environmental risks. See for instance Mayer (1980).) Glick (1982) explores spatial analysis techniques in relation to cancers in the USA, with the idea that change of scale may assist the formulation of causal hypotheses.

Surfaces and Positive and Negative Anomalies

Figure 5.2 is a series of representations of male lung cancer in Victoria, Australia for 1961–4 (Learmonth 1972a): (a) is a relatively straightforward contour or isopleth map of the SMRs, demanding only acceptance that it is worth while as one cartographic option to transform the point pattern of dots or crosses on the map into 'hills and valleys' of cancer for some analyses. But (b), (c) and (d) as a group are much less maps and much more 'models' in that further generalization and abstraction have been attempted. In this particular exercise a very simple arithmetical method of generalizing the 'surface' was selected, averaging, for each centre point of a census recording unit, the several values that fell within a radius of 55.4 miles, yielding circles of 10 000 square miles – an arbitrary figure that seemed in scale with the country's large dimensions. This is really an analogy to using a 'moving average' of say seven years' iron and steel production figures or export data to show broader trends over time than do annual figures, which tend to have peaks and troughs due to ephemeral factors. There are much more sophisticated ways of generalizing from point data to surfaces, and indeed this simple exercise was conducted a good many years ago now in order to encourage this way of thinking about spatial trends in medical geography (Learmonth 1972a following Haggett 1965). The idea is borrowed from a sister science, geomorphology or the study of landforms, where the researcher may wish to identify a broad regional surface, smoothing out the detail of minor valleys or upstanding residual heights. Again by analogy, the cancer study aimed at identifying any broad regional trend or 'trend surface' of cancer mortality. One such did emerge – a broad and simple ridge of cancer deaths, running north–south across Victoria, and much broader in the south so that it included much of the Yallourn valley. This was in itself suggestive of relations with urban and industrial settlements in greater Melbourne and the brown-coal and electricity-generating area around Yallourn. There followed two further stages, representing positive and

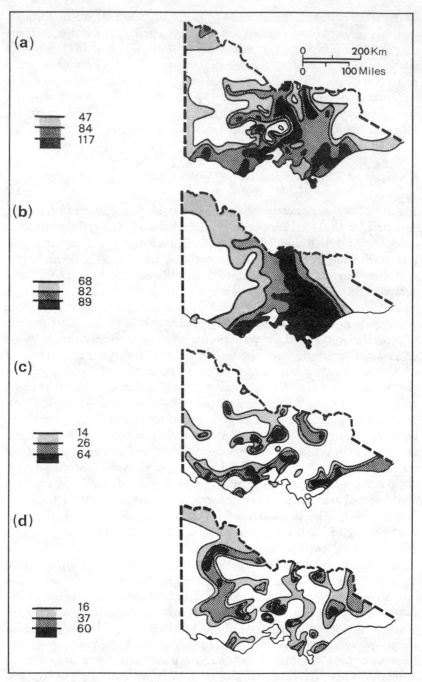

Figure 5.2 Lung cancer, males, Victoria, Australia, 1961–1964: (a) isopleths ('contours'); (b) regional trend; (c) positive anomalies; (d) negative anomalies
Source: Learmonth (1972)

negative anomalies, where the isopleths or contours of (a) were substantially above or below the regional trend surface of (b) respectively – residual heights of cancer, as it were, contrasted with valleys cut into the trend surface. This seems not to have been followed up directly – the author left Australia soon after it was done – but some much more advanced linking of statistical and cartographic thinking has followed from N.D. McGlashan who arrived in Tasmania at about the same time, and this will be referred to in several places.

Isomells (Lines of Equal Probability)

McGlashan, too, wished to draw attention to the idea of positive and negative anomalies, but chose a quite different approach based on probability theory and, of the several means available, selected the Poisson method of calculating probabilities as particularly useful where small numbers are involved, as they are often in mapping comparatively rare diseases or in sparsely peopled areas like much of Australia. With a medical scientist colleague, he first worked out the technique using data for cancers in black goldminers in South Africa, a population showing quite different proportions of cancers of different sites from those applying to the white population (McGlashan and Harington 1976; Bradshaw et al. 1985). While the technique can be used for administrative areas, they also used isopleth or contour maps of the Poisson probabilities, christening these lines 'isomells' from the Greek words for 'equal probability'. McGlashan applied the technique to administrative units in Tasmania, to complement the approach in figure 4.3 (McGlashan and Chick 1974). He later extended this work to cover the whole of Australia for selected causes of death: figure 5.3 shows both a choropleth and an isopleth map of male ischaemic heart disease mortality for 1970–2 (McGlashan 1977a). It has already been pointed out that isopleth maps draw attention to *general* patterns or spatial trends, avoiding risk of over-emphasis on a particular place showing high or low rates. Steep gradients are worth examining in more detail as suggestive of rapid change in incidence over a short distance, and possibly indicating where field investigation may yield useful results. Mapping of statistically significant departures from general expectation overcomes the weakness that most isopleth maps of SMRs take no account of the statistical significance of the lines on the map. On the other hand concentrating on the extreme values – the positive and negative anomalies – also involves neglect of the greater part of the data, namely all the middle values. It often seems best to use different ways of looking at data as complementing each other – a choropleth map in case there is an occupational or local environmental link, an isopleth map of SMRs for the whole population, or for age

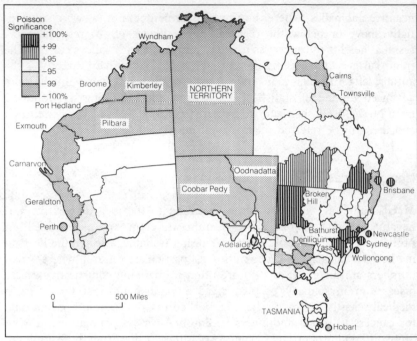

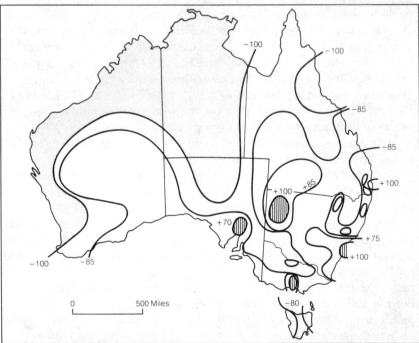

Figure 5.3 Ischaemic heart disease, males, Australia, 1970–1972: (a) choropleth map (by administrative or census divisions); (b) isomell map (with lines of equal probability or risk)
Source: McGlashan (1977)

groups at high risk or representing premature deaths, and isomells to see if anything can be learned from areas of high or low probability of death from a particular disease. One of his pupils has studied high-risk areas of Tasmania for Hodgkin's disease, using the case-control technique comparing matched pairs of patients and controls in terms of life history: as often, this research raised more questions than it answered, but it did point to two specific areas that seemed to be linked with the disease – environment at time of birth, and farming environments (Giles 1983).

An Application of Trend Surfaces in Japan

Kagami (1983) uses mathematically elegant methods to derive trend surfaces of cerebrovascular disease SMRs for Japan (figure 5.4(a)). The seven maps represent different ways of representing the general slope using different formulae to smooth out local variations. Kagami's IV, V, VI and VII all are acceptable generalizations from the conventional map (compare with figure 4.5). However, the trend surface VI was selected for mapping of the residuals from the trend surface (figure 5.4(b)) and for a map of types of this disease, combining the trend surface with positive and negative anomalies (figure 5.4(c)). A large number of environmental and health variables are being further analysed to see if explanations can be found for the spatial variations and types.

An Urban Model

A study of simple chronic bronchitis in adult females in Leeds uses surfaces to an extent, but interestingly wedded to a well-known, almost venerable urban model (Girt 1972). This was a combined Burgess–Hoyt model of concentric zones and sectorial segments of characteristic socioeconomic structure, derived originally from Chicago at a time when sociologists were interested in analogies with biological–ecology ideas of plant and animal succession, dominance, co-dominance and so on (Burgess 1925; Hoyt 1939); the model was modified for England by Mann (1965) and further for Leeds by Girt himself because the coal-mines to the west of the city have inhibited the normal west-end development of high-class residential areas (figure 5.5). Sampling by quadrats, varying in size to give approximately equal populations, yielded 'observed' figures for terrace-like 'surfaces' from the zones-and-sectors model (figure 5.6). Correlation exercises with data on smoking, air pollution and past and present environment were used to produce 'expected' levels according to appropriate hypotheses on causal factors, and results tested for closeness

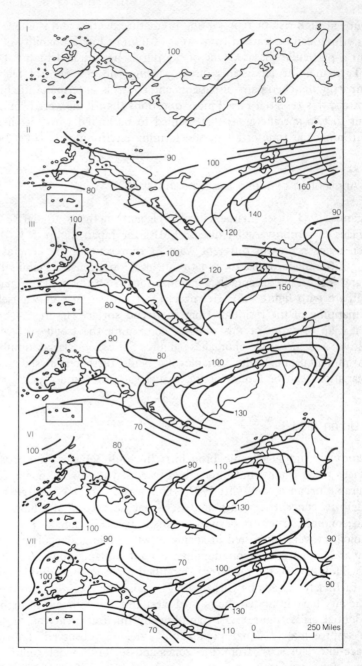

Figure 5.4 (a) Cerebrovascular diseases, both sexes, Japan, 1968–1974: seven different types of trend surface (or mathematically generalized 'contours');
Source: Kagami (1984)

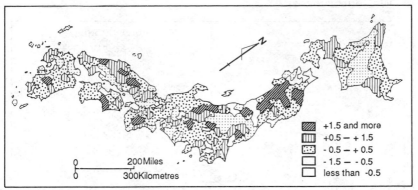

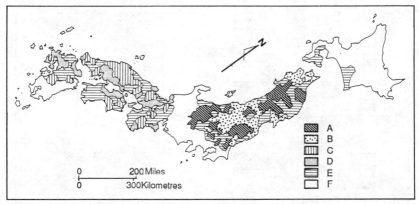

Figure 5.4 (b) Cerebrovascular diseases, both sexes, Japan, 1968–1974: residuals from the 6th trend surface (comparable with the anomalies of figure 5.2),
Source: Kagami (1984)

Figure 5.4 (c) Cerebrovascular diseases, both sexes, Japan, 1968–1974: regional types, combining trend surface values and residuals, for further study of environmental characteristics or possible relevance to the disease
Source: Kagami (1984)

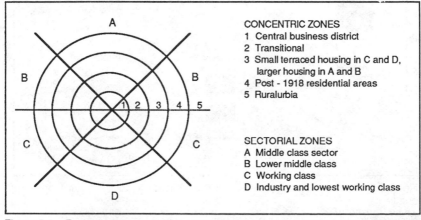

Figure 5.5 Ecological structure (i.e. socioeconomic characteristics) of a British city, as applied to Leeds
Source: Girt (1972)

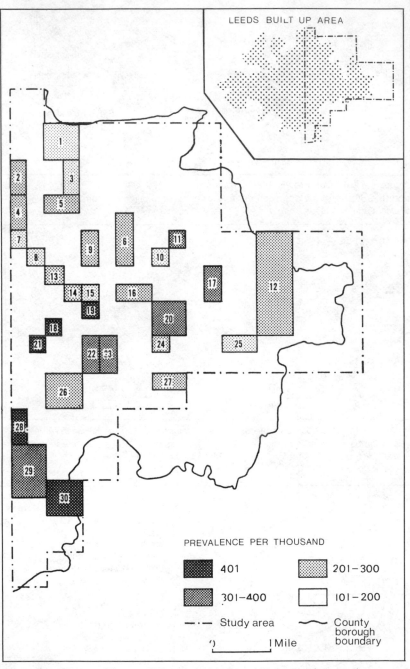

Figure 5.6 Observed figures of simple chronic bronchitis in adult females, from sample quadrats
Source: Girt (1972)

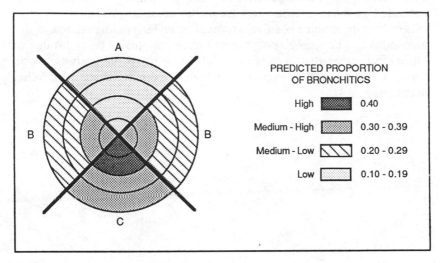

Figure 5.7   Prevalence of the bronchitis as predicted from the 'ecological' model
Source: Girt (1972)

of fit. Smoking (past and present), living conditions (past and present) and past (rather than present) environments *combined* gave the best fit of expected levels (in Girt's words, predicted on the basis of the model), as compared with the observed levels (figure 5.7).

Surfaces used in Forecasting

Lastly under this section on geographical method, it is worth noting that in chapter 16 of this book, on health care, a work by Pyle (1971) is cited as combining mapping of present need and future need with sophisticated analysis of optimal or at least sub-optimal location of facilities adequate to meet the future needs; and that Pyle uses trend surfaces of cancer, stroke and heart disease in Chicago at two past periods in order to produce *forecast* trend surfaces (a) of total need, and (b) of unmet need, for a future year.

Conclusion

In this chapter the idea of generalized surfaces of incidence or prevalence of mortality (generally) or – more positively in many ways – of morbidity where data permit, is related to positive and negative anomalies 'above' and 'below' the surface generalized on a particular model, and this is extended as far as McGlashan's 'isomells' of equal probability or risk. There have been some positive advances in understanding related to this methodology. Few geographers would claim any major breakthrough or discovery, rather that here is one useful tool of spatial analysis, worth using hopefully for appropriate problems, perhaps along with other techniques.

6 The Spatial Diffusion of Disease

Introductory: Hägerstrand to Haggett

Geographers have for generations been interested in spatial diffusion of ideas, techniques, ethnic and racial groups etc., in terms of mapping the movement of a particular variable across a country, a continent or the world. In 1952, however, came a fresh viewpoint on the phenomenon of diffusion across area: Professor Torsten Hägerstrand of the Royal University of Lund pioneered a generalizing and abstracting model that has proved surprisingly robust in contexts far removed from the original studies of innovations diffused in farming populations spread across southern Sweden – some were hardware innovations such as the telephone, others took the form of information networks leading to the adoption of services like anti-tuberculosis vaccination of cattle. Considered aspatially, the adoption of an innovation in a population, say television sets, is widely recognized as starting slowly, gaining speed in a middle phase, and then tailing off towards saturation point for that particular innovation. This may be generalized, still aspatially, in a 'logistic' curve, the shape illustrated in figure 6.1 (Cliff et al. 1981). Turning to a spatial view of the phenomenon, Hägerstrand suggested that four stages may be identified: (1) a primary stage, with a centre of adoption, from which the innovation is diffused outward, areas close to the centre rapidly acquiring comparatively high rates of adoption, while there is a steep fall in the adoption rates towards the periphery; (2) a diffusion stage, with a strong centrifugal effect, rapid adoption at distant points, and a reduction in the strong regional contrasts of stage (1); (3) a 'condensing' stage, with relative rates of adoption equal in all locations, regardless of distance from the centre; and (4) a saturation stage, slowing and eventual cessation of adoption, with uniform total adoption rates or at least minimal regional contrast. Hägerstrand went on to develop a grid of 25 grid-squares in 5 × 5 formation, each of 5 km², within which a probability was assigned to

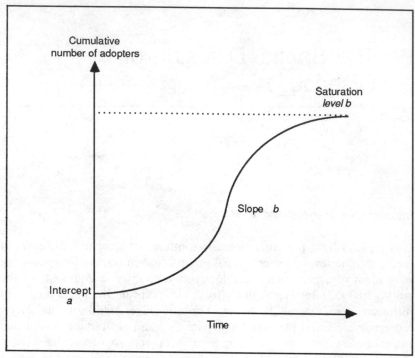

Figure 6.1   'Logistic' curve, an S-shaped curve representing slow initial growth, then more rapid growth, followed by retardation to slower growth, then stability, here representing adoption of an innovation over time. ('Logistic' implies computation but also the supply side of, say, a military campaign: here calculation is obviously involved, and the supply aspect may have been involved in its naming by Verhulst in the early nineteenth century, in the period of Malthusian concern for ultimate control of population growth by food supply).
Source: Cliff et al. (1981)

each grid-square, a probability based on adoption data from migration and telephone traffic statistics. As an example of the use of his model, figure 6.2 illustrates a model-based prediction of the areal diffusion pattern of improved pasture subsidy compared with the actual adoption rates in the same grid-squares placed over the actual map of this part of southern Sweden. (For a sceptical view, by one who has used the approach to good effect, see Blaikie (1978).)

Measles in Iceland

Cliff, Haggett, Ord and Versey, whose 1981 book is a main source for this account of Hägerstrand's contribution, provide in that book perhaps

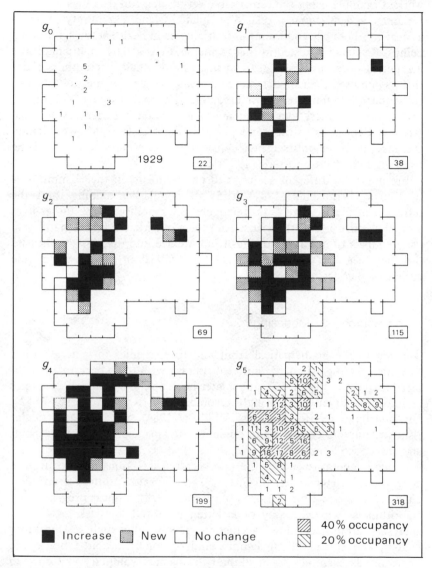

Figure 6.2 Spatial diffusion of improved pasture subsidies in part of southern Sweden, after Hägerstrand
Source: Cliff et al. (1981)

the most complete and mathematically sophisticated account ranging between Hägerstrand's contribution and the considerable body of theory (and practical experience too concerning epidemics and their spatial diffusion), from biomathematics and biostatistics. They also provide a worked example using the remarkable set of long-run data on measles in Iceland – and of course a relatively isolated island community provides as near to laboratory conditions as is attainable in health studies of human beings. Readers interested in this theme, and particularly mathematically competent ones, are urged to read it in the original. The authors claim that having used their model and data from earlier epidemics to 'forecast' subsequent but now long past epidemics for comparison of 'observed' and 'expected' rates, they could now with reasonable accuracy forecast *future* epidemics as to time and place, but not as to scale of epidemic: this may, however, in itself be a considerable contribution, as two of the team argue in Cliff and Ord (1985).

From a quite different society and environment, in the Kisumu area of Kenya, Ferguson's (1981) study of population mobility and the diffusion of measles links the relatively low mobility of the under-fives with slow diffusion of the virus. And for a remarkable if schematic map of the impact of immigrant routes from Mexico into the USA on measles diffusion, see *MMWR* (1981). Katz et al. (1983) provide a world-wide review of measles.

Some Sources on Modelling

Turning to the mathematical front and to epidemics in general rather than measles in particular, some readers may wish to go back to a bench-mark text like Bailey (1967), and a later book on the population dynamics of infectious diseases is strongly recommended (R.M. Anderson 1982). On modelling, see, for example, Mollison (1984), and on the particular issue of studying endemic and epidemic streams at the same time point and place, see Souza (1982).

A good general review of the non-vectored infectious diseases from a geographical viewpoint is in Girt (1974). Girt also proffers a different approach to space–time diffusion of disease (1978): a linear programming algorithm is used as a way of isolating high and low risk groups for analysis – groups with low vaccination rates or other high susceptibility factors; and spread of chickenpox and of gonorrhoea in Ontario are presented as examples of involuntary as against voluntary exposure to risk of infection. Haggett (1976) has also used a hybrid model involving the autocorrelation idea in measles studies, while his use of the planar graph model will be referred to later. Pisani et al. (1984) apply studies of variola minor (mild smallpox) to the problem of reconstructing the chain of contagion, and Angulo et al. (1979) to hierarchies of frequency of contact for the same infection. Elton (1982) raises the possibility of measuring 'contagion distance' as against linear distance. Returning to the work of Cliff and Haggett, and to measles, there is their (1985) monograph on island communities with a much more recalcitrant data set, in the south-west Pacific; see also their (1984) article in *Scientific American*.

Meantime, this chapter will continue with some quite simple ideas of diffusion, of various diseases, in some sort of historical sequence; as with the bronchitis study mentioned in chapter 5 (Girt 1972), the data are on morbidity, not mortality, and most of the material drawn on concerns infections.

It has already been noted that infectious diseases are relatively more important as causes of death in the Third World than in developed countries, but developed country studies are nevertheless justified. Infectious diseases remain important causes of morbidity, and some, such as infectious hepatitis, as causes of prolonged loss of efficiency and enjoyment of life; perhaps, as has been suggested earlier, geographical contributions in this kind of disease have been more successful in academic and practical terms than have most similar studies on degenerative diseases. Finally, methodology found useful in developed countries may prove so in developing countries also, wherever the quality of data permits of its use. (This last point does not imply that the Third World, in this field as in others, carries no lessons for the developed world: the reverse is true, in the author's experience.)

Diffusion of Hepatitis A

Virus hepatitis, or hepatitis A, is sufficiently important in Australia – and a notifiable disease there – to persuade the author to present a very simple and crude model of its diffusion in 1968, actually along with the cancer model of figure 5.2. This hepatitis diffusion model (not reproduced here) was based on virus diffusion between towns along the transport network; it is not further discussed here because it was soon supplanted by better models, thus fulfilling its purpose. Some of those better models are discussed presently, after some description of the disease.

Hepatitis A, hepatitis B and hepatitis non-A non-B – all these are virus diseases affecting the liver or hepatic system. Hepatitis A is the infectious or infective hepatitis of older references cited, and the main topic discussed in this section. Hepatitis B is the serum hepatitis transmissible by blood transfusion in a fashion analogous to malaria, AIDS and other blood diseases, by accidental cuts in hospital or laboratories involving infected blood in test-tubes etc., by dirty shared needles of drug-addicts – and as noted in chapter 1 by vegetation scratching an infected and then a susceptible fell-runner (Vellar 1964). Hepatitis non-A non-B is still being characterized; it seems to be responsible for a good deal of the very widespread hepatitis and antibodies from past infections in India, for example. It is hepatitis B that is suspected as synergistic with aflatoxin moulds on maize and groundnuts, especially in causing liver cancer in many Third World areas. On the complex and rapidly changing field of hepatitis studies, a bench-mark survey is in Sherlock (1980).

Hepatitis A is primarily an intestinal infection, offering many analogies to poliomyelitis – though the vaccines of Salk and others now protect many developed country populations from polio. In contrast is naturally acquired immunity: many Third World adult populations seem to have a high degree of immunity to these viruses at the cost of much suffering (and, for polio, permanent disability) and many deaths in children. In developed countries hepatitis A is mainly a cause of illness rather than death, but often quite prolonged and impairing both efficiency and enjoyment. In warm countries, on Australian findings, hepatitis A does not have a clear seasonal pattern, and probably this is true of tropical areas also. There is some evidence from developed countries of an epidemic cycle of about five years, probably related to the availability of non-immune people; and epidemics tend to affect susceptible individuals in all age groups. For a recent review from the USSR of viral hepatitis as a world health problem (but without data from that country!) see Tkacheva et al. (1981). Two environmental studies offer significant contrasts: in Sydney hepatitis A was linked with areas of low standards of hygiene and frequent soil and water pollution, comparable with those in Wollongong, New South Wales to be cited later (Baczkowski 1980); whereas in Spain a researcher found relatively few cases in unhygienic areas, and indications rather of spread by personal contact (Arroz 1979).

The spread of the infection can be followed in detail from some fascinating community studies. Thus Brownlea's diagram (figure 6.3) speaks for itself on the chain of infection in a small rural community in New South Wales; it is entirely in the tradition of an interpretation of a similar tree-diagram by the celebrated Dr William Pickles of Wensleydale some sixty years ago which, with other evidence, led to his establishing the incubation period of the disease. He had suspected that the common link in early cases in an epidemic in his rural practice must have been attendance at the village fête on 28 August, and goes on to describe how a young girl who went to it in defiance of doctor's orders eventually caused thirteen cases of jaundice or more:

After a prolonged search I found that a young girl who had begun with the disease on 23 August had been at the entertainment. I had actually seen her in bed in the morning and never dreamt she could have left it. She must have eluded me with great skill throughout the afternoon, since I was there myself and never set eyes on her.

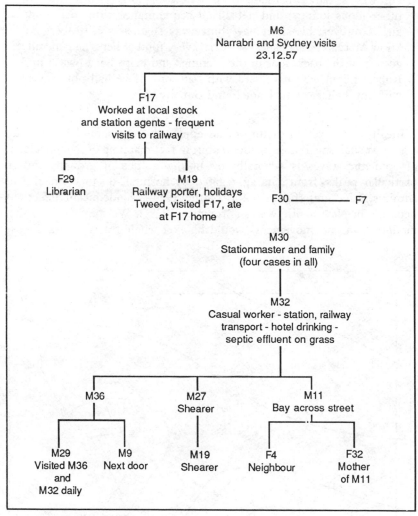

Figure 6.3 Flow of hepatitis virus between members of a small rural community in New South Wales
Source: Brownlea, personal communication following on Brownlea (1967)

She spent the afternoon with E, another young girl, and was in the house of Mrs C, so that I think it is a fair presumption that she infected them and the other three. This young girl E, a maid in another village, infected four others. One was her employer's small son, another his friend, and another her own great-aunt. All this was reasonably clear. Of the fourth – M – there was some doubt.

He was a rather pathetic little fellow of forty (since dead of tuberculous kidney) and denied all acquaintance with this young girl. However, his sister gave him away shamelessly. 'Robert not know Margaret?' said she. 'Why he's very fond of her – he generally goes in at the back door in the evenings and helps her to wash up.' Robert might well have said with Samson, 'If ye had not plowed with my heifer, ye had not found out my riddle.'

(Pickles 1948)

Ideally, any over-all picture of an epidemic wave should be built up from just such small-scale incidents, but in fact mapping of the movement of epidemic waves is generally by noting graphs of growth, and in particular peaks, from data aggregated by hospital, doctors' practice or administrative unit (figure 6.4(a) of the 1954–8 epidemic of infectious hepatitis in New South Wales (Brownlea 1978)). We might expect that modern transport movements would blanket whole tracts with a disease

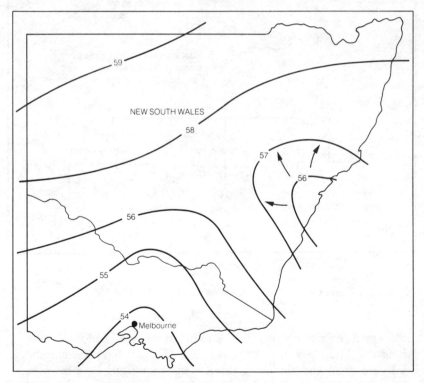

Figure 6.4 (a)   Passage of wave crest of hepatitis epidemic of 1954–1958 in New South Wales
Source: Brownlea, personal communication following on Brownlea (1967)

at a stroke, but in fact the *crest* of many epidemic waves rolls slowly across a country or through its people, even though there may be many individual splashes of infection far ahead of the crest in its early stages (the 'seeding' of many epidemiological studies), and also far to the rear in its later stages. Figure 6.4(a) may be compared with figure 6.4(b) (Chappell and Webber 1970). These two, then young, colleagues of the writer responded to his earlier, very crude, diffusion model of the State by constructing an electrical network with nodes proportional to populations and channels proportional to traffic flow in New South Wales (figure 6.5). An electrical impulse was passed through the network and the timing of the wave-crest at the nodes was recorded on an oscilloscope, timed, and multiplied up to approximate to the timing of the actual epidemic in figure 6.4(a); their map shows a rather faster passage, and fails to show the incursion from Melbourne, which they did not include in their model, across the State border from Victoria. Assessing their

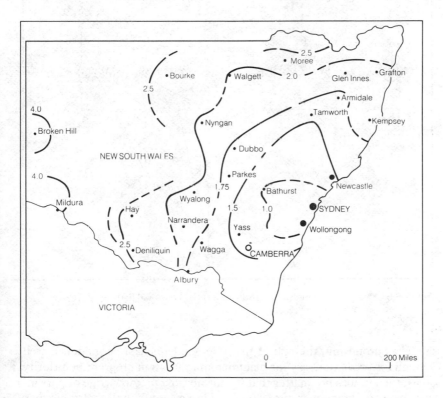

Figure 6.4 (b)   Passage of simulated diffusion of wave crest
Source: Chappell and Webber (1970)

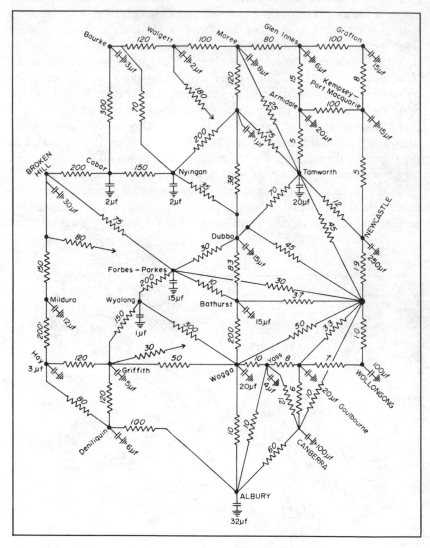

Figure 6.5 The electrical network used to produce figure 6.4(b)
Source: Chappell and Webber (1970)

model as promising, they plead that if an epidemic can be modelled well enough for prediction, say for planning immunization programme priority areas, then it does not matter that it adds nothing to knowledge of person-to-person transmission – interesting and important though that topic may be in its own right.

A Diffusion Model of Wollongong after Hägerstrand

On a scale intermediate between the micro of figure 6.3 and the macro of figures 6.4 and 6.5, Brownlea (1967, 1972a) simulated the diffusion of infective hepatitis in the steel city of Wollongong in New South Wales (figures 6.6(a) and (b)). A grid of 100 squares (10 × 10) is centred on central Wollongong: it has five distance belts from the centre, in each of which the grid squares carry a common *range* of numbers decreasing from belt 1 to belt 5 to represent the friction of distance, but cumulative from square 1 in belt 1 to square 100 in belt 5; random numbers of an appropriate total range are generated (from a table or by computer) and 'diffused' in simulation of spread of the virus (here assumed as random, qualified only by distance decay). 'Hits' are registered for each random number falling within a particular, unique, grid-square range, at least up to a certain proportion of the total population assigned to the grid square, when saturation is assumed. With that exception all numbers dispersed and falling within a grid-square range are hits, that is, it does not allow for the gradual building up of community immunity as in more sophisticated mathematical models of epidemics. Brownlea's leap forward, however, was to re-interpret some of Hägerstrand's thinking to the particular context, by modifying the chances of successful transmission in particular grid squares, some to as low as 90 per cent, some as high as 120 per cent: hence in figure 6.6(b) the decreased chances of transmission in an area of light sandy soils and in an area of old families, and the increased chances in an area of young families and another adjacent to a coastal lagoon, sometimes polluted from badly maintained septic tank sewage, where children swim after school. The chances of success were altered by changing the grid-square ranges, with appropriate adjustment of the cumulative sequence of numbers from square 1 to square 100. Testing by random walk was successful, complementing other studies of transmission in a particular street, a particular school, immigrant hostel and the like. The study as a whole was at least one factor in persuading the city authorities that future suburbs should be fully sewered rather than provided with septic tank disposal.

A Planar Graph Model of Hepatitis in Tasmania

A different and complementary way of viewing the spread of hepatitis A has been used in a very penetrating study of its diffusion in Tasmania (McGlashan 1977b); this was based on a pioneering paper on measles in south-west England by Haggett (1972). As in the electrical network

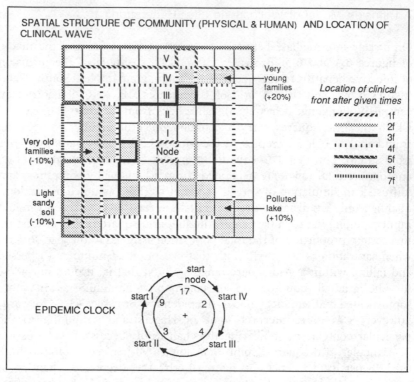

Figure 6.6 (a)   Simulation of hepatitis epidemic diffusion in Wollongong, New South Wales: assuming random diffusion in distance belts (uniform surface)

model, this approach focuses on a hierarchy of towns and cities, but viewed graphically as vertices or nodes, and on transport links referred to as 'edges' in the mathematical literature – in many networks transport links can usefully be envisaged as the edges or sides of triangles by taking an abstract and generalizing view of the map of towns and transport links. The *planar* graph of Haggett's title implies that the network is all on a plane – there are no fly-overs, tunnels or hops by air travel. Plotting fresh cases week by week, vertices with at least one case are marked, then links are plotted as active if cases are recorded in adjacent vertices. As in all models the assumptions of the model have to be noted, but accepted for purposes of investigation to see if the particular model sheds light (or casts darkness!) on the problem or phenomenon being studied. Thus, here the connections between adjacent active nodes are assumed not proved – the infection might have been derived from some quite

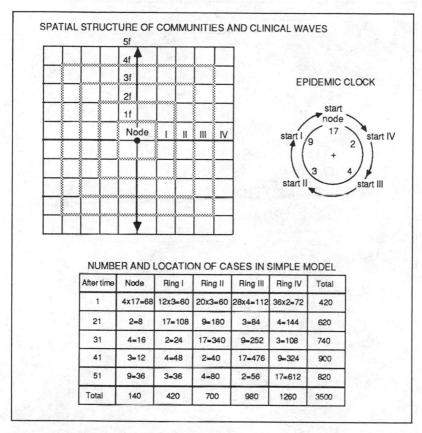

Figure 6.6 (b) Simulation of hepatitis epidemic diffusion in Wollongong, New South Wales: assuming random diffusion in distance belts but now modified by environmental characteristics of parts of the city (differentiated surface)
Source: Brownlea (1972)

different source. However, the method offers one way of viewing in perspective – as it were from a satellite – the overall pattern or system of diffusion in a network: *does* the group of nodes and links function as a whole, as a system, or are there sub-systems in the disease diffusion patterns? Moreover, probabilities of infection can be assigned to vertices, usually decreasing at a distance from the initial point or points of the epidemic. McGlashan, then, plotted hepatitis notifications for Tasmania for 163 weeks from 1 June 1970 to 7 July 1973 and analysed them following this model. Figure 6.7 maps the data for weeks 37–42, for example, in terms of outbreaks in a fresh node, additional cases in a

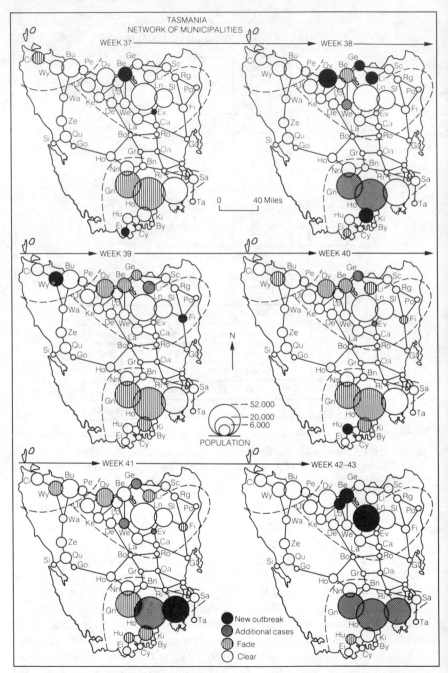

Figure 6.7 Sequence of six weeks' hepatitis A notifications in Tasmania, 1971, in maps assuming a planar graph format of links between human settlements
Source: McGlashan (1977)

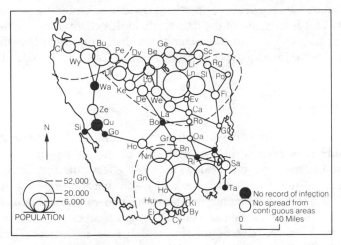

Figure 6.8 Discrete hepatitis regions, Tasmania, 1971
Source: McGlashan (1971)

node already infected, and nodes with infection assumed as fading after
an arbitrary period of four weeks from first or later notification, and
totally clear nodes. The diffusion proved to have a very substantially
repetitive pattern in three successive epidemics, and showed that, as with
the measles study in south-west England, the chances of infection decrease
sharply, comparing nodes only one link distant from an outbreak with
those two and three links distant (falling from 57 to 11 per cent chance
of infection in McGlashan's study). And he demonstrated what he
regarded as 'discrete hepatitis' regions (figure 6.8). While McGlashan did
not claim that the study is translatable into terms of vaccination campaigns
or the like, he was perhaps understating his claims in order to avoid
provoking any hostile reaction in local health authorities: applicable
monitoring systems clearly could be evolved building on the foundation
of this research undertaken for academic purposes. It is worth noting too
that McGlashan also conducted more detailed local surveys of the ecology
of the disease in the sense of pinpointing places where the virus seems
to be transmitted – school, swimming pool, canteen, etc. – with
implications for periods off school, off work etc. of those affected by the
disease, though he grants that sub-clinical cases are common and would
reduce the effectiveness of any attempts at prevention along these lines
(McGlashan 1977b).
    It should perhaps be noted that there is no attempt to model the
geography of hepatitis B, the virus of which is mainly spread in blood,
or the still controversial non-A non-B hepatitis. The hepatitis viruses as
a group are of course by no means confined to developed countries; they

cause much illness, probably particularly among children, in the Third World. This is true also of the next study in this chapter, on the diffusion of influenza, also a virus disease and one that, more than hepatitis, is a killing disease in both types of country in at least some epidemics.

Influenza

Influenza derives its name from Italian for 'influence' – of the stars? of the cold? It is a virus disease, primarily of the air passages with local pain and congestion but also widespread effects on the body: fever, headache, often back pain, weakness and depression, also frequent complications by pneumonia for instance. The virus at present appears to be one parasitic on human beings, though sources of swine fever and birds, for instance, have been suspected, at least as carriers (Pensaert et al. 1981). There are at least several strains of the virus, some perhaps from animals, some arising by mutation, and one strain is generally thought to appear dominant in a particular outbreak though recent records suggest that more than one strain can occur in a community; there is little or no cross-immunity between strains, so up to now vaccines prepared against one strain are ineffective against another. Shortridge and Stuart-Harris (1982) ask if there is an 'epicentre' of influenza dispersal in southern China, while there is some evidence of 'herald waves' before epidemics (see e.g. Glezen et al. (1982); Fox et al. (1982a,b) using household data from Seattle); and a researcher from general practice in England suggests that when, as in some outbreaks, an epidemic seems to spring up at several or many scattered points, latent infections (already 'seeded' as it were) may be activated by seasonal factors still to be identified (Hope-Simpson 1984). The selective discussion of geographical work on influenza, in this chapter and in chapter 8 on some historical geography of disease, assumes that the strains are due to mutation rather than to the spread of zoonotic infections to people (though that can not be ruled out).

On this reading, the mutation process yields the strains that seem generally to dominate particular epidemics. The classification of these has changed over the last generation or so, as virologists have acquired new tools such as the electron microscope to add to knowledge of the detailed structure and physiology of viruses. The old classification was primarily epidemiological though differences in protein structure became known later: A, associated with pandemics; B with more localized epidemics; and C with sporadic cases or outbreaks, and readers will find these terms used in some of the older but methodologically still valuable sources cited here. The modern classification uses combinations of the letters H and N and numbers, H2N2 for the 1957 pandemic of the following paragraphs. H stands for haemagglutinin antigens (as the name implies able to adhere to red blood cells, erythrocytes), N for neuraminidase (meaning able to destroy the neuraminic acid of cell surfaces during attachment, so preventing haemagglutination); and the numbers are in sequence of identification of strains of the virus types (for a brief outline, see Pyle 1980). The almost world-wide pandemic of 1918–21 is discussed in chapter 8, including the necessarily controversial classification of the virus responsible.

Influenza in England and Wales, 1957

The H2N2 epidemic of 1957 was analysed for England and Wales in an important paper by Hunter and Young (1971) the virus being then referred to as A2. The virus appeared early that year, caused an epidemic in south-central China in February, reached Hong Kong by mid-April, and was then diffused directly along world communication routes including early 'seeding' by air travellers, and indirectly by leap-frogging movements with transmission at intermediate points such as European holiday resorts and seaports. Air travellers were then comparatively few, and probably lived mainly at low room densities with less possibility of transmission. Ships' crews and, before the domination of passenger air travel, passengers too, were important. Infected crew members landed at Tilbury, Avonmouth, Sunderland, Jarrow, Manchester, Southampton (including passengers) and Liverpool, and so on to a total of 35 infected ships by October. An infected Pakistan Navy crew flew to London in mid-June and lived on a ship at Tilbury from which the virus spread. Concurrently with this pattern of increasing seeding, the main epidemic wave was advancing across Europe, reached Britain by August, in time to spread with the renewed close contacts of school classrooms in the autumn term.

As often during influenza epidemics, mortality directly from the virus was greatly increased by supervening pneumonia, mainly from bacteria normally commensal such as *Pneumococcus* (now strictly *Streptococcus*) *pneumoniae*, even though antibiotics had radically reduced the impact of bacterial pneumonia since the 1918–21 pandemic. Hunter and Young found the 6000 or so epidemic deaths unsatisfactory for *spatial* analysis, and in any case aimed to analyse morbidity rather than mortality during the crucial autumn months; they were driven to use a multiplier of influenza-to-pneumonia cases as a surrogate for influenza morbidity data, based on national insurance sick claims (of course covering only part of the total population) for the two diseases – in fact 417 influenza claims to one for pneumonia. They then analysed the movement of influenza across the country using pneumonia notifications multiplied by 417 to give estimates of influenza morbidity susceptible to statistical-cum-spatial analysis. As always, the use of a surrogate variable had to be very carefully considered and justified.

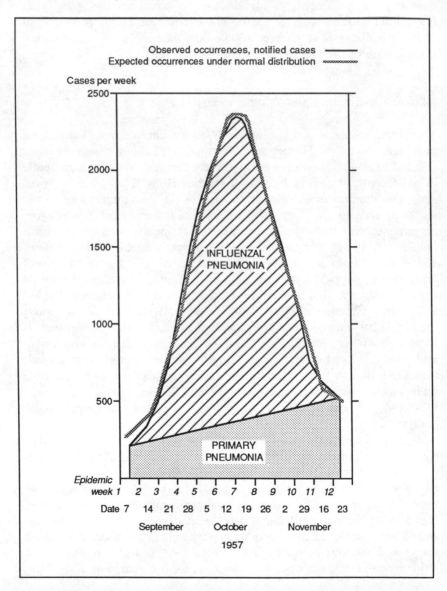

Figure 6.9 Graph of influenza and pneumonia, England and Wales, September–November 1957
Source: Hunter and Young (1971)

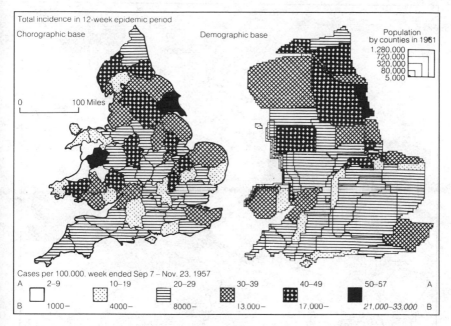

Figure 6.10   Influenza in England and Wales 1957, maps of weekly rates for 12 epidemic weeks
Source: Hunter and Young (1971)

Figure 6.10 shows the total impact of pneumonia and influenza, thus estimated, on a conventional base map on the left, and a demographic base map on the right. (On the virtues and defects of these methods see chapter 3.) As in several of the atlas maps of respiratory diseases there is a distinct bias towards higher rates in the north and west of England and Wales. Overall some 11.5 per cent of the population were affected, but 20 per cent in the North, the Midlands and South Wales. Figure 6.11 shows the pattern, on the demographic base, for the twelve crucial autumn weeks of the epidemic, and figure 6.12 the flow pattern using arrows in one map and five shadings in the other: the important role of west Yorkshire and the industrial north of England in the early weeks (and with the higher total rates of figure 6.10) is clear, with the late onset areas in south-central England and much of rural Wales. In the north the major seaports of Liverpool and Hull, as well as Middlesbrough, were early foci, but inland manufacturing cities were important too, especially those with large immigrant populations including many textile workers with contacts with the East. The pattern was of early infection, rapid spread and early peak mainly among factory workers, overlapping with a slower upsurge of infection in the general population and a second

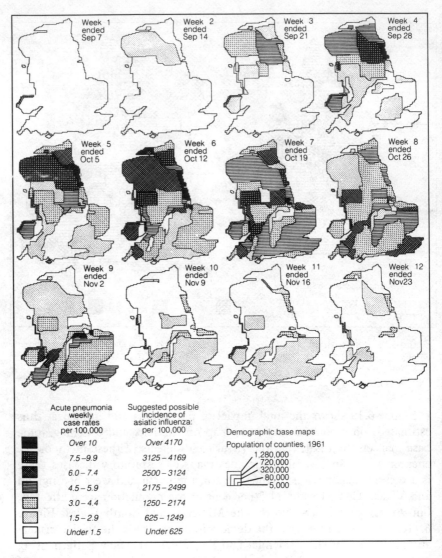

Figure 6.11   Influenza in England and Wales 1957, map of overall pattern for the 12
epidemic weeks
Source: Hunter and Young (1971)

peak peculiar to this type of city. The spread was not necessarily by a
wave outward from the early foci and washing across the whole of the
north. The epidemic spread north to Newcastle, then back southward to
County Durham but leaving industrial Tees-side comparatively lightly
affected despite the early role of Middlesbrough.

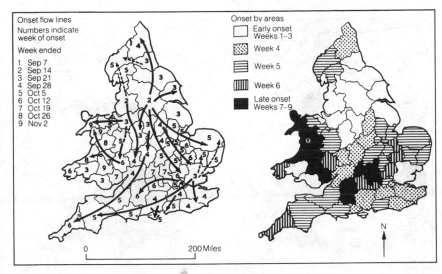

Figure 6.12   Influenza in England and Wales 1957, maps of epidemic flow-lines: (a) by arrows; (b) by five shadings for five groups of weeks during the epidemic period *Source*: Hunter and Young (1971)

So far the study had used mainly quite conventional methods in use in geography for decades. On forecasting they moved to the concept of the gravity model, in which by analogy with Newton's gravity formula, the 'population potential' takes account both of the relative sizes of populations and the distances separating them. They found that early in the epidemic this method could have forecast the areas to be severely affected, and less obviously the pathway along a ridge of high potential from north-west to south-east. High room densities were a better indicator of rapid spread than population density in relation to administrative areas. Greater London, much of which has high room densities, was relatively lightly affected, despite early seeding and massive population, maybe because of relative prosperity and of course large swathes of urban landscape *not* at high room densities.

Influenza in the USA, 1943–1944

Figure 6.13 is from one of a series of studies of influenza by a leading American worker, cited in several parts of this book (Pyle 1980). His conclusions include the following comments: (1) this very lethal epidemic affecting the USA in 1943–4 was not hierarchical, in the sense of diffusing through the urban network in order of size of city and order of importance

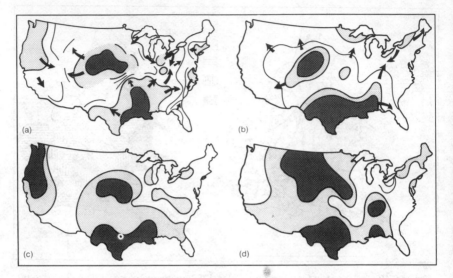

Figure 6.13   Influenza in the USA 1943–1944: (a) clusters during the 'spring seedling' 1943; (b) concentration of peaking, spring 1943; (c) diffusion paths, early fall 1943; (d) concentration of peaking, winter 1943–1944
Source: Pyle (1980)

of 'connectivity'; (2) it can be considered multi-nodal, with the earliest outbreaks in the central part of the country; (3) assuming that the 'spring seeding' of figure 6.13(a) is justified, the areas of fall and winter outbreaks later in 1943 could have been predicted; (4) forms of diffusion appear to be contagious (in the spatial rather than the medical sense), that is the epidemic tended to spread across adjacent areas, rather than along principal lines of movement, already dismissed in (1) above; there are radial patterns, but also some quite marked linear or tentacle-like shapes visible in figures 6.13(a) to (d). Pyle notes that in the modern classification of influenza sub-types, the 1943–4 epidemic is now considered as 'some starting point' for type H0N1 of the virus (as evidenced by the fact that a vaccine against earlier epidemic influenza was ineffective against H0N1); and since the origin was in the centre of the country and not imported (in contrast to the England and Wales study just discussed), it seems possible that H0N1 was some sort of variant of a prevailing virus endemic to the USA.

Legionnaires' Disease

An apparent diffusion pattern may in fact reflect increased or even first recognition of an infection or other disease: thus Legionnaires' disease, caused by *Legionella* spp., was named from an epidemic at a residential conference of the American Legion (a veterans' association) in Philadelphia in 1976. It is now recognised as a worldwide infection (EURO Reports 1982). Thus it was identified in 15 per cent of pneumonia patients in Nottingham over a 13-month period (Macfarlane et al. 1982), and in almost 7 per cent of those in Scotland in 1977–81 (Fallon 1982). However its association with institutional hot water, ventilation and cooling systems brings occasional epidemics in hospitals etc. like that in Glasgow in 1985, attracting great attention from broadcasting and the press. See also Fallon (1983).

Conclusion

Geographers do not profess or possess any monopoly over diffusion analysis or simulation, but can claim substantial geographical contributions to this field of endeavour, and some of the work cited in this chapter has led to modest improvements in disease prevention, while other work has potential applications for instance in forecasting and immunization campaigns.

7 The Challenge of Disease Patterns

Geographical Opportunism? – Primary Acute Pancreatitis in Greater Nottingham

'Opportunism' in the title is of course used in the best sense: that discovery comes to the prepared mind able to seize the opportunity when it presents itself! Primary acute pancreatitis is a relatively rare but serious disease: as the name implies it is an inflammation of the pancreas with an unknown cause, although it is strongly associated with certain other conditions such as alcoholism and gallstone disease; it can lead to pain, sickness and sometimes death. A team in Nottingham was able to gather data on 214 patients over the period 1969–76 (Giggs et al. 1980; Giggs 1984). Mapping revealed the ward rates shown in figure 7.1, and significance testing was done using the Poisson statistic already noted as appropriate to rare occurrences, resulting in figure 7.2. It happens that the city has six water supply areas drawing on different sources (figure 7.3) – this is where the opportunism comes in! – and there are statistically significant relations with one source in particular. Chemical analyses of the six water sources show that particular source to be high in calcium and magnesium carbonates, for instance, and in sulphates; the other sources sharing these characteristics in lesser degree also tend to have higher-than-average incidence of the disease. No causal link has yet been established, but further investigation seems warranted. Six years after the work first appeared, this work had not been initiated by the responsible authorities, as far as the original authors knew. A complication in the city is that, apart from normal migration movements – a common bugbear in epidemiological or ecological studies! – two substantial areas have been virtually cleared of population in housing improvement schemes. Studies allowing for these movements have been undertaken to try to establish lengths of exposure to the different water sources, and conceivably the exposure time likely to produce symptoms in a proportion of the people

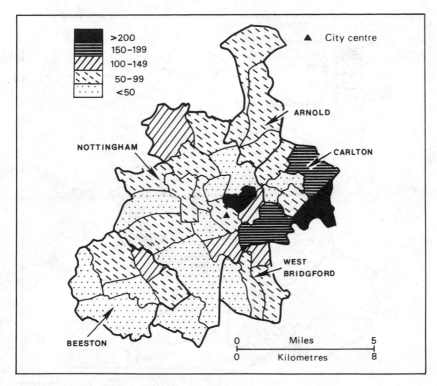

Figure 7.1 Primary acute pancreatitis in Nottingham
Source: Giggs (1984)

with that migration history – another piece of commendable and instructive opportunism?

Change of Scale in Mapping: Schizophrenia in Nottingham

This is such a simple tool that its comparative neglect is surprising. The study by Giggs et al. just cited certainly makes the case for micro studies, and elsewhere in the book the use of larger-scale maps of small areas in order to illumine a smaller-scale map perhaps of a whole country, is exemplified, as in the studies of Tasmania that go deeper than the all-Australia atlases could. We owe to Dr Giggs again figure 7.4, a map of schizophrenia in Nottingham (Giggs 1973a,b, 1975, 1983); the gain in insight as compared with the large units and broad spectrum sometimes necessary in nationwide mapping is indicated by comparing figure 7.4

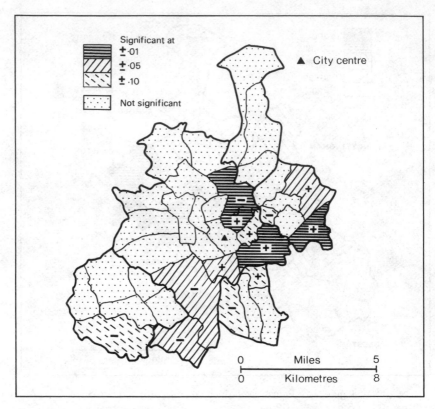

Figure 7.2 Primary acute pancreatitis in Nottingham, significance testing
Source: Giggs (1984)

with figures 7.5(a) and (b) – in which note the intriguing differences between the areas rich in beds for male and for female mental patients. Even so, the use of aggregate data even for wards or census enumeration areas within a city notoriously gives rise to the 'ecological fallacy', or better, 'aggregative fallacy' as mentioned in chapter 1. Moreover, here as often, there is the problem of which comes first, or which causes what? In this context the latter problem is acute: is there an inference in the map and subsequent analysis that inner city conditions *cause* schizophrenia? Such an inference is liable to challenge, on the ground that the inner city may not cause schizophrenia at all, but rather attract people with schizophrenia tendencies into 'bed-sitter land'. As one of the very small group of geographers venturing into this difficult field, Dr Giggs was concerned to use his maps with all due caution, but even so the 1973 paper was the subject of criticism and controversy, some of

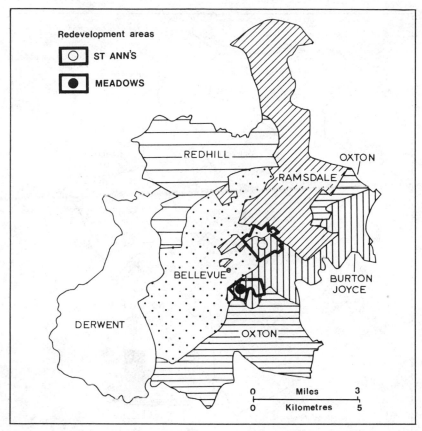

Figure 7.3 Water supply areas, Nottingham
Source: Giggs (1984)

which is in print in the 1975 reference cited. In Giggs (1983, see also Giggs and Mather 1983) we have a retrospect ten years after the first paper: he makes a case that the approach has potential both for research and in planning appropriate facilities, appropriately located; and that the trend in many countries towards the decentralization of psychiatric provision, and towards community involvement wherever possible, greatly strengthens the need for studies of this kind. Indeed there is a growing stream of studies of this general theme, including a major international comparative study (WHO 1979a).

Selecting only from those with some spatial component, Golledge et al. (1979) make important points on the need to understand and assess the 'spatial competence' of retarded people in community care; Hall et

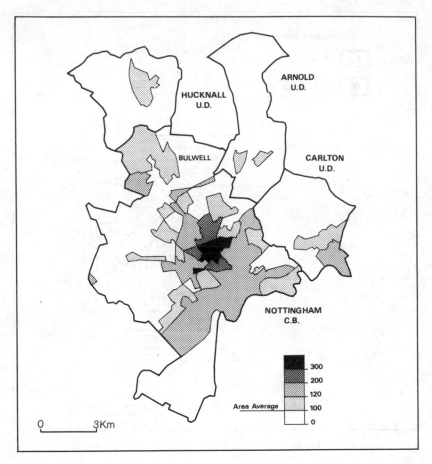

Figure 7.4 (a) Schizophrenia in Nottingham: standardized attack rates
Source: Giggs (1983)

al. (1984) comment on the impact of attitudes and reactions to locating mental health facilities, (see also Joseph and Hall (1985), Radford (1984)). Smith (1978) proposes that environmental characteristics of urban neighbourhoods may offer opportunities to predict rates of return to institutional care. The tendency for areas closer to mental hospitals to use institutional care more does not seem to apply to most diagnoses given the long distances of Western Australia (Stampfer et al. 1984) whereas in Tasmania areas distant from hospitals are under-served, and nearer areas over-served (Davey and Giles 1979). Joseph and Boeckh (1981) analyse the impact of diagnosis on distance decay, which is small for diagnoses of severe illness, but with users of institutional care clustered

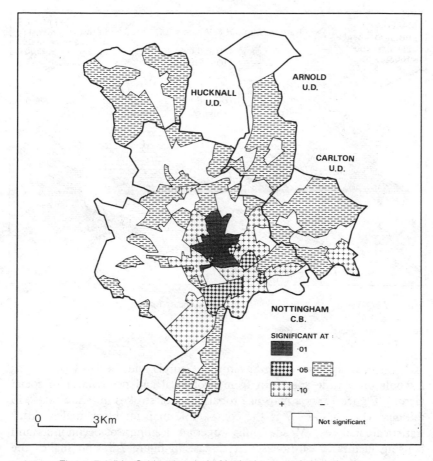

Figure 7.4 (b) Schizophrenia in Nottingham: statistical significance
Source: Giggs (1983)

nearby for people with less serious diagnoses. Aspects of the historical geography of institutional as against community care are brought out in Hunter et al. (1985b).

Scale and Cardiovascular Diseases

From quite a different medical problem, the cardiovascular diseases, Melinda Meade makes the point quite explicitly that micro-scale studies reveal likely causal variables in a way impossible with macro-scale studies (Meade 1979, 1980b, 1983). She invites comparison between mapping

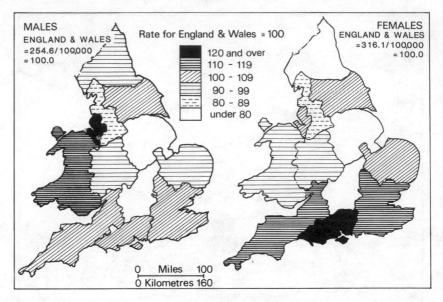

Figure 7.5 Residence rates, males and females in mental hospitals, England and Wales, c.1966
Source: Coates and Rawstron 1971

and statistical analyses from Savannah, Georgia and the USA picture as a whole on a wide spectrum from geological and pedological to social factors. Figure 7.6 is a map of probabilities of strokes in white males in the city while figure 7.7 is the comparable map for black males. After statistical analyses, Meade pulls together leading socioeconomic and housing factors in cardiovascular disease in figure 7.8, and makes the case that work at this scale, important locally, also assists in interpretation of national, macro-scale mapping. Earlier studies by Sauer (1962) and colleagues are still relevant, and see Ziegenfus and Aesler (1984) in parallel studies in north-eastern USA. Howe has pointed out the virtues of Glasgow in testing hypotheses about cardiovascular including cerebrovascular diseases in a city which draws all its drinking water from one (soft-water) source in Loch Katrine and yet has substantial within-city variations (Howe et al. 1977), and this has been followed up by his students including Gatenby (1982) for the surrounding region, and Rachel M. Tyndall (1983) for the city itself. See also Innes (1979) studying Windsor, Ontario, on working class rather than executive suburb incidence. Studies of water hardness and cardiovascular disease show somewhat inconsistent results: workers in New Zealand question the assumption that people using the same source of drinking water consume

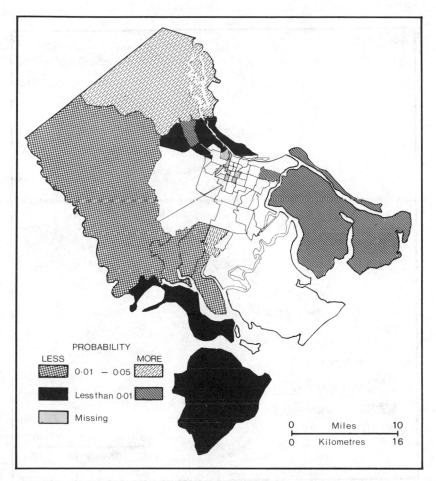

Figure 7.6 Probability map for stroke, white males 15–64, early 1970s, Savannah, Georgia
Source: Meade (1983)

similar amounts of minerals dissolved in it, and found wide variations in individual practice, for instance in boiling hard water before use (Gillies and Paulin 1983). This factor, again, does not seem to influence ischaemic heart disease in eastern Quebec, and socioeconomic factors like age of housing, or income, appear to be more important (Thouez 1979). Studies of this general type have increased in several countries in recent years, while papers like Shannon and Spurlock (1976) reach out to new concepts and methods of analysis, exploring the links between what they call urban ecological containers, involving the identification of urban activity fields,

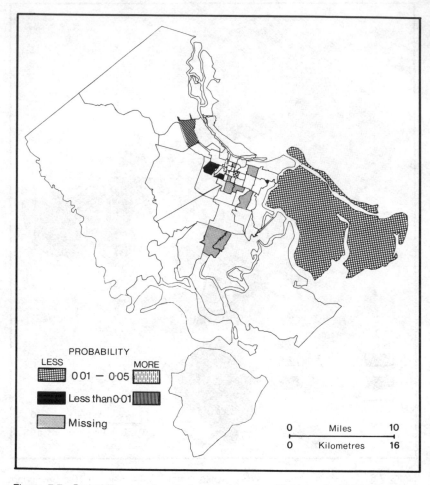

Figure 7.7   Probability map for stroke, black males 15–64, early 1970s, Savannah, Georgia
Source: Meade (1983)

environmental risk cells, and the use of health services. While these concepts must be difficult and expensive to make operational – one really is confronted with the task of observing and quantifying in some way the innumerable movements and interactions relevant to the health of, as it were, the urban molecules – it may well be that in this path lies the defeat of the 'ecological fallacy'. See also Armstrong (1973) on Hawaii and, for somewhat parallel thinking from Third World studies, Roundy (1978b) on Ethiopia.

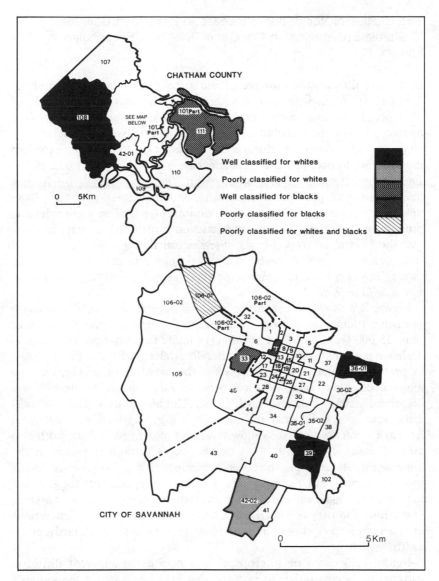

Figure 7.8   Type areas (by census tract) in which housing and socioeconomic factors are associated with strokes
Source: Meade (1981)

Two Studies of Vector-borne Disease in Developed Countries: 'California Encephalitis' in Ohio, and Tick-borne Encephalitis in Europe

Both these illnesses are now recognised as part of a worldwide family of 'arboviruses' often with animal–arthropod cycles as the main mode of existence, but where people may become involved through blood-sucking by infected arthropods including mosquitoes and ticks. A biogeographer's view of arboviruses in Europe is in Aspock (1979). An excellent introduction to bacterial and viral zoonoses is in WHO (TRS 682 1982). Encephalitis (Greek, inflammation within the head) may arise from a large number of pathogenic organisms, and the illness may vary from mild and unpleasant to very severe, disabling or fatal in a considerable proportion of victims. This short discussion is included in order to show that the kind of arthropod-borne diseases usually regarded in developed countries as 'tropical diseases' can and do occur in mid-latitudes, even though not at present of major importance as public health problems; in fact it *is* One World!

Figure 7.9 shows the scattered dots for encephalitis cases in relation to main settlements, to flood-plains and to the extent of the glaciation of some 15 000 years ago; the glaciation is a major factor in upsetting normal drainage patterns to this day and therefore, along with the flood-plains, in providing water bodies suitable for the breeding of certain culicine mosquitoes able to carry the virus between wild animals, farm stock and occasionally man (Pyle and Cook 1978). The mosquito is *Aëdes dorsalis*, a member of a genus that includes *Aëdes aegypti* which we shall meet later as the vector of urban yellow fever and of dengue in Asia, both also virus diseases (Pyle 1979). Pyle points out that another species in the same genus, *Aëdes caspius* has been incriminated in a similar encephalitis in similar terrain in Czechoslovakia. Laboratory experiments suggest that in temperate zone areas endemic for this virus encephalitis, over-wintering of the infection may be via transovarial transmission between generations of the vector mosquitoes; in turn birds may be infected (Hardy et al. 1980).

Figure 7.10 could be interpreted as a map of an apparent diffusion pattern, but seems rather to map the first evidence – hence the author's cautious caption – of a serious, sometimes fatal arbovirus encephalitis in Europe (Velimirovic 1984). This study also includes a map of high and low incidence in the USSR; see also Wellmer and Jusatz (1981). This is a classical case of a zoonosis into which people sometimes blunder, a European analogue for the forest cycle of yellow fever described in chapter 9, in some ways more complex, in some ways less so. The tick

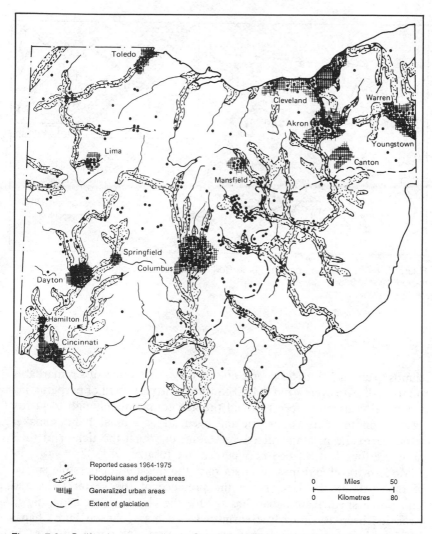

Toledo

Cleveland   Warren

Akron

Youngstown

Lima

Canton

Mansfield

Springfield

Columbus

Dayton

Hamilton

Cincinnati

• Reported cases 1964-1975

Floodplains and adjacent areas

Generalized urban areas

Extent of glaciation

0   Miles   50

0   Kilometres   80

Figure 7.9 California encephalitis in Ohio in relation to flood-plains and settled areas
Source: Pyle (1979)

Ixodes ricinus undergoes three stages, all blood-sucking but from different main hosts: the larval stage, climbing vegetation in forest clearings to a height of about 30 cm and parasitic mainly on fieldmice such as *Apodemus flavicollis*, the 'maintenance hosts', which become viraemic but not ill; the nymph stage climbing to about 1 m and with larger animals like foxes and hares as main hosts, not suffering from the infection but developing antibodies, as do the main hosts, such as deer, of the adult stage that

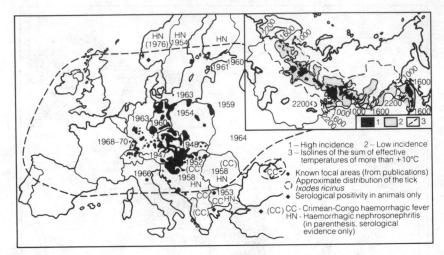

Figure 7.10 Tick-borne encephalitis in Central Europe, year of first published information 1934–1976
Source: Velimirovic (1984)

climbs to about 1.5 m. So people are the only real victims of a remarkably complex disease cycle – but a dead end from the viewpoint of perpetuating the cycle! – affecting foresters and the like commonly enough to justify vaccination in some countries, and even an occasional holiday-maker attracted to the pleasant mixed vegetation in which the ticks and their hosts are found, described in Wellmer and Jusatz (1981).

Modern travel and mass tourism raise the question of possible spread of the cycle to the UK, given the presence of the vector ticks and susceptible small mammalian hosts – for the closely related louping ill virus in sheep is similarly transmitted (see e.g. Johnson and Chanas (1981)). An interesting survey ranging across tick-borne diseases in developed and developing countries brings out social factors in the changing picture including the use of the countryside for leisure pursuits that bring people into contact with ticks and the various disease cycles (Hoogstraal 1981; Jusatz and Wellmer (1982) citing 62 cases in Bäden-Wurttemberg in 1978–9; from Czechoslovakia, Korenberg et al. (1984); and from Finland detailed recommendations for vaccination of travellers to a wide range of places from the Baltic to central Europe and Siberia, in Brummer-Korvenkontio et al. (1984)).

Rabies Diffusion and the Urban Fox

Rabies, also a virus disease, was well-known and much dreaded as 'hydrophobia' by older people, say in the early decades of this century, in Britain. (The name implying 'fear of water' is because water or the sound of water is one of many external stimuli that seem to arouse distressing convulsions in this disease of the central nervous system, usually fatal prior to Pasteur's classic work in evolving one of the first and most dramatic vaccines.) Yet nowadays it is not uncommon for pet-lovers to evade or try to evade the very strict quarantine regulations affecting the importing of animals that are likely hosts of the virus. For again this is a zoonosis, a virus causing illness in dogs, hence the regulations about pets, other domestic animals, and quite a number of wild animals including foxes and bats (though only a Central American species of bat is known to suck human blood!). Discussed here along with tick-borne encephalitis, it could equally well be in chapter 6 as a diffusion problem.

Many readers will recall having seen maps showing the advance of rabies from east to west across Europe and, unlike the 'movement' of tick-borne encephalitis, this does seem to be happening. Hence the reinforced stress on the animal quarantine regulations, and this is heightened by the change in fox ecology and bionomics so that there is now a considerable urban population of foxes living by scavenging in many cities rather than hunting.

The UK, the Atlantic and Pacific Islands, Australia and New Zealand are able to maintain a fragile freedom from rabies, but the virus must be taken as a worldwide zoonosis and human rabies as a universal disease: it is then easy to accept that it is fairly common, and too often in the Third World the victim of a bite from a rabid wild or more probably domestic animal is not able to obtain or maybe sustain the course of protective vaccinations. Modern studies include conference papers on rabies in the Tropics (Kuwert et al. 1985), and a very evocative paper on rabies in India. The dog population is estimated at 50 million, many not really cared for and liable to infection from wild animals; some 3 million people are vaccinated annually but there are some 14–20 000 deaths per year, mainly in village men (Trivedi 1981; Singh 1980). Control measures, familiar enough in cantonments, would meet many cultural and socioeconomic obstacles in the nation as a whole. Comparison with the note on Tinline's (1982) work on rabies in Ontario affords a dramatic illustration of the vast gulf between developed and developing nations; see *Archives de l'Institut Pasteur de Tunis* (1982).

In Canada, as in mainland Europe, the fox is a major reservoir of the virus, though other animals such as the skunk are also involved. A dauntingly imaginative project envisages that a combination of measures against the zoonosis might be effective, but with prophylaxis against the virus *in animals*, using baits containing vaccine, as a main plank. It is clear that close knowledge is needed of animal movements, and also of movements of rabies among animal populations, as the virus moves across susceptible populations as a wandering epizootic (the equivalent term to epidemic in people). Animals' movements, daily and in migrations, were studied using small radio transmitters fastened round the necks of animals trapped and then released. Intensive efforts were made to keep track of rabid animals and animals dead from rabies. (Tinline and Pond 1981). Tinline, already a geographer and biostatistician of animal disease of repute (founded on research on the last great epizootic of foot-and-mouth disease in England and Wales) has for some years been in charge of a geographical use of a modern computer technology as imaginative as is the project as a whole. Data on both animal movements and rabies infections of animals are processed quickly so that a constantly moving picture of the phenomena can be built up and displayed in table, graph or map form on demand. It is remarkable that a set of linked techniques of immense potential for human health monitoring should have been pioneered for an animal disease. First findings are of practical value. The prophylaxis using vaccine in baits can usefully be complemented by trapping ahead of the epizootic wave, and by 'hot spot' campaigns to protect rural populations. This is a remarkable and an inspiring study. The urban problem is different because of the crucial role of raccoons and possums adapted to suburban life and dear to the hearts of city dwellers, which may have to be trapped and individually vaccinated. Large cities are often thought of as concrete jungles, as impoverished in ecological webs as actual jungles are rich: in many western cities the new importance of urban foxes – as main actual or potential carriers of rabies – sufficiently counters that idea. For a review of a much wider range of risks in a total urban ecology (in Belgrade) see Popović and Tadić (1979).

Some Methodological References

Wilson (1978) suggests the analysis of variance as helping with the problem of small numbers in small or sparsely peopled administrative units – an approach perhaps superseded by McGlashan's advocacy of the use of the Poisson statistic (McGlashan and Harington 1976); Miyawaki and Chen (1981), concerned with the same problem, think of merging administrative units, an expedient often used, but by geographers reluctantly, for it takes the presentation of the data farther from the actual 'disease topography'. Glick (1979a,c) writes on space–time clustering in cancer research, with broader discussion in his 1979b and 1980 papers. Craft et al. (1985) analyse cancer in children in northern England by electoral wards, and Mangoud et al. (1985) with a geographer in the team, apply space–time cluster analysis fruitfully to the incidence of Hodgkin's disease in Greater Manchester. Philippe (1985) writes on the generation and evaluation of hypotheses in our field, and Mayer (1983) on spatial analysis in general and the detection of disease causation. Cumper (1984) is on the whole reassuring that the 'ecological fallacy' need not lead us to discard correlation exercises using grouped populations, in a thirteen-region study of infant mortality in developing countries. Fox et al. (1984) find socioeconomic variables more meaningful than spatial analyses – but spatial analysis standardized for social class etc. has not been tried.

Conclusion

This chapter, indeed the book, is necessarily selective, and as always the selection could have been a different one. It moves from Giggs' opportunism in the study of pancreatitis in Nottingham, and his study of schizophrenia in the same city – heightening local understanding and a stimulus to other workers, through Meade's broad-spectrum and very sophisticated thinking about the long-standing problem of high incidence of cardiovascular disease in the coastlands of south-eastern USA, to three infections, two of them vector-borne and all zoonotic, that are still significant in the developed world. Some of the techniques are very much of the computer age, and on these exemplars young geographers who have grown up with that technology can look forward to useful and relevant research in ecological medical geography.

8 Between Two Worlds: The Historical Geography of Disease

Introductory

This chapter must be restricted to quite specific aims related to those of the book as a whole. Some readers may be interested in the historical geography of health and disease in general, and so far as Britain is concerned there is an admirable and readily accessible source (Howe 1972a, 1976); and leading libraries will be able to give access to older classics (e.g. Hirsch 1881 and 1883–6; Creighton 1894, 1965). Third World medical history increasingly overlaps with historical geography, see, for instance, Ransford (1983), Clyde (1980, 1985). Here, however, the main aim is to further the idea that we all share One World by showing how relatively close we are in time, in developed countries, to conditions of health and disease quite similar to those in Third World countries today. This involves some change in balance of interest and presentation as compared with most other chapters in this book: there is more stress on contributing to a general understanding of the comparison just suggested, and relatively less on trying to indicate ways in which an interested student of geography might find his way into research in the field. However, there are interesting points of technique, and some readers may be interested in the ancestry of some geographical techniques that we are too apt to assume as the contributions of today or yesterday, rather than say of the nineteenth century. So from the wealth of material available in primary or secondary sources in archives and libraries, the author has selected only a few readily accessible studies relevant to this One World theme.

When the writer first came to study the medical geography of late colonial India, the three great epidemic diseases of that great country were cholera, plague and smallpox. The infant mortality for many areas

was over 25 per cent and the expectation of life at birth, partly because
of those high infant death rates, was only 27 years. Yet within the last
two or three centuries in Britain cholera, plague and smallpox have all
caused major epidemics, infant mortality rates for many communities
have approached the figure for inter-war India, and the expectation of
life at birth was only 40–45 years in England and Wales as late as the
1860s (Banks 1959); and infant mortality was still about 150 per thousand
live births until about 1900, of course with marked local concentrations
in underprivileged areas (Woods and Woodward 1984). Similar or even
closer comparisons can be drawn for many developed countries, while
several other diseases that we tend nowadays to class as tropical have
been important at particular times or in particular places in Britain and
elsewhere, including, for instance, malaria, yellow fever and leprosy.
Louse-borne typhus was an important killing disease during the potato
famine in Ireland and north-west Scotland in the 1840s, in Napoleon's
retreat from Moscow, and in the terrible famines in south-west USSR
soon after the Revolution. One could go on, but it is perhaps better to
refer to some of the vivid historical accounts that are widely available
(Zinsser 1935; McNeill 1977, 1979; Woodham-Smith 1964).

Plague

For many people, the Great Plague of the 1660s in England is perhaps
the landmark that best reminds us how relatively close we are to Third
World conditions – the Black Death of the mid-fourteenth century making
much less impact? Yet these are now thought to be linked, as we shall
see. Many English people have known from schooldays stories of London
under the plague, and perhaps visited the Derbyshire village of Eyam
and read of the dramatic efforts to contain the disease within the village
and so avoid spreading it into nearby communities (Creighton 1894,
quoting Wood 1842). Shannon and Cromley (1980) assess the London
data from a geographical viewpoint, while a demographic history of a
parish in the West Midlands throws light on the impact of the Black
Death (Razi 1980). Accounts of plague in seventeenth-century Amsterdam
and eighteenth-century Switzerland and Russia, especially Moscow, are
in Alter (1983), Eckert (1982) and Alexander (1980). For some thoughts
on the disappearance of plague from Britain, see Bayliss (1980). It is less
familiar, perhaps, that this is thought to be one indication of the 'burning
out' of the second great world epidemic or 'pandemic' – another being
the catastrophic plague epidemic affecting Marseilles and Toulon in 1720
(see also Slack (1981) on the possible role of *cordons sanitaires*, quarantine
etc.). This second pandemic – the first occurred as a series of great

epidemics affecting the classical world between 1100 BC and AD 644 –
had lasted since the spread of the Black Death across Europe in the
fourteenth century (see figure 8.1). The direction of movement from
eastern and southern Europe is best interpreted with a broad picture of
plague in the world, and the link between figure 8.1 and 8.2 and the
next paragraph is that the outbreak north of the Black Sea in 1347 is
thought to have been associated with incursions by Tartar or Mongol
armies from central Asia.

Plague is primarily a zoonosis, an animal disease in which people
become involved, in fact an infection of rodents, and in particular of
marmot and ground squirrel in central Asia – hence the link with the
Tartar warriors. It is an enzootic or constantly present animal disease
and one of 'wild' rodents rather than of 'domestic' ones like rats – a four-
or five-factor complex in May's terms, involving wild rodents, rodent
fleas, the 'domestic' rodents, people and the pathogen *Yersinia pestis*
(Yersin was a Swiss bacteriologist). This world home of plague is shown
in figure 8.2, along with other areas of enzootic plague in southern Africa,
in central Madagascar and in south-western USA. These are considered
as probably secondary in that human movement has carried the infection
from Asia, subsequently to settle down as an enzootic in wild rodents

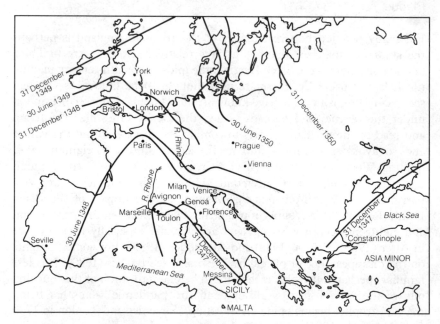

Figure 8.1   Black Death, Europe, 1348–1350
Source: Open University 1985 (II p. 44)

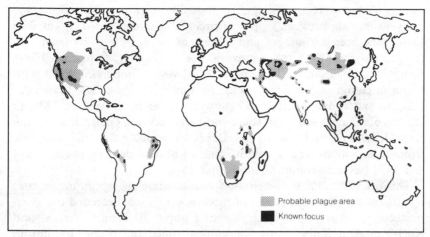

Figure 8.2 Contemporary plague foci
Source: Open University 1985 (II p. 49)

analogous to those of central Asia, occasionally affecting, say, camping children and very rarely domestic animals – cats in two recent cases (Mann et al. 1982). In Soviet Central Asia, plague in animals has been classified according to temperature and rainfall relations into continuous enzootic areas (those with epizootics with 2–4 year lulls) and those areas with long lulls of 8–12 years (Serzhanov et al. 1982). From the wild rodent enzootic conditions of central Asia, at long intervals across the millennia, the infection seems to have moved from 'wild' to 'domestic' rodents, notably rat populations in a ring of ancient market cities round the semi-deserts of central Asia, in India, China and what is now Soviet Asia. With minor and major cyclic variations, probably related to the degree of community immunity, and in turn to the proportion of a particular human population that has survived an earlier wave of plague, the infection tends to cause epidemics, first in the ring of market cities, and then, since markets involve transport of people and commodities, along lines of communication, and out into the world to affect both rodent and human populations with low immunity to the particular pathogen. As already noted, this movement outward is thought to have originated the enzootic foci of plague outside central Asia. (Learmonth 1958; Open University 1985, Book I, chapter 5).

The third pandemic began about 1890 and may be thought of as dying away in the years since the 1939–45 war, its departure perhaps accelerated by campaigns against agricultural pests or against malaria using DDT (at least initially), though with occasional flaring up of epidemics under conditions of population movement under stress, for instance during the war in Vietnam. Human plague is thought to have spread with trade caravans moving between Upper Burma and Yunnan, flared up in cities there, then been encouraged and spread, as often, by war, by troop and refugee movements in the suppression of a rebellion. It reached Hong Kong in 1890, Bombay in 1894 – there was an important trade with China in cotton yarn – Formosa or Taiwan in 1896 and San Francisco, Glasgow and Sydney in 1900. There were deaths in Glasgow in 1900, in Liverpool the next year, and there was a smouldering epidemic along the river Orwell in Suffolk until 1918. But it was in India that this pandemic wrought enormous tragedy, with some 13 million deaths between 1894 and 1938 (see also comment in chapter 15).

This pandemic, important in itself, was additionally significant because it came as the next generation of medical scientists succeeded the great pioneers, Pasteur and Koch. Pasteur's pupil, Alexander Yersin, and Koch's student Shibasaburo Kitasato identified the plague bacillus in 1894, and, after a time when it was known as *Pasteurella pestis* its current scientific name is *Yersinia pestis*. Then a French epidemiologist P.L. Simond suggested that the flea was the vector of the infection, and this was conclusively demonstrated by J.A. Thompson in Australia in 1900. A vaccine was developed in 1897, and an improved version in 1938. We can now see plague as presenting a particularly complex pattern of interactions within the four- or five-factor complex.

As a disease of wild animals, the bacillus, *Yersinia pestis*, circulates between rodents like the marmot and the ground squirrel, carried by fleas, as an enzootic. In some years, perhaps because of warm humid conditions favouring the fleas, or because of animal migrations, it moves out as an epizootic (animal epidemic) disease into more or less 'domestic' rodents like the rat or Indian bandicoot. The fleas desert the dead rodents, and seek fresh hosts. Depending on the climatic conditions in general, dry heat being hostile to most insects and other arthropods, and in particular on the microclimates of, say, rat burrow and of clay walls and straw roofs of village or slum huts, the flea may carry the infection to a human host. Even in the frequently affected ring of market cities round central Asia, to take the Old World case, there are likely to be some people, mainly young, who have low immunity to the infection, and even more so if the disease cycle moves out along lines of migration and commerce, to produce epidemics, sometimes pandemics, as in the historical outbreaks outlined earlier. The limits of an outbreak may be due to change in climate or more likely in microclimates like those mentioned above, or because of a spatial variation in the dominant species of rodent and human flea. Some species of flea are more 'efficient' vectors of plague than others: *Y. pestis* in ingested blood multiplies in the flea's digestive tract, causing 'blocking', so that the flea begins to starve and to seek fresh blood-sucking the more inexorably; since the gut *is* blocked, some blood from earlier attempts to feed is regurgitated, and this may inject some of the now multiplied *Y. pestis* organisms into the new host's blood stream. This seems to occur more readily in some flea species: thus in at least the later stages of the Indian epidemics in the third pandemic the concentration of the disease in the less humid parts of the country may have been due to the dominance in those areas of an efficient vector, *Xenopsylla cheopis*, and of other species of flea such as *X. astia* in more humid areas (Learmonth (1958) based in particular on Sharif (1951)). Plague is often known as bubonic plague, from the common swellings in lymph glands in the groin and armpit given the name bubo (from the Greek for 'groin'), but in some epidemics it changes, probably by mutation in *Y. pestis*, to the septicaemic form, also transmitted by fleas, and to the pneumonic (better 'pulmonary') form, important in cold countries and cold seasons in the Black Death, for instance. As with much historical medical geography, there is much controversy about the nature of long-past epidemics – some workers, for example, suggest that the Black Death was actually anthrax – and this issue is debated more fully in a recent teaching text (Open University 1985). World reviews of plague include Christie (1982), and regional or country accounts include Mitchell (1983) on its arrival and settling down in South Africa, *WER* (1982b) on Bolivia, and an *Epidemiological Bulletin* (1981a) on the Americas as a whole.

Cholera

Cholera – along with typhoid which is not discussed in this book to any extent – is perhaps familiar to most people in western countries as playing a major role in the public health movement in the nineteenth century (Longmate 1966; Morris 1971). Compared with the discussion of plague above, there is more on the evolution of classical geographical techniques, and some modern geographical analysis too. For an overview of cholera pandemics, see Jusatz (1982).

Cholera is caused by a bacillus known as *Vibrio cholerae* (*V. comma* in older literature). It belongs to a genus of which several species appear not to be pathogenic, while some are pathogenic to animals including livestock, and one or two to people. So far as is known *V. cholerae* is an infection only of humankind and so on present knowledge is in a two-factor complex, and it can survive for comparatively short periods outside the human gut, in water, in moist foodstuffs, in human faeces, on soiled hands, etc. The world endemic home of what one might call classical cholera lies in South Asia, in particular in its deltas, notably the Ganga (Ganges)-Brahmaputra delta. (The main organism involved in the present wide spread of cholera in the world is of a different strain or sub-species known as El Tor cholera, and this is discussed in chapter 9 of the book.) Like plague, cholera appears to have a short-term cycle of rise and fall of about five years as well as longer-term crests and troughs, and even in its endemic home in West Bengal it almost disappears for the final two years before a fresh epidemic starts. An alternate host has been suspected, but never proved, and the phenomenon may be related to greater community immunity in the populations in endemic areas, or perhaps to changes in virulence of the organism or a temporary dominance of a non-pathogenic strain or *vibrio* species (see also chapter 9).

Britain and indeed western Europe suffered severe cholera epidemics, sufficiently catastrophic to give very effective ammunition to the public health campaigners in the mid-nineteenth century, as noted above. The scourge was long and recurrent enough to justify the term pandemic, and figure 8.3 illustrates its spread from South Asia, across South-west Asia, into and across Europe with branches moving up the Nile and across the Atlantic, in the years 1827–31. Figure 8.4 was drawn about 20 years afterwards, in 1852, by the distinguished German cartographer Augustus Petermann, then resident in an England still sharply reminded of the importance of cholera, as we shall see. An inset map in the original

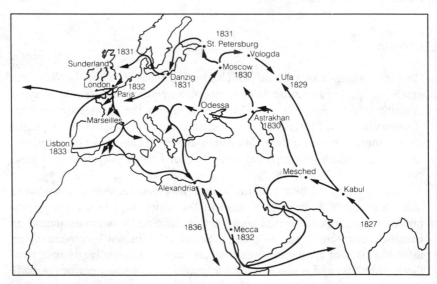

Figure 8.3   Cholera advance, India to Britain, 1827–1831
Source: Howe (1972a p. 171)

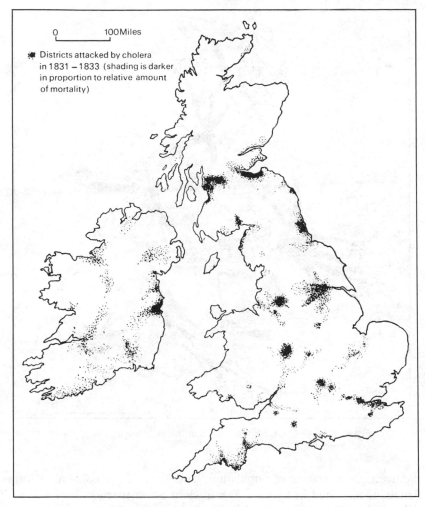

Figure 8.4 Cholera, British Isles, 1831–1833, dot map by Petermann
Source: Gilbert (1958 p. 177)

shows London's forty-three registration districts on a larger scale, with dense shadings for the higher *rates* of cholera in the City, Southwark and Bermondsey. Figure 8.4, in contrast, is of the character of a dot map, with two disadvantages: (1) in the densest patches of the disease the dots fuse so that they cannot be counted for purposes of further analysis; and (2) it is difficult from this map to see if particular concentrations of population were at abnormally high (or low) risk, again for purposes of further analysis – in fact the distribution quite closely approximates to

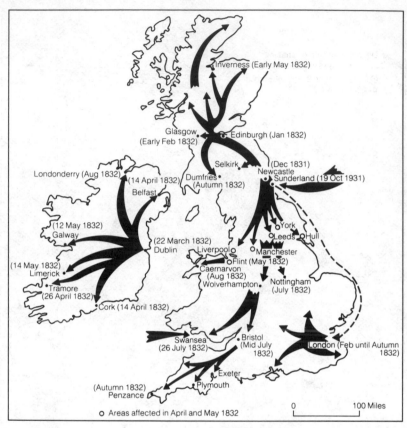

Figure 8.5 . Cholera advance through the British Isles, 1831–1833
Source: Howe (1972a p. 173)

the main concentration of population. The route of the epidemic within
Britain is indicated in figure 8.5, a modern reconstruction by Professor
G.M. Howe (1972a). It arrived in Sunderland with the first case notified
on 19 October 1831; it succeeded in 'overwintering' there, a comparatively
rare event in a cool climate, it is thought in heaps of night soil piled on
the Town Moor. It then spread, mainly on land, but with some coastal
movements by sea, to London, perhaps with coal ships, from Dumfries
to Liverpool (not mapped) and of course across the Irish Sea; there is
some indication of what one might call hierarchical rediffusion, from
main centres of trade and traffic – London, Bristol, Liverpool the mid-
lowlands of Scotland and notably Dublin.

One of the last of the linked series of epidemics in Britain was in the
early 1850s, and this brought a flurry of contemporary cartography using

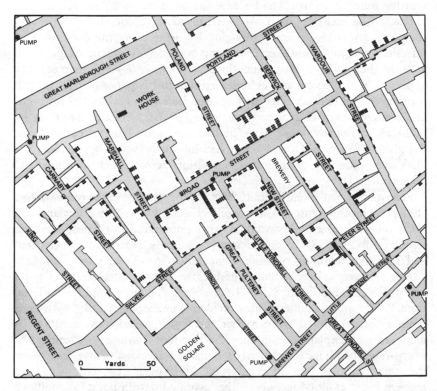

Figure 8.6   Cholera, Snow's map of Soho, 1854
Source: Gilbert (1958 p. 174)

various techniques, lovingly assembled in an important paper by the late
Professor E.W. Gilbert (1958). One of these was a celebrated dot map
by Dr John Snow of the 1854 epidemic in Soho in London, centred on
a pump used for drinking water in Broad Street, now Broadwick Street
(figure 8.6). Snow claimed that this outbreak proved that cholera is water-
borne, and indeed it is widely accepted that *explosive* epidemics usually
are so (as distinct from a smouldering epidemic like that overwintering
in Sunderland, where polluted tools, vessels, hands etc. and, in warm
damp conditions, houseflies also, are more likely routes of infection).
This map is sometimes claimed as an example of the use of cartography
as a research tool; Snow had already formed his views on the importance
of sewage-free water when he wrote the first edition of his paper (1849);
however, the outbreak in Soho in 1854 gave him fresh ammunition: he
claimed that only people who had drunk water from the Broad Street
pump fell ill in that area, and that a woman from some distance who

sent for water from that well because she liked the taste also fell ill, and that when he had the pump handle removed the epidemic ceased. (This is not to say that Dr Snow thought that water was the *only* route of infection, a point recently reviewed and argued with vigour by Feachem et al. in their 1981–2 papers mentioned in chapter 9.) The map actually appeared in his second and enlarged edition of his paper (1855), though it cannot be quite established that he used it as an actual tool of research. His contemporary detractors maintained, probably justifiably, that the outbreak was on the wane when he had the pump handle removed (see Creighton 1894 p. 854); and yet he had hit on the water-borne nature of explosive epidemics of cholera a generation before Koch identified the organism in 1883.

Petermann had pointed out from contemporary and retrospective studies including figure 8.4 that while cholera was mainly a lowland and river valley disease its association with population concentrations was strong (Gilbert 1958). The epidemic of the early 1850s brought detailed and sensitive mapping of cholera incidence in several cities including Exeter (Shapter), Leeds (Baker) and a particularly interesting series on Oxford by Acland (figure 8.7(a), (b) and (c)): Acland's emphasis differed from Petermann's, linking valley incidence and relative relief with poor drainage and polluted rivers rather than with population density. His maps are self-explanatory in that the five-foot contours, revealing the micro-relief of Oxford very well, are marked in steps of five feet below the high point of the city at Carfax, itself measured, confusingly to modern eyes, at 49.64 feet above the 'assumed datum point' at Sandford Weir. Anyone who shared a field excursion on cholera in Oxford with the late Professor Gilbert will remember Gas Street as the other Oxford, and the realization of the immanence of Third World conditions in the city of dreaming spires that reinforced the consciousness of the One World model that I am advocating, of the closeness of Victorian England to the Third World of today.

Lastly on nineteenth century cholera is figure 8.8, from an important diffusion study by Professor G.F. Pyle (1969). While important epidemics have often been thought to spread by water-borne routes, e.g. downstream in rivers, this is not always so – it is not uncommon for cholera in India to advance from the endemic home in Bengal *up*stream along the Ganga plains. Here Pyle is suggesting that while some movements are suggestive of waterborne movement, e.g. along the Mississippi system, hierarchical movement between main cities and along main transport routes may be important, that the epidemic leapfrogs between centres rather than progressing in a wave-like pattern. This concept has already been encountered in this book in the discussion of hepatitis A and its diffusion patterns. On ethnicity and the 1849 cholera epidemic in Buffalo, see Cotter and Patrick (1981).

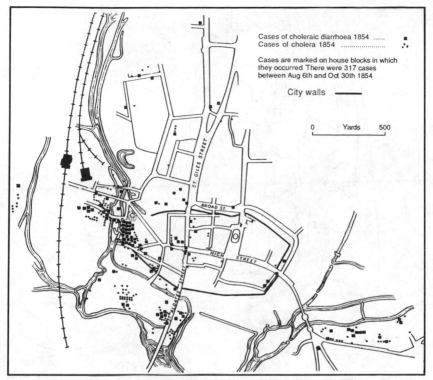

Figure 8.7 (a)   Cholera: Acland's map of Oxford, 1854
Source: Gilbert (1958, figs 7–9)

Smallpox

Smallpox, happily, is one disease that can be said to be historical in a particular sense, for the World Health Organization declared it eradicated in 1980 after over two years with no report of any outbreaks despite continued surveillance in its last strongholds like Somalia where the final documented, naturally occurring case occurred in October 1977. Smallpox or variola was a severe, often fatal, virus disease, highly infectious, probably contagious, and typically with spots or pustules on the skin, especially on the face and often leaving disfiguring pockmarks in people who recovered from an attack. Severe attacks were often haemorrhagic, with bleeding into the pustules including those on the air passages. Death was commonly caused by invasion of the skin lesions by bacteria, or by pneumonia. Spread of the virus by droplet or by contagion, and with only humankind and the virus involved on all the vast accumulation of

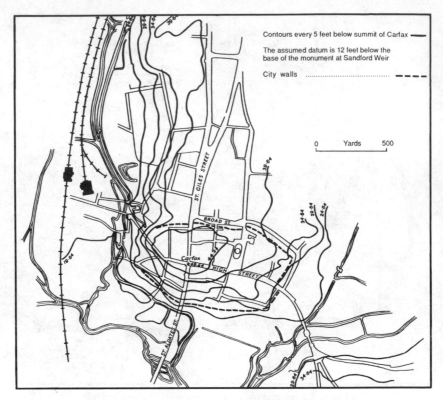

Figure 8.7 (b) Cholera: Acland's contour map of Oxford
Source: Gilbert (1958, figs 7–9)

evidence, implies that the disease was associated with overcrowding in
dwellings, historically almost universally, and in recent times in Third
World countries, rather than with particular macro-climates (Learmonth
1958 p. 47), though a within-city study of Patna, not long before
eradication, suggested illiteracy and agricultural work as correlates, rather
than overcrowding as such (see Singh and Dutta, 1981). Still, crowded
rooms seemed to favour the spread of the virus whether in humid Bengal,
arid Sind or Somalia, or in Victorian London or Liverpool. Inoculation
– often into the nose rather than the eye as inoculation literally implies
– had for centuries been practised using material from pustules on
smallpox patients; however, the procedure was quite hazardous and many
fatal attacks resulted from such heroic early immunization methods, as
well as the protection of survivors. Revolutionary change in immunization
for smallpox came from Dr Edward Jenner's country practice at Berkeley

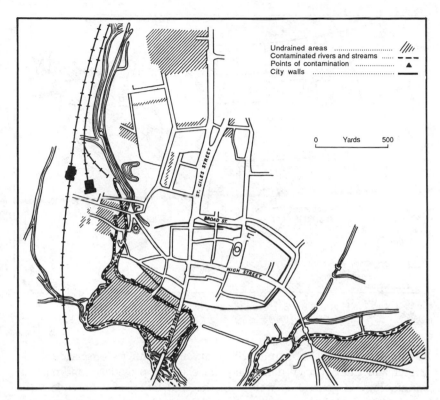

Figure 8.7 (c)   Cholera: Acland's map of undrained areas of Oxford
Source: Gilbert (1958 figs 7–9)

in Gloucestershire, north of Bristol: he noticed that dairymaids who had picked up vaccinia or cowpox from milch cows in their care appeared to be immune to the smallpox virus during a local outbreak of that human disease. This was the beginning of the worldwide adoption of vaccination against smallpox, which, though not without risks, is widely accepted as one of the medical or public health interventions that was almost certainly crucial in the protection of large populations, initially in industrial or industrializing countries in temperate climates, followed by mass vaccination campaigns, then carefully targeted ones in populations at risk from reported outbreaks. Once a large proportion of a population has acquired immunity, one way or another, it is possible to contain outbreaks of an infection, given good reporting and surveillance. It was by this more selective campaign, assisted by some technological developments like the bifurcated immunization needle, that eradication

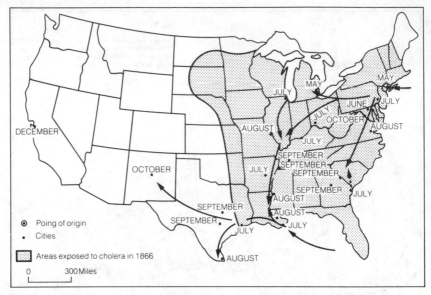

Figure 8.8   Cholera in the USA, diffusion pattern 1866
Source: Pyle (1979 p. 131)

was finally achieved, not quite 200 years after Jenner's observation. So Jenner and the Berkeley dairymaid can claim to provide a landmark in immunology in general as well as in the eradication of a horrible virus disease (Open University 1985, Book VII, p. 43).

From the time of wide acceptance of Jenner's vaccination onwards, the geography and history of the disease can be generalized. There were of course many minor variations in space and time as the battle against the virus here won new territory, there sustained a temporary defeat where vaccination came to be neglected by too large a proportion of the population. Figure 8.9 shows a crucial period in England and Wales, 1840–1920; from 1840 to the end of the century a large part of the general decline in death rates is generally accepted as due to vaccination, but since then the further decline of smallpox has been associated with under two per cent of the twentieth-century reductions in death rates (McKeown 1976). Though the timing of events, the degree of legal compulsion etc. varied from country to country, broadly comparable changes occurred in most modern industrial nations, so that by the 1950s and 1960s smallpox, once a well-nigh universal disease, became, as it were, a tropical disease in the sense that it had retreated largely to the tropics, and to Third World countries, though with occasional, quite alarming sallies back into temperate and developed countries, causing a handful or a score of cases,

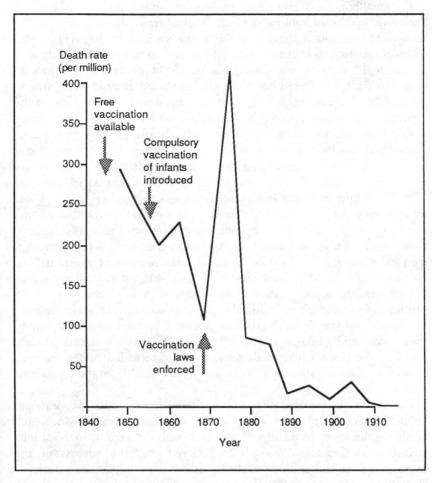

Figure 8.9   Decline of death rates and of smallpox, England and Wales 1840–1920
Source: Open University Reader (1984 p. 111)

a few deaths, and a flurry of vaccinations in affected localities and in international travellers (with rare cases of complications from the vaccination lesions). The association with the Tropics was not one of climate, as we have seen, but related to health care and particularly preventive medicine. Measles occupies something of the same niche today, with very widespread immunization campaigns in some countries, and comparatively few serious illnesses and fewer still fatal ones in countries not adopting mass prophylaxis, and yet still a scourge in many Third World countries.

For smallpox the WHO world eradication campaign began in 1967, in the teeth of considerable scepticism arising from the faltering of the attempt to eradicate malaria from the world (see chapter 10). There were 130 000 reported cases that year, but the real incidence was thought to be about 10 million, with many thousands of deaths. More than 30 countries were considered endemic, with imported cases in twelve more; the main endemic reservoirs of the virus were Brazil, Africa south of the Sahara, South Asia as a whole, and the Indonesian archipelago (Strassburg 1982). Mass immunization campaigns no doubt played their part, but in many countries these are very difficult to implement because of difficult climate and terrain, of social barriers, traditional attribution of the disease to the intervention of God, or a god or goddess of illness of this type (like Mariamma in South India), or sometimes to witchcraft, spells cast by an enemy etc. In the early 1970s workers in West Africa showed that the time was ripe for the more selective 'surveillance and containment' policy referred to above. This was adopted by the whole WHO campaign with excellent results. By 1981 India, a main reservoir for centuries at least, was able to advertise widely offering a substantial cash reward to anyone able to report a case of smallpox, with few takers. By 1975 eradication was confirmed in Brazil and Indonesia after two years carefully monitored and free from the disease. South Asia was well on the way to eradication, and all Africa except Ethiopia and Somalia – the last already noted as the place where the disease was last recorded under 'natural' conditions, that is, laboratory stocks and 'break-outs' from these excepted (Christie 1977).

The tale is an inspiring one, and it is tempting to apply it as a model for the elimination of other infectious diseases. Complementary accounts of the eradication of smallpox will be found in various publications including Behbehani (1983). It is believed that the success of the surveillance and containment strategy was due to particular characteristics of smallpox: (1) it normally spreads comparatively slowly, one active case infecting only two to five other people; (2) it tends to cluster within a village or street or area; (3) humankind are thought to have been the only source of the virus; and (4) immunity after an attack or immunization is of long duration (Strassburg 1982). Policy on surveillance after the eradication of smallpox (and on human monkeypox) is surveyed in the *Weekly Epidemiological Record* (WER 1983).

To sum up on smallpox, the story is not a strongly geographical one, but it is included for its valuable perspective on different types of epidemic disease, some already discussed in this chapter, some to be mentioned later. Some knowledge of the history of this terrible disease and its elimination is vital, I believe, to the kind of overview attempted towards the end of this book.

Influenza

Influenza, a very different virus disease in its symptoms and course, and yet mainly spread by droplet and soiled hands etc., has been discussed in chapter 6 – indeed some of the material cited there is already a generation old and in a sense historical. However, a further brief retrospect here is relevant. Britain experienced moderate to severe epidemics in 1803, 1831, 1837 and 1847–8. For a geographical study of the period 1830–48, see Patterson (1985). There was then a comparative lull until 1889–94 and 1895, with recurrence in 1900 and 1908. Pyle and Patterson (1983) give a European context. There followed another ten-year lull, including the 1914–18 war, but 1918 saw the beginning of one of the greatest of all pandemics, lasting until at least 1921, spreading over very large parts of the globe, and causing some 20 million deaths, more than the war itself, largely from pneumonia, just as in the 1957–8 epidemic discussed in chapter 6 (Howe 1972a). A geographer's viewpoint on the possibility that the pandemic may have originated with swine fever is in Pyle (1979 p. 149, 1980 p. 227). It is regarded as a winter disease, made worse in this pandemic by wartime chaos, overcrowding and undernutrition. But it spread to many tropical countries. In India, for instance, it caused millions of deaths, mainly in and around Bombay where there was and is much overcrowded industrial housing and many slums too, and in the Punjab where winter can be quite sharp; the warmer and wetter parts of the country were much less affected. The diffusion of the pandemic influenza in Japan was first from the seaports, then into urban areas, and then down the urban hierarchy from Tokyo (Sugiura 1977). A geographical view of the impact of the pandemic in Africa is in Patterson and Pyle (1983), stressing the overwhelming importance of the railways in its diffusion (cf. Hogbin 1985). See also Pyle (1979). The writer attempted some broad mapping for British data some years ago, and concluded that the distribution of the disease, and of influenza and pneumonia deaths, corresponds very closely with the population map. Figure 8.10 however, for the years immediately preceding the 1914–18 war, shows that urban death rates were higher in the north and west of England and Wales, in sympathy with what we know of the distribution pattern of bronchitis, tuberculosis and other respiratory diseases (Learmonth 1972b). Immunization against influenza remains a difficult problem because of the several strains involved – immunity conferred against one strain is apparently of little effect against another – so at present influenza remains one of the universal diseases most liable to remind us sharply that we do share One World.

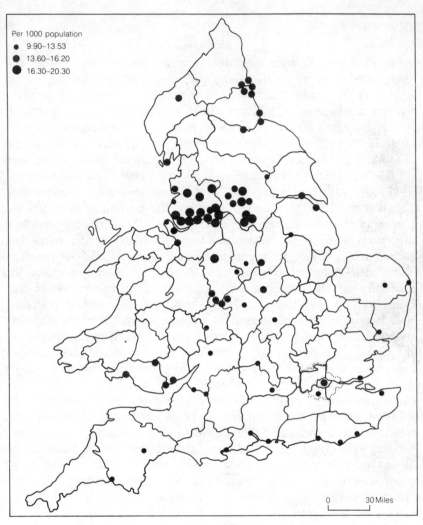

Per 1000 population
● 9.90–13.53
● 13.60–16.20
● 16.30–20.30

0   30 Miles

Figure 8.10 Influenza in urban England and Wales *c*.1910
Source: Learmonth (1972b p. 26)

Malaria in Europe including England

It comes as a surprise to many people that malaria was common in parts
of Europe until after the 1939–45 war, including the Rhine delta, low-
lying parts of the Mediterranean countries and through the Balkans into
the south-west of the USSR. The story of the various ways in which the

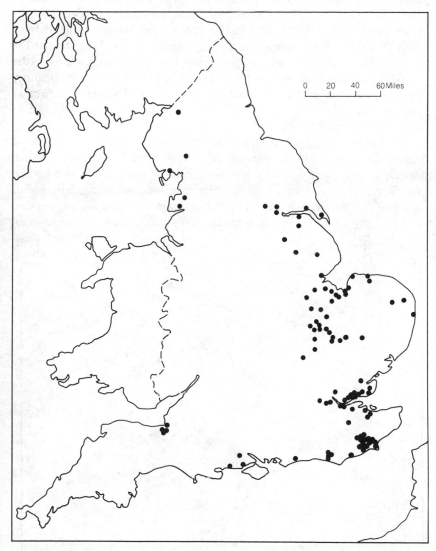

Figure 8.11   Ague in England in the nineteenth century
Source: Darby (1940b p. 181) (based on Nuttal et al. 1901); Dobson (1982 p. 97)

disease came to be eliminated is a fascinating one, the more so since
there are two classic books on the subject separated by a generation
(Hackett 1937; Bruce-Chwatt and de Zulueta 1980).

For England the equally classic historical geography of the fen country
includes figure 8.11 and many interesting references to the ague as

affecting life and death there prior to the great drainage projects, (Darby 1940a,b; 1983). In fact it lingered on there for many years – some ten years ago a retired banker in Lincoln told me that he had suffered from malaria without ever leaving the country. In discussion I mentioned the fact that one of the main vector mosquitoes has some preference for cattle blood rather than human, though ready to bite humans when opportunity presents itself, and it then emerged that his duties had included inspecting farm steadings in the course of assessing the credit-worthiness of farmer clients of the bank!

Until at least the eighteenth century there was a sufficient reservoir of one species of the malaria parasite, *Plasmodium vivax* for this protozoal disease to remain at a locally serious degree of endemicity, and several vector mosquitoes were common. The main one as an efficient vector often in contact with human populations prior to draining of marshes and the separation of rural housing from cattle-sheds was *Anopheles*

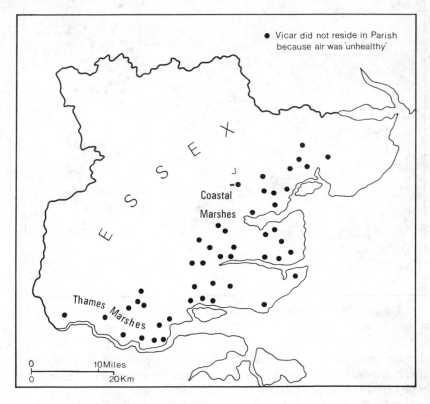

Figure 8.12 Unhealthy parishes avoided by vicars
Source: Dobson (1982 p. 97)

atroparvus; this was a marsh breeding mosquito, including salt-marshes since it could tolerate brackish water. A flood-plain mosquito, *A. messeae* was less important while two other species were capable of transmission, indeed still are. Vector species have been found as far north as Lochinver and Forres in northern Scotland. The marsh ague discussed by Darby may not all have been malaria, of course, but much of it does seem to have been so, on various pieces of admittedly fragmentary evidence (Bruce-Chwatt 1976). Recently much historical geography research on malaria has been done, some of it published in a popular journal (Dobson 1980, 1982). Figure 8.11 is similar to Dr Mary Dobson's map of malaria as late as the 1860s. Much patient sifting of parish register data gave her evidence, from vicars avoiding actually living in unhealthy parishes (figure 8.12), topographers' characterization of parishes as healthy or unhealthy (figure 8.13), excesses of deaths over births (figure 8.14), to graphing death rates in warm summers likely to encourage the disease cycle, as compared with cool ones.

There was active transmission of malaria from servicemen returned from malarious theatres of war after both the 1914–18 and the 1939–45 wars, though the disease cycle was fairly soon broken. And perhaps most surprising of all was an outbreak in a London square, the vector mosquito

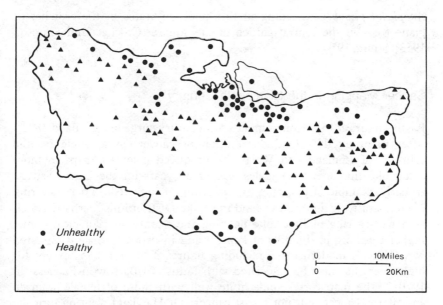

Figure 8.13 Unhealthy parishes in Kent according to contemporary topographers
Source: Dobson (1982 p. 98)

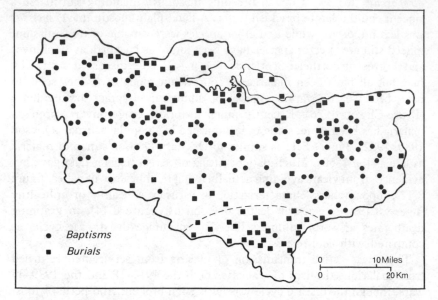

Figure 8.14   Unhealthy parishes in Kent judged by excess of deaths over births
Source:- Dobson (1982 p. 98)

Anopheles plumbeus breeding in tiny pools of water in the crotches of plane trees in the central garden of the square (Crockett and Simpson 1953; Shute 1954).

Cancer Mapping in the Nineteenth Century

Lastly, figure 8.15 is from a nineteenth-century surgeon (Haviland 1892). After mapping the broad distribution of cancers as a whole for the counties of England and Wales, he produced coloured maps in more detail like this one, for females of over 35 years for the Lake District, an early example of mapping by age-group at high risk. There is a ring of comparatively light rates round the Lake District hills, perhaps associated with a ring of limestone flanking the Cumbrian geological dome; higher rates are in the hills of Penrith and in urban Carlisle. Compared with Howe's modern maps including figures 3.14 and 3.15, except for high rates that may be associated with industrial Barrow-in-Furness, in 1970–2, the map corresponds quite well with those of female stomach and uterus cancer, but not breast cancer. Dr Haviland went on to make recommendations about choice of residence, presumably for those able to afford such a choice! He suggested that children of cancerous parents

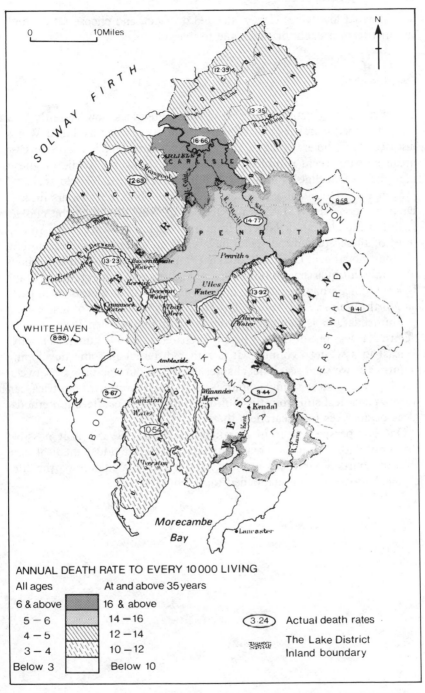

ANNUAL DEATH RATE TO EVERY 10 000 LIVING

All ages   At and above 35 years

6 & above   16 & above

5 – 6   14 – 16

4 – 5   12 – 14

3 – 4   10 – 12

Below 3   Below 10

(3·24) Actual death rates

The Lake District
Inland boundary

Figure 8.15 Cancers, females at and over 35 years, Cumberland and Westmorland
1851–1870
Source: Haviland (1892, map 2)

should avoid low-lying, clayey, flooded districts, and choose rather high dry districts on chalk or limestone formations.

Conclusion

This brief and selective historical chapter illustrates how recently it is that developed countries shared what are now regarded as Third-World diseases, like cholera, plague and smallpox. Smallpox is a special case because of its recent complete eradication in the world, while plague is in a phase of decline as a public health problem on the world scale.

More must be said about cholera later in the book, but readers in, say, Dumfries or Merthyr Tydfil may feel more sympathy with the cholera victim of Bangladesh or Nigeria from even such a brief account. And all three of these epidemic diseases have value in adding to understanding of other infections. The study of cancers in the Lake District is perhaps of mainly antiquarian interest, but the high rate of cancers in the Lake District hills perhaps recalls the modern and persistent high rates in parts of North Wales. And surely Dr Haviland's readiness to make bold recommendations is thought-provoking; perhaps Dr Allen-Price in 1960 (figure 5.1) was one of the last people prepared to back a hunch as boldly, at least in a western country. It is rather different in some developing countries as we shall see. This chapter illustrates our one-ness as between developed and developing countries. But we in western countries can learn a good deal still from the Third World as well as offering methods, ideas or analyses to researchers there.

One last perspective from Herzlich and Pierret (1985): is it possible that only with the end of mass epidemics was individual medical care able to flourish? Or then, as now, was it rather a matter of the life-chances into which one happened to be born?

Conclusion to Part I

This part of the book has contained material on what I have called the ecological medical geography of developed countries, naturally with no claim to comprehensive coverage. Discussion of the nature of health and the disease burden in developed countries stresses the importance of the so-called degenerative diseases like heart disease, stroke and certain cancers, as compared with quite a different, as well as heavier, burden of disease in the Third World. Some of these seem to be at root genuinely degenerative diseases associated with ageing, and of increasing importance in recent decades simply because of the longer life-expectancy that has evolved in developed countries in the last few generations, say from the turn of the century but not much before. Some, on the other hand, appear to be associated with infections, often viruses, and some are certainly associated with environmental factors such as occupation, and with air pollution including self-pollution or family-pollution by cigarette smoking. Some are probably associated too with the interaction of a number of life-cycle factors like diet, including fat consumption and alcohol intake, exercise and the lack of it, obesity, and in some cases the nebulous and yet immanent factor or group of factors that is called stress. (For an attempt to disentangle the effects of pollution from other variables, see Bozzo et al. (1979).)

The discussion became more geographical with the chapter dealing with maps of cancers: while it is still in the main descriptive, it is clear that mapping can open up lines of inquiry that may prove useful in further research.

Some of the studies cited suggest probable correlations with socioeconomic variables such as poor housing, probably in interaction with other aspects of deprivation; it is sometimes suggested that if socioeconomic factors are clearly or even probably crucial, there is no real point in mapping, and that it is better to proceed straight to statistical correlation between disease data and groups of socioeconomic variables to bring out the diseases and the variables that are interactive. In some types of study this is surely true. In many, however, there seem to be at least three answers to this argument: (1) There is often a logistic gain from mapping, if rational location of health facilities is a matter of concern: I have heard a statistician claim that one table is worth a thousand maps – it depends on the table and on the maps! – and no doubt partly because the decimal points can be read on tables, hence ideally both table and map should be used; the late Professor P.C. Mahalanobis FRS claimed that he could visualize a map of India, say of the 400 districts, while reading a table, but he was a remarkable man, and for more pedestrian thinkers help in pin-pointing with appropriate scale of mapping cannot but help in planning preventive campaigns or provision of health care facilities. (2) Mapping can be invaluable in heightening public awareness of disparities in health and disease. In the early days of the Open University, I recall the sharp impact on the mature citizen-students, by no means an unaware group of people, of such a simple challenge to complacency as the map of infant mortality, much along the lines of figure 4.9. (3) If socioeconomic variables are indeed crucial, there may nevertheless be significant regional or spatial factors at work: the ideal response by a geographer to this criticism is perhaps to design mapping projects so that socioeconomic variables are standardized – thus one would map age-standardized data for, say, heart disease for the United Kingdom for social classes IV and V (using the Census definition of social class based on socioeconomic groupings, based largely on occupation). There are problems, hence no doubt the lack of studies of this kind, apart from that just hinted at in defining social class and socioeconomic groups: the so-called ecological fallacy will remain, and aggregate data may yield deceptive results and may conceal causal factors related to individual behaviour. Indeed, map analysis of this kind should by common consent be complemented by individual case histories wherever possible; again the problem of small sample size, particularly in sparsely peopled areas, will be compounded, and if one responds by taking longer runs of data over time, trends over time may invalidate any findings. Nevertheless research to establish whether there are or are not significant spatial patterns within particular social groups is a field for further research. Some of the problems are discussed, though without grasping the nettle of mapping data in this way, in a recent paper using United Kingdom census data (Fox et al. 1984); in the absence of mapping exercises it is difficult to accept their view that social factors are more likely to yield significant findings than spatial factors.

The chapters mainly based on descriptive mapping nevertheless seem cumulatively to give a distinctive perspective view; even quite simple mapping, as in the series on stomach cancer, does make a case for the importance of within-country variations. Less intensive discussion of maps of other cancers, of other degenerative diseases like heart diseases and stroke, etc., then of diabetes, and finally one or two maps indicative of general conditions in a society, inevitably make less impact, but are examples of the wealth of material available to gain a great deal of knowledge of existing conditions and as a perspective within which further research may be planned.

Mapping as such, then, seems to be the beginning of wisdom rather than an end in itself, but yet invaluable in suitable contexts. And given the potentialities of computer mapping today – and more tomorrow – there should be much more mapping in future, much more closely following on events, much more like a kind of weather mapping – not perhaps daily except for epidemics or the like, but with, say, weekly and monthly pictures of changing, moving and evolving patterns of disease. Indeed some of this is already available from international agencies.

Part I continued with chapters about geographical tools beyond cartography and visual inspection of maps. Surfaces, or hills and valleys of disease were discussed to see if there are techniques useful in ecological medical geography, culminating in the idea of hills and valleys of risk of particular causes of death. Spatial diffusion studies were illustrated from work on hepatitis and on influenza, with some challenge as to potential applicability. Chapter 7 included studies of change of scale as an analytic tool, and – a reminder that we are in one world! – two examples of vector-borne disease in developed countries.

A historical chapter, designed to link with Part II on the developing world, ended the first part, on developed countries. It ranged freely between developed countries yesterday and developing countries today, from the great epidemic diseases of colonial India as the author knew them, cholera, plague and smallpox, to their former importance in much of the developed world, used malaria in England and elsewhere, and the worldwide influenza pandemic of 1918–21 too, to stress the 'One-Worldness' of health and disease, and cited some nineteenth-century cancer geography of England as a link between the relatively good data of chapters 3 and 5 and the much cruder data-bases used in chapter 13.

As noted earlier, geographical findings seem up to now to be a little firmer, a little more confident and at home, in dealing with infections than with degenerative diseases. Not many geographers make dramatic discoveries, but modest applicability in practical affairs may well be claimed for some of the diffusion studies of hepatitis and influenza, and indeed of the workers cited both Brownlea and McGlashan can point to specific changes in environmental health in their different parts of Australia to which their work has contributed in significant degree.

Part II The Third World

9 Jacques May's Classification and 'Tropical' Diseases

Introductory

This chapter does not consider the question of how far the complex of interacting diseases in many Third World countries is due to the post-imperial (and neo-colonial?) world economy, but has the more limited objective of helping new students of the field towards a first understanding of a number of diseases often regarded as 'tropical' even though many of them were formerly widespread outside the tropics; to this end it employs May's one-factor, two-factor etc. classification of chapter 1, but also loosely follows recent WHO sources indicating the main sources of ill-health or premature death in the Third World (WHO Scientific Working Group on Social and Economic Research 1983; *World Health Forum* 1981a).

First, however, it is worth stressing again that universal diseases such as influenza and pneumonia, measles and the like are important in the Third World, indeed kill a larger proportion of those affected than they do in the developed world. Tuberculosis is one of these given space later in this chapter. Moreover, infections like the measles virus or various intestinal organisms seem to interact with poor nutrition (Whittle et al. 1980); from the difficult conditions of post-revolution Maputo, Mozambique, see Cliff and Zinkin (1983); and from a geographer McGlashan (1969)). On the other hand leprosy, malaria, cholera and even a disease-complex like yellow fever have formerly been widespread outside the tropics, and even today various dysenteries and other enteric infections including typhoid are by no means unknown in developed countries though seldom as major public health problems. Table 9.1 is an attempt to show the premature deaths, or years of useful life lost through various causes in Ghana, very roughly matching table 2.1 for Canada, and the mixture of 'tropical' and universal diseases is clear (Morrow et al. 1982; Morrow 1984; cf. Meade (1980a) on Malaysia; Epidemiological Bulletin

Table 9.1   Years of healthy life lost by people of Ghana of all ages, with causes
including causes of disability

Rank order	Disease	Percentage of total healthy life lost
1	malaria	15.4
2	prematurity	9.1
3	sickle-cell disease	6.2
4	measles	6.2
5	birth injury	6.0
6	pneumonia (child)	5.5
7	malnutrition	5.1
8	gastroenteritis	4.5
9	neonatal tetanus	3.7
10	accidents (all kinds)	2.9
11	tuberculosis	2.7
12	stroke	2.4
13	pneumonia (adult)	2.3
14	psychiatric disorders	2.2
15	neonatal respiratory disease	2.1
16	congenital malformation	1.9
17	pregnancy complications	1.6
18	cirrhosis	1.3
19	cancer	1.2
20	hypertension	1.2
21	hepatitis	1.2
22	hernia	1.1
23	schistosomiasis	1.1
24	umbilical sepsis	1.0
25	leprosy	1.0

Source: Open University 1985, III, p. 18

(1984) on Brazil). Measles, for instance, has a huge literature, partly
because of the possibility that it could be eradicated by a vaccination
campaign like that successful for smallpox – it has almost been eradicated
from the USA. Without in any way underplaying these mainly two-factor
disease complexes, then, I attempt outline sketches of the complexes,
often involving three or four factors, at a minimal level for some
understanding of the classic questions of geography: what is it? where is
it? and why is it there (and not elsewhere)?

The brief outlines in this chapter are derived mainly from standard
medical works such as Lucas and Gilles (1984), Peters and Gilles (1981)
and the older but still useful Davey and Lightbody (1956). See also
Service (1980) or Muirhead-Thomson (1968, 1982) on medical entomology

and R.A. Wilson (1979) on parasitology. It is not possible to quote comprehensively from current work in the biomedical sciences: the biomedical literature is so rich that material analogous to citations in later chapters could be found for almost every one of the 'tropical' diseases discussed in the present chapter, and a student interested in gaining a biomedical perspective on any of the diseases discussed should refer to current indexing or abstracting journals such as the *Tropical Diseases Bulletin*, as well as to standard texts like those just cited.

Malaria

Malaria, already encountered historically in chapter 8 as a disease in England and in western Europe, still affects some 200 million people in many parts of the tropics, and may cause a million deaths, mainly of children. As already noted, it involves a three-factor complex: the life cycle of the mosquito-borne protozoa *Plasmodium* spp. includes a phase in the human body and a phase in *Anopheles* mosquitoes of many species. It is discussed further in the next chapter.

Schistosomiases (Bilharzia)

The schistosomiases are debilitating infections affecting the well-being, and efficiency too, of perhaps 500 million people, the urinary form alone accounting for some 200 million, mainly in Africa and Latin America rather than the Asian and Pacific tropics: only one or two per cent are treated. They are named from the genus of trematodes or flukes causing the disease, *Schistosoma*, from the 'split body' shape of the male, folded over to contain the long, slender female in the mature worms. The diseases, especially in the urinary form, are also known as bilharzia from Theodor Bilharz's discovery of the cause in 1851, involving *Schistosoma haematobium* ('living in blood', suggestive of the symptoms of blood in the patient's urine): people become infected by the mobile cercarial ('tailed') free-swimming final larval stage of the fluke while they are working, bathing, wading to fill water-pots and so on, the cercariae having the ability to penetrate the human skin. The adult worms live in the veins, *S. haematobium* in the veins near the bladder, and the eggs are discharged with the urine – often in the Third World in or near water, where, after hatching, a free-living larval stage swims in search of the alternative host, water-snails mainly of the genus *Bulinus*, where it undergoes several stages until the cercariae emerge. There are three other schistosomes important in human disease, all intestinal rather than bladder infections and so discharging eggs in the faeces: *S. mansoni* (from Sir Patrick Manson 1844–1922), also widespread in Africa and at least the east of Latin America and in the Caribbean, has also aquatic snails as alternative hosts, mainly *Biomphalaria* spp.; *S. japonicum*, still important in China and parts of south-east Asia, has an amphibious – rather than aquatic – snail as its main alternate host, *Oncomelania* spp. ('black mass'); *S. intercalatum* (Latin, 'inserted') circulating mainly between animals and snails, but with occasional human infections, mainly in eastern Congo and Gabon (Doumenge et al. 1983; Doumenge 1984). Schistosomiasis, then, is a three-factor complex, discussed as such in a little more detail in chapter 11.

Filariases

Filariases, of many kinds, form a very varied group of diseases affecting about 300 million people; it is hard to generalize but many at least seem to be three-factor complexes involving an animal reservoir of small to minute worms, arthropod, including insect, vectors of immature forms or micro-filariae, and people – so often four-factor complexes (animal host, worm, vector, people) but sometimes three-factor if no vector is involved or indeed no animal host. Thus bancroftian filariasis is a three-factor complex causing, if untreated, the swollen lower extremities popularly known as elephantiasis; the cycle involves people, anopheline and culicine mosquitoes, and *Wuchereria bancrofti* (from Wucherer, a German physician in Brazil, and Bancroft, an English physician in Australia). (Elephantiasis is now known to occur also through absorption of fine clay soil particles in wet climates through the sweat glands on the soles of barefooted farmers, see Price et al. (1981); Price and Bailey (1984).) A similar filariasis is now distinguished as caused by *Brugia malayi* (from Brug, a parasitologist), and carried by *Mansonia* mosquitoes such as *M. annulifera* ('ringed'), a species associated with breeding close to certain aquatic plants and therefore highly localized, for instance in the coastal lagoon belt of Kerala in south-western India. And *B. timori* is important in Timor and other Indonesian islands. A number of important global or biomedical surveys of this important group of diseases have appeared including WHO (1984d) and Southgate (1984). A biogeographer's view of filarial diseases in Sri Lanka, including important historical discussion, will be found in Schweinfurth (1983, 1984); other geographical surveys include Petit et al. (1982) on eastern Malagasy. For the massive control projects in China, see C. Zhong and Zheng (1980), H.L. Zhong et al. (1981). On crucial mosquito densities, Webber and Southgate (1981).

The large Guinea worm or Medina worm *Dracunculus medinensis* ('little dragon') circulates in a three-factor complex involving the worm, infective larvae discharged into water bodies from an ulcer-like lesion on the human skin formed by the head of the gravid female worm, and the animal host *Cyclops*, a small crustacean or 'water-flea' common in wells, reservoirs, canals etc. in the body of which the worm larvae mature and mate. The cycle is completed when water is drunk by people who swallow the *Cyclops* along with it. Dracunculiasis is difficult to map, but occurs in parts of the tropics and sub-tropics, usually arid or semi-arid, where drinking water is obtained by women (usually) wading into step-wells, reservoirs, pools etc. while discharging infective larvae from the ulcer-like lesions on their legs. Guinea worm is estimated to affect over 50 million people, mainly in India – which has an eradication programme – and West Africa which so far lacks a concerted campaign (WER 1985b). For an interesting attempt to cost the impact of this worm in lost work-days etc., as against costs of treatment, see Guiguemde et al. (1983), though of course good water supplies would prevent the disease; and on population mobility interacting with this helminth, see Watts (1984).

Onchocerciasis (River Blindness)

Onchocerciasis ('tumour' + 'tail') causes subcutaneous fibroid nodules that may – and in thousands of people do – cause blindness, the River Blindness discussed in chapter 12; this is a four-factor complex, for there is an animal reservoir in cattle and game (antelope and buffalo), the black fly *Simulium damnosum* that breeds in well-oxygenated 'white water' in cataracts etc., the worm *Onchocerca* and lastly the human host. (See figure 12.1 and further discussion in chapter 12.)

Hookworm and Roundworm: the Burden of Helminths

Hookworm is another of the diseases that causes many millions of people to be debilitated and apathetic. The principal pathogens are *Ancylostoma duodenale* (Greek, 'crooked mouth' + duodenal) and *Necator americanus* (Latin, 'murderer'), nematode worms differing in morphology but epidemiologically similar. Formerly Old World and American organisms, both are now widely distributed through the tropics, forming a two-factor complex involving only humankind and the worms; transmission occurs when a fairly short-lived free-living larval stage of the worm is able to penetrate the skin of bare feet on damp ground polluted with infected faeces, especially in warm, humid climates and where there is decaying vegetation. As often, the extent of exposure has to be qualified by some kind of pre-disposition to infection, whether genetic or somehow environmental (Schad and Anderson 1985).

The roundworm *Ascaris lumbricoides* (The Greek name for the worm + 'like an earthworm') is an all-but-universal worm wherever soil polluted with faeces contaminated with eggs from adult worms in the human intestines may be ingested from soiled fingers or food: they hatch in the duodenum, move as minute rod-like forms via the blood stream to the lungs, and after two larval moults there migrate via the windpipe and gullet to mature in the intestine.

Along with other helminths, some of course from animals, the total burden on human health of these infestations makes some workers think that the helminths ought to be the next target for a world-wide eradication campaign. For economic and nutritional implications of widely ranging studies in the tropics, see Stephenson et al. (1980). Diesfeld (1965a) gives a picture of the interaction of various kinds of intestinal parasite in Addis Ababa.

Some Intestinal Diseases

Significance, especially in Infant Mortality

The main intestinal diseases are of course not confined to the tropics or to developing countries, but are proportionately more important in those areas both as killers and as causes of inefficiency and economic loss. The intestinal infections contribute a very large proportion of the tragically high infant mortality of the Third World. Bahrain has halved infant deaths in three years, and while oil-rich Middle East countries have funds not available to poor countries some of their methodologies may well be widely applicable (see Farrag (1983), linking these infections with child nutrition issues). Recent studies in Bangladesh, the USA and Guatemala show that improved hand-washing can reduce child diarrhoeas by between 14 and 48 per cent (Feachem 1984).

Dysenteries

The dysenteries are very widespread, debilitating and on present technology difficult to eradicate except by improved sanitation. They are caused by several different organisms such as *Entamoeba histolytica* ('tissue-dissolving') (amoebic dysentery) and several species of bacilli, mainly of the genus Shigella (named from a Japanese physician). The dysenteries are common causes of severe diarrhoea, acute or chronic, and severe debility, sometimes with wider, even fatal, effects on the body. Direct faecal pollution, flies, and bad water are all involved, more or less so with different organisms and in particular outbreaks and environments. Mixed infections are not uncommon, and this may partly account for the fact that some organisms are usually harmless or commensal (literally 'sharing a table'!) but occasionally cause diarrhoea, sometimes with complications. Thus *E. histolytica* raises difficult problems because the organism is almost universal as part of the commensal organisms in the human gut: a major general book is Martinez-Palamo (1982). Some workers believe that its change to pathogenicity depends on the nature of the bacterial population in the intestine, and the dietary and endocrine balance of the host; see also Diesfeld (1965b) on possible seasonal triggers to amoebiasis in highland Ethiopia. As with other infections, there are reports of the pathogens developing resistance to drugs (e.g. Khan et al. 1984).

Typhoid

Typhoid, typhoid fever or in older literature simply 'enteric' arises from a two-factor complex comprising people and *Salmonella typhi* or *typhosa* (*Bacillus typhosum* in older literature). (Salmon was an American pathologist, typhosa is from the Greek for smoke, implying delirious.) While typhoid occurs in almost all climatic zones, the heaviest toll of severe illness and death is probably among young children in the Third World. The genus is a very large one, including the parasites of poultry and livestock animals which occasionally cause quite severe epidemics in developed countries, especially in closed communities or at large social functions sharing a meal including undercooked or re-infected meats.

Cholera

Cholera, already discussed in chapters 6 and 8 tends to occur in cycles, but affecting many millions of people in epidemic years. It is associated with a two-factor complex, as far as is known, involving only people and the spiral and motile bacillus *Vibrio cholerae*, causing very severe diarrhoea and dehydration so marked as to cause heart failure – hence the early twentieth-century break-through in therapy using Rogers's intravenous saline, and a recent technique, less demanding of skilled personnel. This oral rehydration, using a solution of salt and sugar, was evolved by doctor with the US naval medical research unit (NAMRU) who worked on cholera in Cairo, the Philippines and Dacca, R.A. Phillips. It is one of the startling simplicities of modern medicine that cholera has now been found to be a self-limiting disease: that given successful rehydration in treatment 'so simple that any twelve-year old boy or girl of average intelligence can give it, the patient will cure himself without further treatment, as if cholera were the common cold' (van Heyningen and Seal (1983); and see the valuable account of the technique by Mahalanabis et al. (1981)). Better-protected water supplies would reduce or prevent explosive epidemics (see Feachem et al. 1981). And better hygiene, faeces disposal and control of houseflies would reduce smouldering epidemics (cf. chapter 8). Nevertheless, widespread diffusion of oral rehydration as a home or community remedy clearly has a large role to play, in cholera and other diarrhoeal diseases too. It is ironic that after a recent BBC television programme on oral rehydration therapy, letters to the press claimed similar solutions of salt and sugar to be long-known family or folk remedies for diarrhoea: the breakthrough in treatment of tropical child diarrhoeas is none the less real and revolutionary.

In the last 20 years or so the dominant pandemic strain of V. cholerae has been the El Tor, named originally from a Muslim pilgrim station in Sinai in 1906 but long endemic in Sulawesi (Celebes) and spreading from there across the world since 1960. A particularly important feature of its spread has been that cholera affected much of Africa in severe epidemics with many deaths after a gap of 75 years, and has apparently settled down in places as an endemic disease. This was such a dramatic instance of disease diffusion that it has been much studied by geographers (Kwofie 1976; Stock 1976; Adesina 1981, 1984a, b, c); Stock's monograph in particular is a model of its kind and essential reading for any student of the geography of cholera. On a different scale, see Ferguson (1977). The Bengal Delta has long been regarded as the world endemic home of the classical strain V. cholerae (see the world atlases of May (1950–5) and of Rodenwaldt and Jusatz (1952–61)). Bangladesh, while newly independent and still suffering from the political and economic chaos following the war of independence with Pakistan, and also a severe food crisis, was hit by a sharp epidemic caused by the El Tor strain in 1974–5: that strain seems to have been completely dominant from 1973 to 1979, but then the classical strain re-emerged so that the two types co-exist at present (Samadi et al. 1983; W.L. Cook et al. 1983). It has long been a mystery and a source of speculation as to how the pathogen survives during the marked lull of 2–3 years between epidemics of classical cholera. A suspicion some years ago about the migratory (and delicious!) hilsa fish has now been discounted; however, estuarine waters seem to be involved somehow, and recent work has provided a plausible though not yet wholly proven mechanism, in attachment of the vibrios to planktonic crustaceans (copepods), varying with temperature and salinity: see the major review of cholera by Feachem et al. (1981–2); also Huq et al. (1984); C.J. Miller et al. (1982, 1985). It may be that it is in some form of seafood that the pathogen gets ashore, bringing first pre-epidemic seeding to fishing communities or fish markets, and it is from these points that the main epidemic mechanisms take over – a point Feachem et al. are much concerned to debate, going back to the views of John Snow and his contemporaries about the 1854 epidemic in Soho and other nineteenth-century outbreaks (see chapter 8). Occasional indigenous cases of cholera around the Gulf of Mexico have brought at least some evidence that the pathogen was introduced in oysters, eaten raw (MMWR 1980; Kaper et al. 1982). Detailed micro-geography of movement of the disease in the Matlab area north of Dhaka is in progress and this may throw further light on the problem (Craig 1985, 1986). Geographical studies from India include Banerjee and Jayati Hazra (1974) on West Bengal, Hyma and Ramesh (1977) on Tamil Nadu and Kumaraswamy (1984) on Madras. Studies of routes of transmission of cholera include Küstner et al. (1981) on South Africa and Mandara and Mhalu (1980–81) on Tanzania, noting the importance of Muslim pre-burial cleansing of bodies.

Polio and Hepatitis A

Polio and hepatitis A, lastly of the intestinal diseases discussed here, are two of the many virus diseases of the intestinal system, somewhat similar in their behaviour. Polio (acute anterior poliomyelitis) is from the Greek for grey matter and for marrow, and hepatitis implies inflammation of the liver. While the Salk and Sabin vaccines have largely removed the polio problem in developed countries – complacency and low immunization rates apart – it remains important in the Third World, while hepatitis remains important as a universal disease, already discussed in the diffusion studies of chapter 6. The two enterovirus infections are both two-factor complexes involving only man and the viruses, on present knowledge, and probably affect millions of people with severe illness and many deaths mainly in children – many adults having acquired immunity. Though polio at least also has a droplet and pharyngeal route of transmission, the main one is by faecal–oral means, sometimes including contamination of drinking water or swimming places. Thus better hygiene will reduce the incidence, but polio in particular is likely to be a target for immunization programmes in the near future in many Third World countries. Most intestinal hepatitis seems to be hepatitis A, though it has recently been claimed that most of India's is from the virus so far classed simply 'non-A, non-B' (Tandon et al. 1984): this latter virus, and more rarely hepatitis A, is thought to be involved in severe liver damage though far less frequently than occurs with with the blood virus hepatitis B (also suspected of a role, possibly synergistic, in liver cancer – see chapter 13). A recent review of viral hepatitis is by Deinhardt and Gust (1982). De and Gollerkiri (1984) offer a first within-city geography of hepatitis in Vadodara (Baroda) in Gujarat – apparently without the high child incidence one might have expected. The South Pacific Commission (1982) plead for research on the serious hepatitis problem in that macro-region. And a remarkably compact world view is in *World Health Forum* (1983).

Sabin (1981) discusses the polio problem in the Third World as a whole, and there are broad reviews by Horstmann (1982) and in papers from a 1983 symposium (Horstmann et al. 1984).

Enteroviruses and the Water-supply Issue

On enteroviruses, a vital survey of rapidly expanding knowledge is in Feachem et al. (1981). There are many studies showing that improved water supply alone may not produce the expected improvements in health, especially if maintenance is not adequately provided from the outset – for example in Ghannoum et al. (1981) on the Brak area of Libya. In a geographical study citing examples from Ethiopia, Malaysia and Liberia, Roundy (1985) pleads for a locally based and people-centred approach to water problems and has also contributed an unusual paper on faeces disposal in Peninsular Malaysia (1978a). Roundy's grasp and mapping of a topic usually avoided is reminiscent of A.C. Chandler's (1926–8) classic review of hookworm and faeces disposal in late colonial India.

Eye Diseases

Significance

Last of this group of major scourges, those affecting hundreds of millions of people, comes the enormous toll of various eye diseases and blindness for many millions. A WHO (1984b) report concentrates on six major causes: trachoma, malnutrition, onchocerciasis, cataract, trauma and glaucoma: depending on the definition of blindness, estimates range from 28 to 42 million actually blind in the world (WHO 1979b). Vitamin deficiency (rather than infection) is one main cause. On May's classification this might be a one-factor disease, intrinsic to humankind; though he seemed to exclude them from his classification, he discussed nutritional diseases at some length in his 1950 paper, and later devoted the last years of his life to research on the geography of diet and nutrition. A major cause of deficient eyesight and blindness arises from insufficiency of vitamin A in the diet, leading to xerophthalmia (Greek, 'dry eyes'), with night blindness and excessive dryness of the conjunctiva, then the cornea, often succeeded by keratomalacia (Greek, horn or cornea + *malakia*, 'softness'), and ultimately blindness. Infections like measles have already been noted as interacting with malnutrition in causing blindness.

Trachoma

Trachoma involves a two-factor complex, an eye infection that may affect some 500 million people. The pathogenic organism is *Chlamydia trachomatis* (Greek *chlamys*, a cloak, presumably from early researchers' interpretation of the somewhat globular shape of these very small organisms, or perhaps the drawing of a sort of veil over the eye); trachomatis has already received a mention in chapters 1 and 2 as a cause of one of the 'new' sexually transmitted diseases. Its taxonomy has been much disputed and subject to change, but a degree of consensus has been reached that it is an atypical virus lying between the 'true viruses' and the bacteria, along with those causing psittacosis (parrot disease) and one of the classic venereal diseases *Lymphogranuloma venereum*: they are unique in multiplying only in the host's cell plasma (the liquid or viscous part of the cell round the nucleus). *C. trachomatis* is found very widely in human populations, and after wide travel and field work in different environments and in communities with different standards of hygiene and of contact, a very geographically minded ophthalmologist, Professor Ida Mann, concluded that the chlamydia usually occur as a mild and self-limiting eye infection. She found that severe cases and ultimately blindness occur in conditions of poor hygiene, community and personal, and, she believed, because of interactions with secondary infections by other organisms, or of the xerophthalmia just noted as due to vitamin A deficiency (Mann (1966), and see also her enthralling, travel-cum-eye-detective story under the pseudonym of Caroline Guy, *The Cockney and the Crocodile*). A geographical survey of marginal changes in the physical or social environment from Northern Australia is in Tedesco (1980).

River blindness or onchocerciasis puts many millions of people at risk, and much blindness arises in severely endemic areas; one of the many filariases vectored by various arthropods affecting human beings, it has been the subject of important geographical research, so has been outlined under Filariases earlier in this chapter, and is also the subject of chapter 12.

Selected References

A major world survey of blindness is by the International Agency for the Prevention of Blindness (1980). A textbook focusing on the Third World is by Rodger (1981), while McLaren (1980) covers eye conditions linked with malnutrition. See also Sommer (1982b.) A special issue of *Social*

Science and Medicine (*17*, 1983) was devoted to Ocular Needs in Africa. The links between vitamin A deficiency and eye conditions are discussed in WHO (1982 TRS 672) as common throughout the Third World but with most of the quarter of a million children annually going blind concentrated in South-east Asia; and on field methods see Sommer (1982a). An account based on a large sample in West Java gives some of the evidence for such an estimate (Sommer et al. 1981). Devadas and Saroja (1980) report on the diet–blindness link in a rural area near Coimbatore in South India. (The last paper provoked Dr R. Passmore to compare the findings with some of his own field notes in 1939, showing little change despite all the nutritionists' efforts.) From Vietnam comes a geomedical model of eye disease (Verin and Peyresblanques 1983). Brilliant and Brilliant (1985) use 'social epidemiology' on factors determining who stays blind and who gets a cataract operation in a rural setting in Nepal, and N. Cohen et al. (1985) in Bangladesh relate the chances of blinding malnutrition specifically to measures of wealth and poverty. An example from Mali of harmful Arab traditional medicine is in Queguiner (1981), 'couching' in cataract treatment involving surgical displacement of the lens.

Before leaving the topic of blindness – chapter 12 apart – it is important to stress the inter-relatedness of phenomena (Inua et al. 1983). Among geographers interested in blindness, McGlashan wrote a number of papers on Zambia (McGlashan (1969) and earlier papers cited there): he brings out the importance of measles, smallpox (since eradicated, of course) and chickenpox as factors, and the importance of childhood blindness as compared with the incidence of much blindness in the developed world after the age of 55. He also stresses the interaction with malnutrition and particularly with vitamin A deficiency and keratomalacia. Given good nutrition, many of the children would not have gone blind: custom, farming and food patterns, and the world economy all play a part.

Other Scourges

The geography of nutrition is further discussed in chapter 14. Meantime I turn to a number of Third World diseases of a different order from those so far considered, affecting populations of millions rather than hundreds of millions – scourges of particular populations or sectors of society rather than major scourges of mankind, but I think essential in understanding the medical geography of the Third World.

Leishmaniases

The *Leishmaniae* form a large and widespread genus of protozoa parasitic on a wide range of animals. Human disease occurs mainly in two forms: cutaneous, affecting some eight million people, and visceral, affecting some 10 million (though some workers put the leishmaniases as second only to malaria among the parasitic diseases). Cutaneous leishmaniasis is widespread in many tropical and Mediterranean countries, mainly in comparatively dry climates, and it forms a four-factor complex: a large animal reservoir in dogs, jackals, gerbils etc.; the pathogen *L. tropica*; *Phlebotomus* ('vein-cutting'!) sandflies; and people. Visceral leishmaniasis or kala-azar (Hindi, 'black fever') is caused by *L. donovani* with again an animal reservoir in dogs, jackals, foxes and the mongoose and so a four-factor zoonosis. In East Africa termite hills are a particular source of risk and there is a skin phase prior to kala-azar. In India, however, an animal reservoir has never been proved, so there it seems to be a three-factor complex: people, *L. donovani* and the peri-domestic sandfly *P. argentipes* ('silver-footed'). (See Chakraborty et al. (1982) on a change in *P. argentipes*' feeding habits from animals to people.) A very similar organism *L. braziliensis* is found in hot wet regions from Mexico to Buenos Aires, again with a sandfly vector, *Lutzomyia* spp. and a reservoir in wild rodents: the disease *espundia* causes lesions of the skin and mucous membrane, often around the mouth and nose, mainly in lumbermen and pioneer settlers in forest clearings but decreasing as wild rodents are driven away from the new settlements. On the world scale a major review of animal reservoirs of Leishmania is in Bray (1982), and a general world survey is in Marinkelle (1980), while workshop summaries in Killick-Kendrick and Ward (1981) give an introduction to their ecological relations. For a general biological approach see Molyneux and Ashford (1983).

Sleeping Sickness and Chagas' Disease (the Trypanosomiases)

The *Trypanosoma* (Greek, borer + body) are protozoa related to the *Leishmania* and cause African trypanosomiasis or sleeping sickness, and Chagas' disease in Latin America (named from a Brazilian physician). The *Trypanosoma* include many species parasitic on a wide range of wild and domestic animals. Sleeping sickness is caused by two species, *T. gambiense* and *T. rhodesiense* (named from Gambia and the former Rhodesia), and is carried by various species of the tsetse fly (*Glossina*, other species of which are vectors of cattle and game animal disease).

Chagas' disease is caused by *T. cruzi* (Cruz was also a Brazilian physician) and vectored by bugs of the genus *Triatoma*: the organism is picked up when the bug sucks blood from an infected person or perhaps occasionally a domestic or wild animal, developing in the insect's gut and so thereafter in its faeces. If a bug then emerges from its hiding place in cracks in mud walls etc. and bites a human being, often about the face and lips (hence 'kissing bug'), the trypanosomes often enter into the body through the bite lesion or the mucous membrane of the mouth or eyes, often migrating to the myocardium where they multiply and later appear as transmissible forms in the blood-stream. There is much acute illness in children and chronic disease in adults, with heart and intestinal complications.

A general biology of *Trypanosoma* (and also of *Leishmania*) is in Molyneux and Ashford (1983) and a series of papers in Newton (1985). On blood-sucking flies (in general), see Muirhead-Thomson (1982).

The Arboviruses (Arthropod-borne Viruses)

The arboviruses, on present knowledge, are in this group of diseases affecting millions rather than hundreds of millions of people; the term was coined in the last twenty or so years as a contraction for arthropod-borne viruses. The group is large and diverse, including yellow fever and dengue (discussed briefly in the later paragraphs) and, for instance, the mosquito-borne encephalitis in Ohio and the tick-borne encephalitis in central Europe outlined in chapter 7. On the arboviruses in general the French armed forces medical school provide a useful conspectus (*Médicine Tropicale* 1980), and *WER* (1980) gives an example of an annual survey of yellow fever. See also Chamberlain (1982). Brazil provides examples of regional surveys (e.g. Pinheiro et al. 1981).

Yellow Fever

In May's terms yellow fever is a four-factor complex: (1) the virus; (2) an animal reservoir in monkeys in the main crown layer of rain-forests in equatorial Africa and (probably) later in similar environments in Latin America; (3) several species of vector mosquitoes of the two rain-forest areas, but also several species of peri-domestic and urban mosquitoes; and (4) humankind, with many and diverse patterns of activity involving contact with infected mosquitoes. The range of mosquitoes' adjustment to different environments is impressive. In central Africa there is an intermediate phase between the forest cycle and the human and domestic one, of mosquitoes feeding on monkeys raiding banana gardens in Africa! The urban mosquito *Aëdes aegypti* is widespread throughout the tropics (and in Asia a main vector of dengue); it is a culicine mosquito, breeding freely in urban waste water of almost all kinds. Large tropical populations are protected by vaccines and anti-mosquito measures, largely thanks to the crusade against the disease some 50–60 years ago by the Rockefeller Foundation; their researchers made crucial discoveries about the real nature of the disease complex, as a zoonosis into which people blunder. The sylvan cycle extends not uncommonly to lumbermen and other frequenters of the rain-forest, who may be bitten by infected forest mosquitoes say as a tall tree is felled; at their home in a clearing *Aëdes* may transmit the virus to their families, the families may carry the infection to the market town, where the urban mosquito abounds, and so out along lines of communication. Nowadays such 'break-outs' from the rain-forest areas are normally quickly suppressed, but historically there were worldwide outbreaks as far north as Bristol and Halifax, Nova Scotia, for *Aëdes* was able to live in ships' water-tanks and the like – indeed slave-ships may have carried the cycle from Africa to South America (Strode (1951) for a post-Rockefeller account).

Dengue

The urban vector *Aëdes aegypti* has already been mentioned as carrying the dengue virus in large parts of Asia (miraculously, it seems, free from yellow fever but for obvious reasons vigilant in quarantine measures of all kinds at seaports and airports), and in the south-west Pacific and large parts of the Americas. Dengue is reported as returning to Queensland after a generation free from the disease (Kay et al. 1984). Traditionally dengue causes an influenza-like illness lasting a few days, with few serious illnesses or after-effects; the name is thought to be from Swahili with 'assimilation' to the Spanish *dengue* ('prudery', perhaps from the stiff-necked attitude of the patient with painful neck and shoulders). However, in recent decades a haemorrhagic form – causing bleeding from soft tissues – has become a serious and often a killing disease in much of South-east Asia, especially among children. Geographical accounts include Aiken et al. (1980), Aiken and Leigh (1978), Meade (1976), and Rhodain (1983) and a major monograph on Thailand by Wellmer (1983), with a summary paper (1984), giving her insights as geographer and medical doctor. Some workers believe that the haemorrhagic form may result from a second attack of dengue of a different virus type from the first attack (for a broad discussion of the immunology, see Halstead (1981)). The *Epidemiological Bulletin* (1981b) carries an account of dengue in the Americas.

Dengue in epidemic form appears to be a three-factor complex involving people, *Aëdes* mainly *aegypti*, and the virus; however, it is possible that as in yellow fever there is an animal reservoir, probably in monkeys. Similarly many of the wide range of viral encephalitis illnesses may be zoonotic in origin. Some, like Japanese encephalitis in much of Asia, are commonly carried by culicine mosquitoes, and this is discussed further in terms of the ecological niches occupied by *Anopheles* and by culicine mosquitoes, in chapter 10. Some writers distinguish the tick-borne viral infections (though the ticks *are* arthropods) including the forest and heath illness of Europe already noted in chapter 7. The California encephalitis of chapter 7 is also an arbovirus.

Tetanus

A disease difficult to estimate in numbers but certainly important in the Third World is tetanus – indeed though very largely preventible it still causes some deaths in developed countries. Tetanus (Greek, 'to stretch' – lockjaw) is caused by a bacterium common in soil in inhabited areas, *Clostridium tetani* (Greek *kloster*, 'spindle'). A recent estimate is that it causes half a million perinatal deaths a year (Stanfield and Galazka 1984), though in the terrible toll of infant mortality as a whole the intestinal diseases must rank much higher. In South Asia the use of a sliver of bamboo by traditional midwives to sever the cord is said to be a major cause of neonatal tetanus (Learmonth 1958), but great progress has been made with the problem in recent years. In southern Sudan a plant used to tie the cord has been incriminated, in Accra a dusting powder used on the wound, and so on (Woodruff et al. 1984; Neequaye 1984). Vaccine has long been available and a simple sterile pack for cutting and tying the cord could avoid thousands of infant deaths. Ityavyar (1984) gives an account of progress in integrating traditional midwives into modern practice in Sokoto state, Nigeria – however the brief review by Haworth (1985) offers a critique of some of Ityavyar's figures and, citing experience in the same area 30 years earlier, suggests that progress can result in regressions as well as advances!

Useful entry points into the related and (geographically) little-explored topic of perinatal *maternal* mortality include the survey by Potts et al. (1983). Similarly a geography student wishing to sample the biomedical literature on child health and nutrition might start with a set of abstracts such as nos 844–54, pp. 205–8, in the *Tropical Diseases Bulletin* 81/4 for 1984, the report by the United Nations Children's Fund (1984), WHO (1980) and Mundo et al. (1983).

Leprosy

Leprosy is caused by *Mycobacterium leprae* (Greek *mykos*, 'fungus'), and is almost certainly a two-factor complex involving only people and the bacillus. Overt leprosy affects some 12 million people, half of them in Asia: comparatively few of them die from leprosy, especially from the neural or tuberculoid form, but the open or lepromatous form can shorten life, if untreated, and also causes much disability and in many cultures much social stigmatization and social and economic distress. Different species of *Mycobacterium* are found over a wide spectrum of hosts, some in several sites in the human host; some are pathogenic and some apparently harmless. Tuberculosis, already mentioned as one of the universal diseases affecting many millions of people in the Third World and generally causing more severe illness and deaths than in developed countries, is caused by *M. tuberculosis*, closely similar to *M. leprae* though behaving differently in the human host; some workers believe that leprosy is tending to decline as epidemic and virulent tuberculosis spreads in many Third World countries (some are perhaps settling to more endemic conditions, possibly India for instance). This remains controversial, even speculative, and is discussed further in later paragraphs (see J.M. Hunter (1973, p. 16); Hunter and Thomas (1984a) and comment by Fine (1986)). The classical view is that the pathogen is not highly infectious, repeated skin to skin contact being the most likely route of transmission. However, the discovery of large numbers of bacilli emerging from the nasal mucosa of people with lepromatous leprosy has led to the idea that initial development of the disease in the nasal and respiratory tract is possible, even likely (Rees and McDougall 1977; Ahmed et al. 1983). So relatively transient contact – as against earlier ideas of prolonged familial contact – may after all be important. Given the slow development of the overt disease – taking years rather than months – either must remain very difficult to prove, and for a geographical analyst to map (Fine 1982)! It is perhaps this change in thinking that prompts Srinivasan (1984) to suggest a catastrophe theory model of leprosy, as against the classical spectrum of types of infection.

The Damien Foundation (1981) have published an atlas of leprosy. Geographical studies in west central Nepal suggest that main lines of travel may be important in transmission of leprosy, with high male incidence. However, there are data problems and on present evidence some ethnic differences are not fully understood as yet, and the author remains tentative in her findings (Pearson 1982a,b, 1984, 1985).

Leprosy and Tuberculosis

Hunter and Thomas (1984a) have already been cited on the possible antipathy between two mycobacterial diseases, leprosy and tuberculosis, as has Fine's (1986) sceptical review of that paper. The idea is by no means a new one – Hunter and Thomas cite medical literature back at least to 1957, but Fine finds no more in the paper than that the two diseases tend to have different spatial patterns – to occur in different places, as he puts it. The assemblage of material on the two diseases is massive and the paper is essential reading for a geography student approaching the problem. The authors' conclusions are modest: they believe that the modern endemic home of leprosy may lie in hot and wet climates (which accords with what we know of its persistence in damp warm conditions in medieval Europe and even in damp soils, including areas of sphagnum moss in Norway (Pearson (1985) and cf. Banerjee and Hazra (1982)); they find some evidence that there is 'some cross-interference between tuberculosis and the milder, paucibacillary form of leprosy; and they explain a negative correlation between urbanization and leprosy in Africa by 'a combination of (urban) influences'. There is some support at least from a medical historian (Manchester 1984) who thinks that just as BCG vaccination (based on *M. bovis* not *M. tuberculosis*) seems to afford some protection against leprosy, so an advance of *M. tuberculosis* may have underlain the retreat of leprosy from medieval and renaissance Europe. Perhaps it is well to note that with another co-author Hunter has warned us, on data from Puerto Rico, that gradients in maps of tuberculosis incidence can be artefacts of the health-care facilities and especially the presence of trained tuberculosis nurses (Hunter and Arbona 1984b, 1985a).

Tuberculosis

In view of this possible interaction with leprosy, some entry points into the literature on tuberculosis, mainly in the Third World, are included here. A bench-mark study of the mycobacteria is in Grange (1980). Chretien et al. (1984) point out that respiratory diseases as a group account for more years of life lost than do heart diseases, yet attract only one-fiftieth of the WHO budget allocated to cardiovascular disease. A WHO review of progress in the control of tuberculosis, particularly in the Third World, coincided with the centenary of the identification of the tubercle bacillus by Koch (WHO 1982 TRS 671); for a critical view, almost dissenting, certainly less diplomatic, see Bignall (1982) on the real reasons for the failure to eradicate the disease, ranging from lack of zeal and inadequate knowledge of control methods in campaign workers, to poverty and the world economy, and also covering the need for integration with general health and development programmes, and the circumstances where tuberculosis is *not* the highest priority. An urban geography of tuberculosis in Ibadan is in Folasade Iyun (1984): she finds the spatial pattern links with poverty and overcrowding. Citron et al. (1981) point out that while the disease is commoner in immigrant groups in the UK the main source of infection lies in middle-aged and elderly men born in Britain; cf. a geographer's view of a single town, Bolton (Gerrard 1981).

The Meningitis Belt

This long and yet very incomplete tale of 'tropical' diseases concludes with the briefest outlines of two disease complexes chosen for rather different reasons – meningococcal meningitis because of its geographical concentration in the well-known 'meningitis belt' south of the Sahara (though focusing on that area may be rather blinkered), and scrub typhus because of the very elegant ecological and geographical analyses of the late Ralph Audy, influential in thinking beyond the immediate problem.

It is possible to map the 'meningitis belt' of West Africa, but this may well over-concentrate attention: the disease is by no means unknown – along with other causes of meningitis – in developed countries: see for example Peltola's (1983) broad survey, *WER* (1981b) on France, Peltola et al. (1982) on Scandinavia, Fallon et al. (1984) and Fallon (1985) on Scotland, noting shifts towards younger age-groups that may presage an epidemic. This meningitis, on existing evidence, has a two-factor complex involving only people and the pathogen *Neisseria meningitidis*, closely resembling the venereal pathogen *N. gonorrhoeae*; it is a delicate organism and so unable to survive for long outside the human host. Apart from the belt south of the Sahara, it is important in many parts of the Middle East, in parts of central Asia, and in north-eastern, mainly semi-arid, Brazil. The African epidemic season has always been linked with the *harmattan* season of dry dusty winds blowing outward from the desert in the dry season, with incidence falling with the onset of the rains (Greenwood et al. 1984, 1985). The medical literature makes it clear that such a delicate organism cannot come with the wind, and sees the ecology as based on symptomless carriers, perhaps as high as 8 per cent of the population: overcrowding (to escape the dusty wind?), fatigue (from the hot season?) and cold spells earlier in the dry season, may cause the carrier rate to rise and when this exceeds about 20 per cent, an epidemic may be expected (Davey and Lightbody 1956). Other nasal infections may play a part and possibly even mechanical damage from dust? In regions other than the sub-Sahara there seems also to be a spring incidence – in the Uzbek SSR, for instance, a winter–spring peak in cities, and spring peak in rural areas (Usmanov and Glinyanova 1982). For a recent workshop ranging from epidemiology and animal models to control, see Klein et al. (1984). Geographical analyses include Limper (1984) who analyses the incidence in relation to the air masses from which such a huge phenomenon as the *harmattan* is derived, but also in relation to deforestation and the end of migratory farming, offering some parallel with the pattern in Brazil. Monnier (1980) also links the disease with deforestation, while Remy (1984) uses this disease complex as one illustration in a stimulating paper on 'epidemiological space', including it in a table of different epidemic patterns in the climate–vegetation belts from the Sahel to the wet savannah and with a splendid flow-diagram of the factors that may affect people and pathogen. Mohammed and Zaruba (1981) briefly review the promising possibilities for control, and also in a series of longer papers starting with Mohammed et al. (1984). There is a gap like a geological unconformity between the epidemiological and the geographical approaches – a not uncommon occurrence! – that may present a challenge to some students of geography: ideally, of course, in team work with biomedical researchers.

Scrub Typhus

Audy's work on scrub typhus has already been mentioned in chapter 1, and this paragraph is a minimal expansion of that reference. In this instance I shall not try to up-date Audy's material from the abstracting journals, though there are current research reports to be found and followed up, but rather rely on his *Red Mites and Typhus* (1968) and his (1949) report from the Institute of Medical Research in Kuala Lumpur. Scrub typhus, like louse-borne typhus, is caused by a rickettsia, an organism intermediate in size between the bacteria and the viruses, in this case *Rickettsia tsutsugamushi* (from an American pathologist, Ricketts, and the Japanese name for a local vector mite); it involves a three-factor zoonotic complex into which people occasionally blunder but, as with the tick-borne encephalitis of chapter 7, people are really a 'dead-end' as far as the perpetuation of the cycle goes. The ultimate reservoir of infection lies in jungle rodents, the pathogen moving between them and larval stages of acarine mites – in Burma *Trombicula deliensis* or in later references *Leptotrombidium deliense* (*leptos*, 'slender'). Under purely natural conditions the interaction between these three factors occurs in what Audy called 'mite islands', often at margins between vegetation types such as monsoon forest and grassy flood-plain. Jungle clearings, however, for permanent or more likely shifting agriculture, simulate this sort of margin, and become, as it were, linear 'mite islands' with attendant rodents. (It was this sort of site that caused a number of military casualties to both sides in the Burma campaigns of 1942–5 – the Japanese of course were already familiar with the disease cycle from home.) Audy traces the human provision of fresh potential mite-island sites through various types of terrain and land use, even to rice-fields where hedges help to simulate the jungle vegetation boundary sites. Mapping, use of air photographs and ecological analyses in Audy's work are of great elegance, and particularly exciting because of the convergence with geomedical insights from USSR, from J.M. May and from Rodenwaldt and Jusatz in Heidelberg, but particularly perhaps with Pavlovsky et al. (1955) on the now widely accepted concept of natural nidi ('nests') of human diseases. (On application of these ideas in the USSR, see Ignatyev (1966).) For an outline account in the context of human interaction with tropical forests see Learmonth (1959). For a developed country example, see Derrick (1961), including a photograph of a holiday hut in coastal bush, and a little grassy glade where a woman holiday-maker put down a blanket and sun-bathed. An overview is in WHO Working Group on the Rickettsial Diseases (1982).

Conclusion

This chapter is an attempt to look at the main disease burden of the Third World – and therefore the leading causes of illness and premature death in mankind as a whole – through the concept of two-, three- and four-factor disease complexes introduced by May in 1950. Each paragraph could be expanded into a monograph, given data, to illustrate much more deeply the ecological web that binds the two, three or four factors together through the interactions with each other, and with the community housing, diet, activities at work and play, that make up the holistic approach that ecology involves. The sketches given can afford only an occasional glimpse of this whole picture. However, it seems worth while to present this overall picture of Third World diseases as a context for the later chapters presenting some mainly geographical research on the distribution and ecology of particular diseases, and by way of comparison with the earlier chapters on the developed world. Let us return to table 9.1, the parallel to table 2.1, representing lost years of life caused by premature or preventable death in one Third World population, namely

Ghana. It seems to sum up a great deal of the foregoing material in this chapter, and like the chapter as a whole, gives a context for later, more detailed discussion of selected diseases and issues in health. Most readers may well be struck by the importance of the universal diseases like measles and pneumonia. However, it fails to bring out the importance of the debilitating and – many believe – apathy-inducing diseases like schistosomiasis and dysentery which cause a comparatively small proportion of lost years through premature deaths. Indeed one has to remind oneself how much is hidden by a table like this, including the fact that much of the wide spectrum of infections and vector-borne diseases is going on in a country like Ghana, year in, year out.

The following chapters include references to some of the great eradication campaigns, and the one against smallpox has already been mentioned in chapter 8. A major study of this topic is in Yekutiel (1980), and there is a brief but very compelling condensation in *World Health Forum* (1981a). And Rosenfield et al. (1984) note the enormous problems of assessing the economics of parasitic diseases and of control and its consequences, for neglecting the natural history of the disease or diseases, on the one hand, or on the other failing to take account of the complex interactions with the society, demography and economy, prove equally to lead to faulty estimates.

10 Malaria and Some Other Mosquito-borne Diseases

Introductory

It was in 1880 that Laveran in Algeria discovered malaria parasites in human blood, and in 1898 that Ross in Calcutta worked out the role of mosquitoes in avian malaria (in sparrows) while Grassi, Bignami and Bastianelli described the cycle of human malaria and *Anopheles* mosquitoes. (A centenary symposium commemorating Laveran's discovery of *Plasmodium* is in *Cahiers ORSTOM* (1980); see also Kreier (1980) and for an Italian retrospect, see de Santis and Grasselli (1983).) There is a huge biomedical literature on all aspects of the disease, its treatment and prevention, including a good deal that is essentially geographical in approach, and at its best excellent in quality of cartography, environmental analysis and regional synthesis. Yet all this accumulated knowledge did not prevent the resurgence of the disease in India from the nearly complete success of eradication campaigns in 1965, spreading back across much of the country as a major public health problem (though happily not as severe as it was before the campaigns). Similar re-advances have occurred in many other areas (*Soc. Sci. and Med* 1986c) and this is one reason why geographers may well find themselves involved in individual or preferably team research on the problem. As chapter 9 has shown, too, malaria on the world scale is sufficiently important as a feature of population and welfare geography to justify geographical commitment. For an essay on unusual breadth on the world malaria picture see Wyler (1983); for an historical view Harrison (1978); and a biologist and a geographer look at the world ecology in Dutta and Dutt (1978). See also the special issue of the *British Medical Bulletin* (Cohen 1982); and on the geography of chloroquine resistance in malaria parasites, Charmot (1983). Chapter 8 has established that on May's classification malaria involves a three-factor complex, between the parasite *Plasmodium*, the vector or alternate host *Anopheles* mosquitoes, and the human host. The ecological

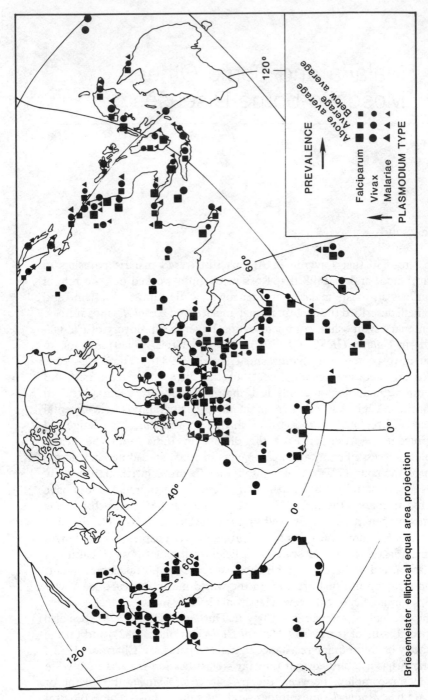

Briesemeister elliptical equal area projection

Figure 10.1 World map of *Plasmodia*
Source: May (1950–55)

interactions that make up the ecology of malaria in a particular region are complex. There are three principal species of *Plasmodium* involved in human malaria, mapped by May in 1951 (figure 10.1). *P. falciparum* is regarded as the most recently evolved as a human disease. It is the most virulent but does not remain in the liver to cause relapses over many years (as *P. ovale* and *P. vivax* may, or in the red blood cells as *P. malariae* may). Paradoxically, in areas long saturated with the parasite, it may cause less severe illness in adult survivors of childhood attacks than the very widespread and less virulent *P. vivax*. *P. malariae* is less widespread, slower in development and notoriously long-lasting. The distribution pattern in figure 10.1 has been altered by anti-malaria campaigns: *P. vivax* has been eliminated from many temperate and even sub-tropical areas, so that its area approximates to that of *P. falciparum* though with re-advances as noted earlier for India. *P. malariae* is reported as eliminated from USSR though long persistent in infected people in nearby Romania. To these three species must be added *P. ovale*, a comparatively mild form in forest communities in West Africa and parts of East Africa, comparatively little affected by the control or eradication campaigns; it may represent the nearest approach to good host–parasite adjustment of the four species. Other *Plasmodia* are parasitic on primates, birds and other animals, also with mosquitoes as alternate hosts. On the evolution of *Plasmodium*, see Bruce-Chwatt (1965) and McCutchan et al. (1984).

The mosquito vector genus *Anopheles* is a very large one including hundreds of species and many of these are actual or potential vectors. While they are mainly involved in the malaria cycle in warm areas with relatively humid seasons, with bodies of still or running water and unpolluted water for egg-laying and the larval stage (some general climatic limits will be suggested later), they have a very wide range of ecological preferences and behaviour. Most prefer still water, but a few running water, for oviposition. Characteristic feeding times are near dawn and dusk, or at night, but resting places vary from room walls in 'domestic' species to sheltered forest sites in 'wild' ones. For all its near-universal character at its greatest extension, malaria is in a sense a local disease, with flight distance from breeding places an important control. These flight distances, often taken as about a kilometre in pre-Independence India, unless wind-borne, are now regarded as commonly up to 10 km or so in African species, and more if wind-blown. One way of synthesizing biomedical knowledge of malaria vectors is by the macro-regional approach of figure 10.2: the original paper gives an account of the progress of anti-malaria campaigns against the principal local vectors, summarizing difficulties arising both from mosquito behaviour and from the development of anopheline resistance to insecticides like DDT and dieldrin

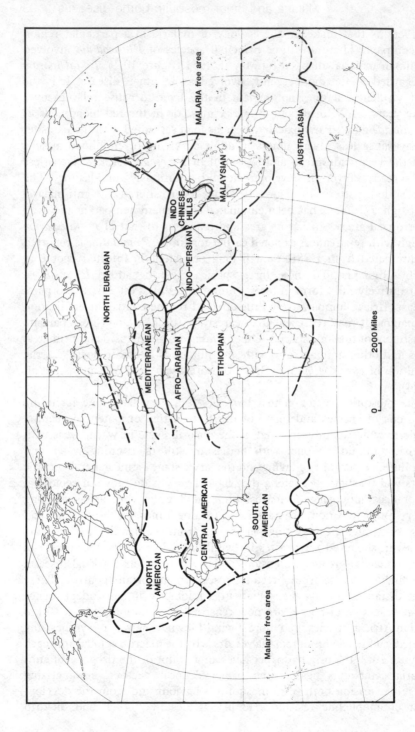

Figure 10.2 World map of *Anopheles* regions
Source: Bruce-Chwatt (1970)

(Bruce-Chwatt 1970). At a completely different level, but with the splendid photography typical of the *National Geographic Magazine*, see Nielsen (1979).

If mosquitoes' behaviour is variable, humankind, though of one species only, presents enormous diversity in patterns of work, housing, cooking, sleeping, clothing, travel and migration, all of which may affect contacts between people and *Anopheles*. Use of protective screens, prophylactic drugs, and acceptance of anti-mosquito spraying or drainage etc. vary widely, as do education and awareness of the disease cycle. Even biogeographers may need to seek biological collaboration in research on geographical distribution of *Plasmodium* or even *Anopheles*, but many of the patterns of human contact with infected mosquitoes are within the competence of human geography. And several areal scales can usefully be applied. Of the interacting life cycles involved in the total disease complex (see figure 10.3) that of humankind is relatively neglected in geomedical research.

A Model of a Hypothetical Malarial Continent

So far the material presented in this chapter has been almost entirely from biomedical sources, though much is clearly of geographical significance. The author some years ago developed a model of a hypothetical malarial continent, really for teaching rather than research purposes. Hypothetical simply because it can be used as a model, it can be manipulated to bring out particular aspects of the changing geography of malaria (see figures 10.4A–10.4M).

What is the present over-all picture? (See figure 10.5.) This is mapped in terms of the progress of anti-malaria campaigns up to a certain date, and shows the generally better progress towards the poleward margins of the affected areas. Along with this map it is necessary to consider one way of classifying malarious areas, that is in terms of varying degrees of endemicity (constantly present) or epidemicity (periodically present with partial or total lulls in fresh cases).

Endemic areas

Hypoendemicity: in areas with little transmission and only slight impact on the population as a whole.

Mesoendemicity: typically in small rural communities in subtropical zones, transmission varying in intensity with local circumstances.

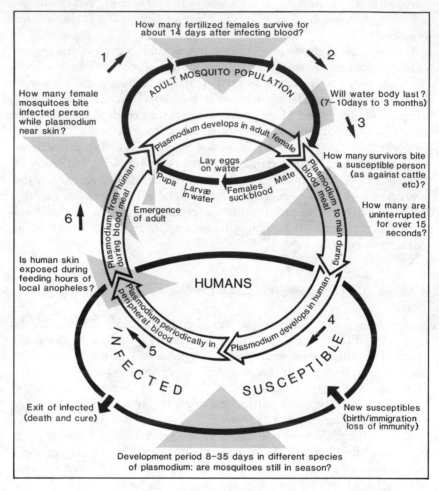

How many fertilized females survive for about 14 days after infecting blood?

1

ADULT MOSQUITO POPULATION

2

How many female mosquitoes bite infected person while plasmodium near skin?

Will water body last? (7–10days to 3 months)

3

Plasmodium develops in adult female

Plasmodium to man during blood meal

Plasmodium from human during blood meal

Lay eggs on water

Pupa

Larvæ in water

Females suck blood

Mate

How many survivors bite a susceptible person (as against cattle etc)?

How many are uninterrupted for over 15 seconds?

Emergence of adult

6

Is human skin exposed during feeding hours of local anopheles?

HUMANS

Plasmodium periodically in peripheral blood

Plasmodium develops in human

4

I N F E C T E D

5

S U S C E P T I B L E

Exit of infected (death and cure)

New susceptibles (birth/immigration loss of immunity)

Development period 8–35 days in different species of plasmodium: are mosquitoes still in season?

Figure 10.3 Interlocking life cycles
Source: Learmonth (1971)

Hyperendemicity: in areas with intense but seasonal transmission, conferring immunity insufficient to prevent illness in all age-groups. (Some of the literature will be found referring to 'seasonal' epidemics.)

Holoendemicity: in areas with perennial transmission of such intensity as to confer a considerable degree of community immunity, mainly in adults. It has long been thought that malaria, like some other infections, tends to increase the spontaneous abortion rate, with important demographic effects especially in holoendemic areas (Learmonth 1958, p. 6): for a recent editorial on malaria and pregnancy see Bruce-Chwatt (1983). Bray (1981) working in Gambia, reports that *falciparum* malaria seems to cause low birth-rate rather than abortion – *vivax* malaria having been the main suspect.

Epidemic areas: are those in which the disease occurs after a period in which it has been unknown, and where therefore immunity is low, and characteristically there are severe illnesses and possible deaths in all age-groups. (Contrast the considerable degree of adult immunity in holoendemic areas.) See Bruce-Chwatt (1980).

Clearly these terms can be quantified, and indeed WHO has defined endemicity in terms of the simple but equivocal spleen index (based on palpation to see if that organ is enlarged – but there may be several causes of this). Details are given, for instance in Learmonth (1977). Since modern authorities tend to avoid quantification, it may be best to apply measures suitable for particular surveys. Epidemics may often be defined in terms of a rise in incidence of say ten or more times the normal.

Other terms will be found: stable and unstable; autochthonous (acquired locally) and indigenous ('natural' to an area – rather like the botanist's use of 'endemic'!); imported (of infections acquired outside the area) and introduced (of secondary cases arising from imported ones). See Bruce-Chwatt (1980), p. 135.

'Airport malaria' is becoming a recognized term in western Europe: two recent cases of *falciparum* malaria 10 and 15 km from Gatwick Airport in Sussex are attributed to *Anopheles* imported on aircraft and then travelling onward by car – rather than to local mosquitoes becoming infected by malarious human travellers (Curtis and White 1984; Whitfield et al. 1984). It may be startling to many readers to know that the same local vector *A. messeae* has returned to cattlesheds near one of Moscow's reservoirs in densities similar to those of 1941 – before the DDT campaign that wiped out malaria and for a time the vector: with much modern use of the reservoir's recreation facilities there is concern that imported malaria from people returning from the tropics might cause fresh incidence (Sokolova and Volegova 1980).

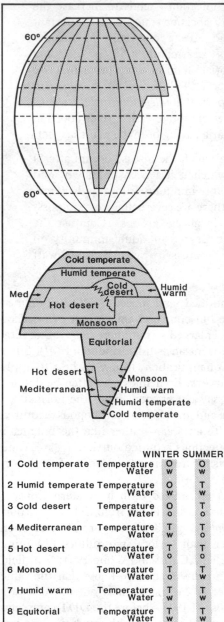

(a) **Hypothetical malarial continent**
It is simple and massive, and, stretching from latitude 75°N to 55°S, it generalizes the broad northern hemisphere landmasses and the more peninsular shapes of the southern hemisphere. Climates as in B below and (at this stage) low to undulating relief are assumed, yielding water-bodies on land varying from still water, some frozen in winter, running water subject to spates and droughts, brackish water in coastal lagoons etc. - a range including the conditions preferred for egg-laying by different species of Anopheles. Uniform distribution of human population and of Plasmodium are assumed, both of a density that would maintain the malaria cycle as a public health problem. Underdevelopment is assumed: the malaria cycle is not inhibited, directly or indirectly, by human technology.

(b and c) **Climates**
These are portrayed much as in a simple textbook on climatology in sequence poleward north and south from the equator, in both 'map' and table, while the latter records winter and summer temperatures suitable for anopheline breeding (T), and similarly for water conditions (W) but with O where either factor is absent. Roughly, breeding and activity occur at temperatures over about 16°C, while relative humidities over some 60% give conditions congenial to mosquito activity for large parts of the day; often under about 16°C by night and at dawn and dusk. Temperatures over about 35°C and relative humidities under about 25% bring conditions unfavourable to adult mosquitoes and they will tend to die off or aestivate in warm damp hiding places e.g. in stables, cow-sheds, irrigation tunnels etc. Rainfall amounts may not be related directly to activity, but a three months' rainy season or more is likely to provide some of the wide range of water-bodies used by different species of Anopheles.
Note: These figures are generalized for purposes of model-building and are not presented as definitive in any way.

		WINTER		SUMMER	
1 Cold temperate	Temperature	O		O	
	Water		W		W
2 Humid temperate	Temperature	O		T	
	Water		W		W
3 Cold desert	Temperature	O		T	
	Water		O	O	
4 Mediterranean	Temperature	T		T	
	Water		W	O	
5 Hot desert	Temperature	T		T	
	Water		O	O	
6 Monsoon	Temperature	T		T	
	Water		O		W
7 Humid warm	Temperature	T		T	
	Water		W		W
8 Equitorial	Temperature	T		T	
	Water		W		W

Figure 10.4   Hypothetical malarial continent
Source: Learmonth (1971)

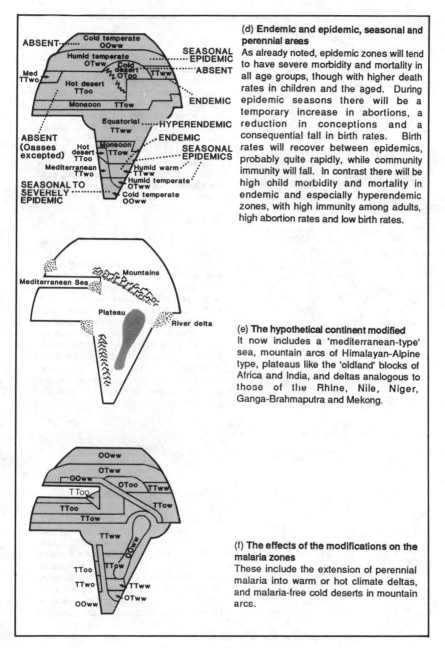

(d) Endemic and epidemic, seasonal and perennial areas
As already noted, epidemic zones will tend to have severe morbidity and mortality in all age groups, though with higher death rates in children and the aged. During epidemic seasons there will be a temporary increase in abortions, a reduction in conceptions and a consequential fall in birth rates. Birth rates will recover between epidemics, probably quite rapidly, while community immunity will fall. In contrast there will be high child morbidity and mortality in endemic and especially hyperendemic zones, with high immunity among adults, high abortion rates and low birth rates.

(e) The hypothetical continent modified
It now includes a 'mediterranean-type' sea, mountain arcs of Himalayan-Alpine type, plateaus like the 'oldland' blocks of Africa and India, and deltas analogous to those of the Rhine, Nile, Niger, Ganga-Brahmaputra and Mekong.

(f) The effects of the modifications on the malaria zones
These include the extension of perennial malaria into warm or hot climate deltas, and malaria-free cold deserts in mountain arcs.

Figure 10.4 (*Continued over*)

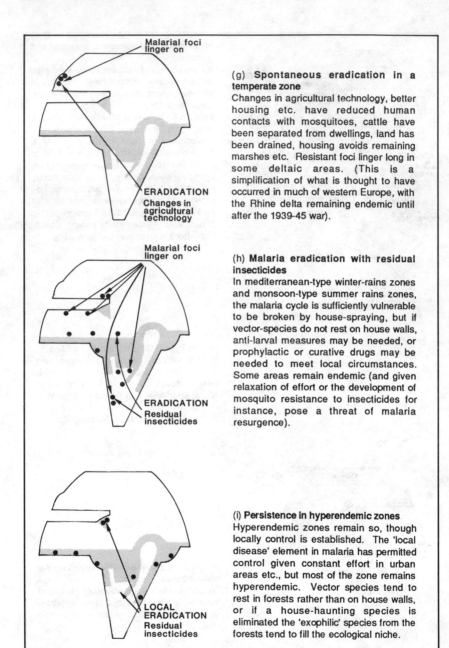

(g) **Spontaneous eradication in a temperate zone**
Changes in agricultural technology, better housing etc. have reduced human contacts with mosquitoes, cattle have been separated from dwellings, land has been drained, housing avoids remaining marshes etc. Resistant foci linger long in some deltaic areas. (This is a simplification of what is thought to have occurred in much of western Europe, with the Rhine delta remaining endemic until after the 1939–45 war).

(h) **Malaria eradication with residual insecticides**
In mediterranean-type winter-rains zones and monsoon-type summer rains zones, the malaria cycle is sufficiently vulnerable to be broken by house-spraying, but if vector-species do not rest on house walls, anti-larval measures may be needed, or prophylactic or curative drugs may be needed to meet local circumstances. Some areas remain endemic (and given relaxation of effort or the development of mosquito resistance to insecticides for instance, pose a threat of malaria resurgence).

(i) **Persistence in hyperendemic zones**
Hyperendemic zones remain so, though locally control is established. The 'local disease' element in malaria has permitted control given constant effort in urban areas etc., but most of the zone remains hyperendemic. Vector species tend to rest in forests rather than on house walls, or if a house-haunting species is eliminated the 'exophilic' species from the forests tend to fill the ecological niche.

Figure 10.4 *Continued*

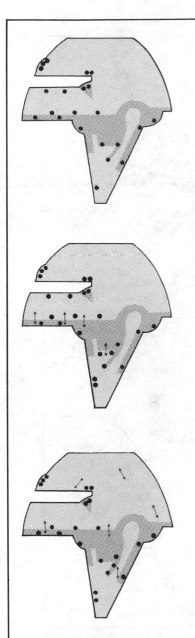

(j) A summary diagram of successes and failures

Eradication has been achieved in mediterranean-type winter-rainfall and tropical summer rainfall zones, mainly by using residual insecticides against adult <u>Anopheles</u>, but leaving some residual foci. In contrast the equatorial rainfall areas show only limited areas of control achieved through intensive attacks at several points of the interlocking life cycles that together make up the <u>whole</u> malaria cycle. Outside these, control is too difficult so far, owing to the presence of myriad water-bodies suitable for anopheline breeding, innumerable retreat and resting places for the adult mosquitoes in the forest,and'wild' strains like those of <u>A.gambiae</u>

(k) Human mobility and malaria

Migration and nomadic movements, like those in Nigeria and elsewhere, documented by Prothero (1965), are known to be major obstacles to anti-malaria campaigns. Such movements of people constantly replenish the reservoir of infection in the human host-population, so permitting resurgence in areas in which control had been achieved. Kondrashin and Orlov (1985) note also the impact of the spread of resistance to chloroquine in <u>Plasmodium falciparum</u>.

(l) Climatic shifts and malaria

Climatic belts can move to and fro, carrying malaria into a previously malaria-free or little affected zone. A wet 'Bombay year' can invade a normally much drier area like the Punjab plains, as happened prior to the great epidemic there in 1912. And conversely - and more surprisingly to most people - an epidemic can arise from a dry 'Deccan-type' year invading an equatorial rainforest climate like that of the Wet Zone of Sri Lanka as in the catastrophic epidemic year in the West Zone in 1935. This was caused by a Dry Zone mosquito <u>A.culicifacies</u> not normally suited to the West Zone conditions - and to the very lethal <u>falciparum</u> malaria.

Figure 10.4 *Continued*

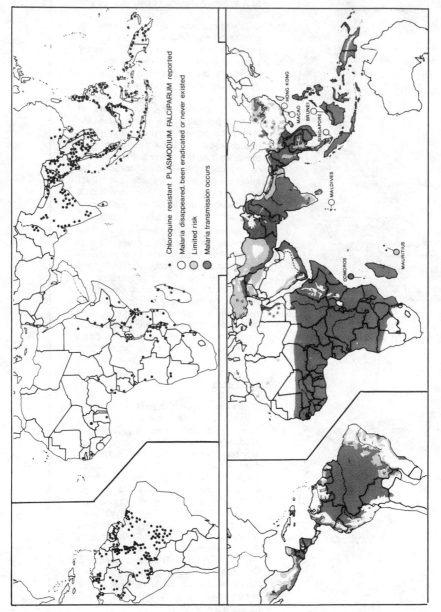

Figure 10.5 World map of malaria prevalence or control
Source: WHO 1987

Control Points in Interlocking Life Cycles

It must already be clear that one of the crucial problems in trying to control malaria is the selection of the point or points at which the interlocking cycles of figure 10.3 can best be broken given the particular and *local* ecological web. After the end of the 1939–45 war for two decades at least the emphasis was overwhelmingly on the use of residual (long-lasting) insecticides like DDT, and later dieldrin and others, in campaigns on spraying of interior walls etc. of houses, that is on attacking the resting adult female, usually after a blood-meal. We have already seen that not all species are so house-haunting, and moreover mosquito behaviour can change over a comparatively short time, since 'wilder' strains are more successful in surviving and breeding (the phenomenon sometimes called 'biological drift' within the same species). Figure 10.3 has been further developed to show half-a-dozen contrasting combinations of points of attack on the interlocking cycles (Learmonth 1977); figures 10.6(a) and (b) are selected as sufficient to make the point here. Figure 10.6(a) from work in Cameroon represents many of the classic problems of campaigns in the equatorial rainforest environment. The two great African vectors were present: *Anopheles funestus* the more closely associated with permanent water-bodies, swamps and marshes, and the notoriously opportunist *A. gambiae* breeding in temporary pools, even those in hollows and containers on relatively dry sites flooded by the rains. Curative drugs had some success, at least in timber camps. Then came DDT apparently as a *Deus ex machina*, and indeed with early successes: *A. funestus* was almost wiped out, and two forest vectors *A. moucheti* and *A. nili*. *A. gambiae* was reduced in and around dwellings and workplaces, but 'wilder' or exophilic strains survive and may cause malaria in lumbermen, hunters etc. Densely peopled plains can be protected, at quite high costs in continued surveillance, and clearly the goal of complete eradication is unattainable on present techniques. If an effective vaccine is evolved, it may prove a more reliable *Deus ex machina*!

Figure 10.6(b), based on work in Israel, illustrates attack on the interlocking cycle at almost every point possible on existing technology and with the complications of immigrants carrying *Plasmodia* and its transmission *via* blood transfusions ('induced' malaria): there is prophylactic and presumptive treatment of immigrants, anti-larval spraying, imagocidal too (i.e. against the adult emerging after pupation), and a certain amount of house-spraying. And an accidental weapon, in the form of escaped aquatic rodents (nutria) changed the character of aquatic vegetation against the bionomics of anopheline larvae.

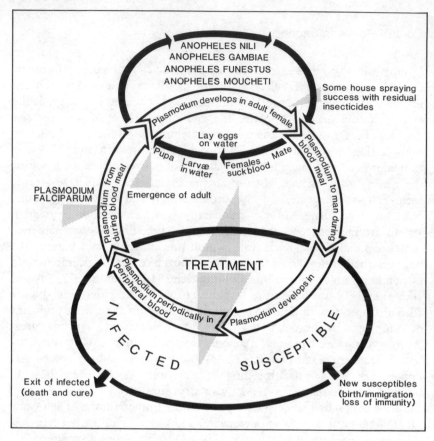

Figure 10.6 (a) Interrupting the interlocking life cycles: Cameroon
Source: Learmonth (1977)

Following Jacques May's (1950) plea to professional geographers, then, this three-factor disease complex has been looked at cartographically, in both static pattern and dynamic: spatial distribution pattern has been considered, by changing scale, in terms of the interlocking cycles involved in the complex; ecological insights can be claimed, though granting that to a purist the ecology of a community is one and indivisible.

India: a Study on the Macro-scale

Malaria Regions and Principal Vectors

Two classic maps by malariologists are perhaps salutary: not only the professional geographer or cartographer can make and use maps, and the

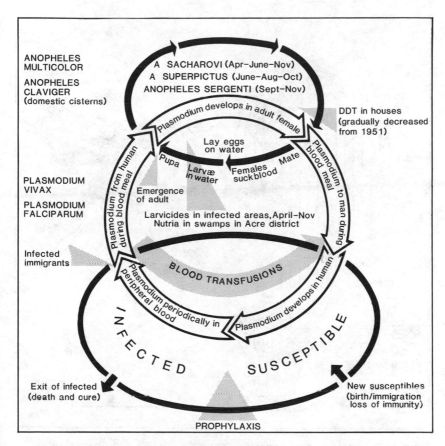

Figure 10.6 (b)   Interrupting the interlocking life cycles: Israel
Source: Learmonth (1977)

original texts accompanying these maps, in common with much of the biomedical literature both before and since Independence, are full of geographical insights, sometimes regional syntheses from the malariologist's viewpoint of remarkable quality. These particular maps of course represent late colonial and undivided India, not the independent republics of today.

Figure 10.7 is a 1938 version of a map dating back originally to Christophers and Sinton in 1926 and accompanied by a regional characterization of great percipience. Sir Rickard Christophers as a very old man wrote to the present author attributing much of its quality to a series of major regional memoirs largely researched before the 1914–18 war, during which some of the authors were killed or died from disease on active service. He and his co-author seem to have taken the 40-inch

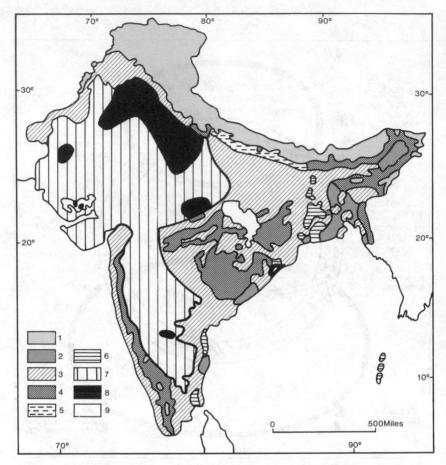

Figure 10.7 Malaria in late colonial India, after Christophers and Sinton 1926.

1 Areas of 5,000ft (non-malarious).

2 Known healthy plains (spleen rates less than 10 per cent). Now somewhat smaller area in East Bengal than shown on map.

3 Moderate to high endemicity of more or less static character, the intensity depending on local surrounding; seasonal variation moderate, fulminant epidemics unknown.

4 Hyper-endemicity of hilly jungle tracts and *terai* land.

5 Probably hyper-endemic hill areas.

6 Hyper-endemicity other than hill areas.

7 Variable endemicity associated with dry tracts, usually showing autumnal rise in fever incidence (potential epidemic areas), spleen rate low except for years following epidemics, or in special local circumstances, and much affected by conditions of irrigation.

8 Known areas liable to fulminant epidemicity (diluvial) malaria. Spleen rate dependent on occurrence of epidemics, high during and immediately after such, slowly falling to low rates in course of half a decade or so.

9 Unsurveyed.

The heavy pecked line marks the broad division between the endemic and epidemic regions of India and Pakistan.

Source: Learmonth (1957)

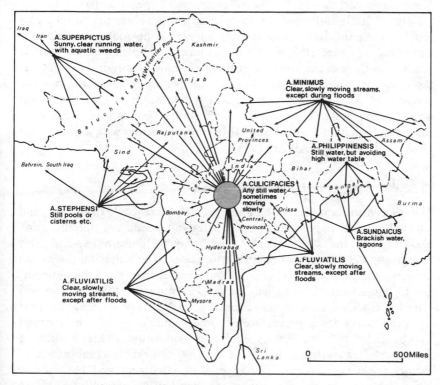

Figure 10.8   Principal malaria vectors of India, after Covell 1949
Source: Learmonth (1957)

mean annual isohyet as a crucial divide, a line on the map familiar to
geographers as roughly dividing humid (rice-eating) India from arid and
semi-arid (wheat and millet-eating) India: here it is similarly taken as the
malariological divide between humid and endemic India as against arid
and semi-arid epidemic India. Within endemic India type 5 comprises
hyperendemic hill tracts where the principal vectors are stream-breeding
forest mosquitoes like the *Anopheles fluviatilis* and *A. minimus* of figure
10.8. For a recent synthesis on the anopheline mosquitoes of India, see
Ramachandra Rao (1984). And type 6 in figure 10.7 is hyperendemicity
of more lowland areas, notably including densely peopled western Bengal
where the principal vector was *A. philippinensis*, a still-water breeder
thought to prefer areas where the water-table was relatively low. In
contrast the hyperendemic area of the Kaveri delta (opposite the northern
tip of Sri Lanka) was dominated by the main and highly opportunist
vector of the whole sub-continent, *A. culicifacies*. The variable endemicity
of the coastal tract and notably coastal towns north and north-west from
Bombay was largely due to *A. stephensi*, recorded as highly urbanized by

Stephens as early as 1915. The sub-continent appears in figure 10.2 as mostly in the Indo-Persian or Indo-Iranian zone while the eastern part touches both the Indo-Chinese Hills zone and the Malaysian zone, as confirmed in figure 10.7 by the dominance of *A. philippinensis* and *A. minimus* in the east; in contrast in the west, now mainly in Pakistan, *A. superpictus* is a Middle East mosquito, aestivating to avoid the hot dry summer in cool dry resting places, including *karez* or *qanat* irrigation tunnels. The 'watershed' position of the Indian sub-continent has been the subject of an interesting study by a surgeon writing with a geographer (Joshi and Deshpande 1972, 1985).

Control Campaigns and Resurgence

Malaria control campaigns began immediately after the 1939–45 war, and naturally gained impetus immensely after Independence, initially using DDT against the adult *Anopheles* by spraying house-walls, and later employing dieldrin and other later insecticides. The following discussion concerns the post-1947 Republic of India rather than the sub-continent. By 1957 the control campaigns were so encouraging that the aim was raised to eradication, with house-spraying as the major strategy. By 1965 the pre-Independence prevalence of some 70 millions had been reduced to about 100 000 and in an increased population. This is quite a remarkable feat, attributable to an equally remarkable combination of factors favouring success: a large pool of intelligent and enthusiastic labour able to do house-spraying conscientiously; supervisors able to negotiate the very limited public cooperation needed – really only access to house-walls, with only occasional problems arising from sacred wall-paintings and the like; a mainly house-haunting principal vector *A. culicifacies*; and in the main sub-tropical rather than equatorial rainforest conditions, so that the interlocking life-cycles of figure 10.3 proved relatively fragile, certainly under the massive national effort of the two decades 1945–65. Then with victory so near the campaigns seemed to falter. In the words of a professor of demography and former Registrar-General of India:

> The very low malaria incidence presumably gave rise to a general feeling that malaria was eradicated and there was undoubtedly premature complacency around the middle of 1965. It needs to be remembered, however, at this point, that should there be even only one positive case of malaria in July–September, theoretically it can generate up to 1120 malarial cases in a chain unless vigorous steps are taken effectively to break the chain. The first setback came that year. The strategy in anti-malarial spraying was based on the

observed course of malaria during the active season of malarial transmission from March to October. The first round of spray must be complete between April and mid-May, which takes care of the next ten weeks. The second round of spray should be undertaken in July–August to depress the peak of malarial transmission, usual in this season, so that the curve goes down fast enough by October. The outbreak of the Indo-Pakistan War in the second half of 1965 and the closure of Suez delayed imports of DDT and other drugs from USA.

(Mitra 1978)

There were a number of other complicating factors. Several species of *Anopheles* developed strains resistant to DDT and apparently able to evolve generations resistant to other later insecticides with even greater speed. See WHO (1980 TRS 655) for a world review of vector resistance to insecticides. Some workers believe that the use of agricultural insecticides has increased mosquito resistance to these, as an unwelcome by-product, and that this is largely responsible for the resurgence of malaria in Central America and India (Chapin and Wasserstrom 1981, 1983). Sharma and Mehrotra (1982b) believe that Chapin and her co-author are mistaken, at least so far as India is concerned: that there anopheline resistance had developed *before* large-scale use of agricultural pesticides, that the residual insecticides remain sufficiently effective and cost-effective, that there is no real alternative to their use; but see also rejoinder by Wasserstrom and Chapin (1982). For a field study see Sharma et al. (1982a). Other species were already 'wild' or exophilic, tending to rest in forest refuges rather than on house walls, and some evolved exophilic strains. The urban vector *A. stephensi* extended its range south from Bombay, and round cape Kanya Kumari to invade many Bay of Bengal coastal towns. Moreover *Plasmodium* was also changing. *P. vivax*, the relatively less virulent though lasting species, always causing substantial illness and loss of efficiency even in hyperendemic or holoendemic areas, had long been the dominant malaria of India. *P. falciparum*, the more virulent though less long-lasting species, extended its area, spreading from the north-east across middle India, fortunately in relatively sparsely peopled areas but still the homes of many millions of people. Moreover resistance of *P. falciparum* to the synthetic drug chloroquine spread from South-east Asia (it had been important to the US forces during the Vietnam war), and the resistant strains spread to many of the areas with falciparum malaria, apparently in leap-frogging fashion following lines of human movement including migration and perhaps service postings. For a geographical view of the development of chloroquine resistance, see Charmot (1983). Urban malaria was increasing, with *A. stephensi* as already noted, and other *Anopheles* were incriminated in cities including Calcutta. There were particular local problems, like the sacred paintings already mentioned, or double-roofed houses in some tribal tracts. Labour migration from tribal areas, relatively sparsely peopled, granted, by Indian standards, is thought to have triggered off the resurgence from several of the 'residual endemic foci' of 1965–6, to diffuse, or re-diffuse across much of the country but *not* so far reproducing the classic pre-control pattern of figure 10.7. (On migration and malaria, see Prothero (1965) and other listed publications, also Kondrashin et al. (1985).) Table 10.1 shows the fall from the 1945 figures to 1965, then the resurgence: though the increase is some 50-fold, even five million shows a remarkable improvement on the pre-Independence and pre-DDT figure of 70 millions. (For comparison, China recorded just over three million cases of malaria in 1981 (China Malaria Commission 1983; Zhou 1981). On South-east Asia see Brandling-Bennet et al. (1981), and on control in China see Pal (1982).) However, the 100 000 cases of 1965 were concentrated overwhelmingly in a handful of 'residual endemic foci': three of these were in forested areas in middle and eastern India, and seem to be linked with stream-breeding and exophilic mosquitoes, including some species in Assam that may have increased in relative importance since the spray campaigns. The fourth, in Cutch, was largely vectored by the urban *A. stephensi*, and there was a small area north-east of Delhi where the mosquito was probably *A. culicifacies*. Figure 10.9 shows how from these residual endemic foci the disease cycle seems to have spread out year by year over

Table 10.1   Malaria incidence in India 1965–1976

Year	Total Malaria Cases
1947	*c.*70 000 000
1965	100 185
1966	148 136
1967	278 621
1968	274 881
1969	348 647
1970	694 647
1971	1 323 118
1972	1 362 806
1973	1 934 485
1974	3 167 658
1975	5 166 142
1976	5 082 467

Source: Akhtar and Learmonth 1977

most, though not all, of India – some differences from the pre-Independence picture have already been noted up to the peak years of 1975 and 1976 (Akhtar and Learmonth 1977, 1979). This suggestion of a spatial diffusion – or re-diffusion – pattern seems to invite attempts to analyse the phenomenon by simulation of the spread, perhaps following the classic work of Hägerstrand (1967) in Sweden outlined in chapter 6. This attempt has been made and is fully reported by Learmonth and Akhtar (1984). The simulation achieved only modest success, indeed as often with similar exercises its chief value may be negative, that is in eliminating some possible explanations for the successful readvance of the disease in face of modern biomedical technology; so only a brief and selective account will be given here. First, though, three points should be made. The steady rise in reported parasite rates from 1965 to 1975 brought agonizing reappraisal of the campaign strategy, and as a result a modified plan of operation of the National Malaria Eradication programme was adopted from April 1977 to hold the disease in check rather than to aim at complete eradication in the near future: the aim is to combine government effort, public participation and scientific research in order to maintain the benefits to general economic development programmes brought by the earlier successes. (See Pattanayak and Roy (1980) and several more popular accounts on the world scale, *WHO Chronicle* (1978), Farid (1980), Bruce-Chwatt (1984); and for some figures on India's recovery from the peak resurgence years of 1975–6, Harinasuta et al. (1982).) Then in the geographical literature of the period when the present author was working under some difficulties on the diffusion problem, a number of Indian workers were undertaking more conventional and often regional studies; some of these are listed in the references, and many readers may well prefer them to the attempts at simulation (Dutt et al. 1980; Hyma and Ramesh 1980; Akhtar 1982; Ramesh et al. 1984; Prasad 1984; Hyma and Chakrapani 1983; Picardat 1982). Lastly there is the large literature on the mathematics of diffusion, as we have already seen in relation to chapter 7: in relation to malaria it extends back to Sir Ronald Ross – amateur mathematician as well as poet! – with intermittent contributions up to the present day including a successful simulation of epidemics in northern Nigeria and Syria (Macdonald et al. (1968) cited in Learmonth and Akhtar (1984); and see Bailey (1982) for an essential biomathematical view).

Towards a Spatial Simulation Model of Re-diffusion

Why attempt to simulate the patterns at all? The case for such an exercise rests mainly on the fact that already the problem is one in historical

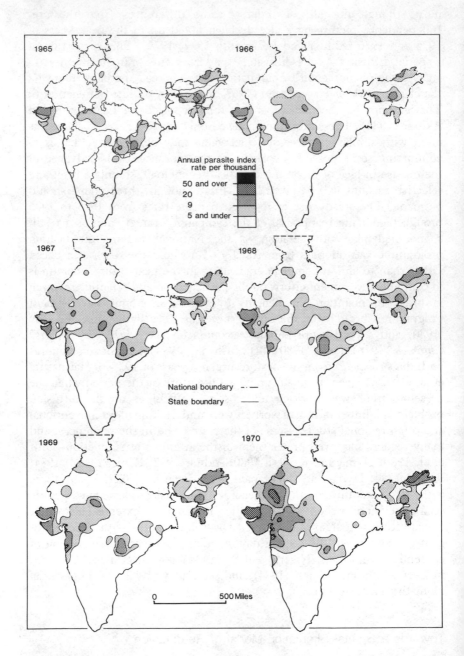

Figure 10.9   India, Annual Parasite Index rates (APIs) by malaria control areas and by years 1965–1976
Source: Akhtar and Learmonth (1977. 1982)

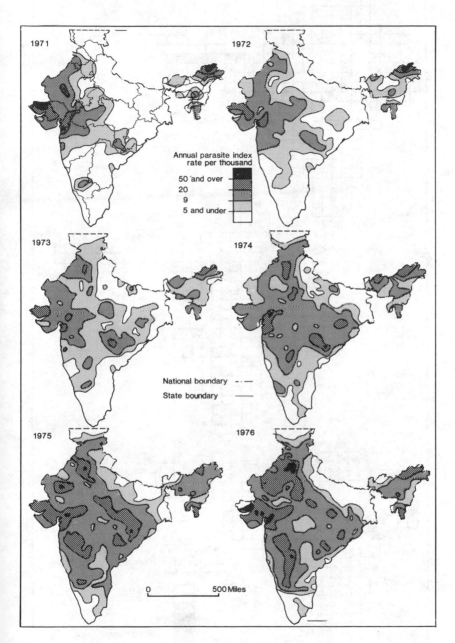

Figure 10.9 *Continued*

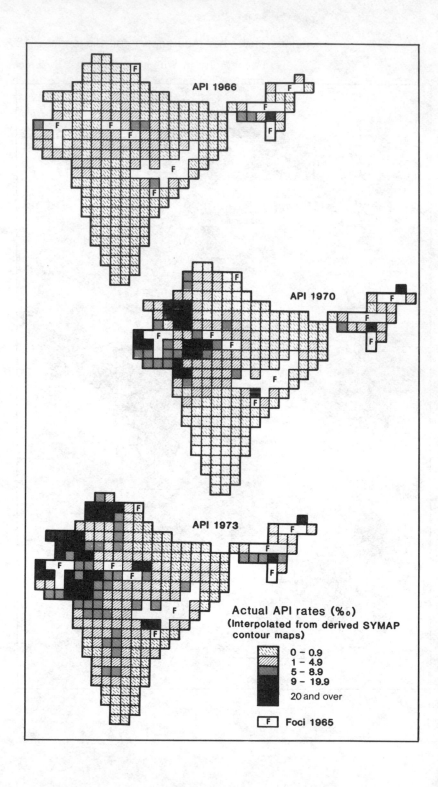

API 1966

API 1970

API 1973

Actual API rates (‰)
(Interpolated from derived SYMAP contour maps)

0 – 0.9
1 – 4.9
5 – 8.9
9 – 19.9
20 and over

F   Foci 1965

geography, and an historical geography in which much of the evidence that might have established firmly what factors underlay the resurgence as such is ephemeral and undocumented, especially the spatial patterns in its diffusion. That the patterns of spread 'must have been' controlled by this or that factor at such-and-such stage may be the limit of what attempts at causal analyses can now achieve.

Assuming, as often in geographical models, an isotropic plain and in this case a population density uniformly sufficient to sustain malaria transmission, the maps in figure 10.9 were stylized into grid-squares (in fact latitude-longitude 1° squares, involving slightly different areas in a country extending over some 27 degrees of latitude) as in figure 10.10 for 1975. Figure 10.11 shows how belts of one grid-square deep at successively greater distances from the residual endemic foci were indicated, and also the ranges of numbers allocated to grid-squares within each of the nine distance belts. These differing distance-belt ranges decrease proportionately to the *general* decrease in annual parasite index rates (APIs); this device was preferred to following the probabilities decreasing with 'distance decay' used in Hägerstrand's seminal paper and by many subsequent authors. (The results are admittedly surprisingly good in studies quite far removed from Hägerstrand's original topics (see chapter 6) such as a recent simulation of the spread of Dutch elm disease in the elm-tree population of England, see Sarre (1978).) Then 10 000 random numbers were allocated in each of ten 'years', recording 'hits' and producing simulated API rate maps as for 1966 to 1975 assuming 'distance decay' only in this 'round' of the simulation. Figure 10.11 is the simulation for 1975, which may be compared with figure 10.10 – figure 10.11 as 'expected' rates on the stated assumption, figure 10.10 as actual rates. The grid-square ranges, and therefore the probabilities for each distance belt, were then modified in turn assuming an important role for a number of possible factors in malaria diffusion: elements in the human or the physical geography were assumed in turn to influence the three key factors of *Anopheles*, *Plasmodium* and people in their manifold movements and activities, ultimately to influence contact between infected people, mosquitoes and susceptible people. In some 'rounds' of the simulation it was possible to make some estimate of the possible influence of the factor: thus for population density the API rates for a range of population densities were calculated, and the distance belt number ranges altered proportionately. For other possible factors, however, in the time available data to assist in this way could not be

Figure 10.10 Actual APIs 1966, 1970 and 1973 stylized to grid-squares used in simulation
Source: Learmonth and Akhtar (1984)

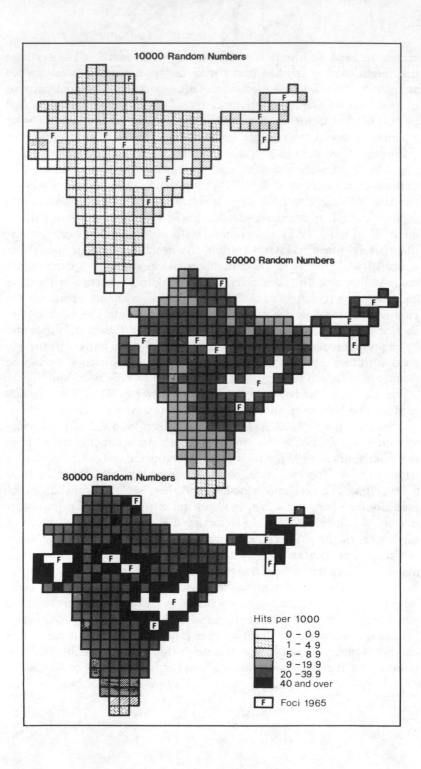

10000 Random Numbers

50000 Random Numbers

80000 Random Numbers

Hits per 1000

- 0 – 0 9
- 1 – 4 9
- 5 – 8 9
- 9 – 19 9
- 20 – 39 9
- 40 and over

F Foci 1965

obtained, and arbitrary decisions had to be made. Thus for tribal population there were no separate API rates; an arbitrary figure of 20 per cent of tribal to total population had to be taken, the API rates for the grid-square above and below that arbitrary figure worked out, and then the distance belt ranges modified for appropriate grid-squares before diffusing random numbers much as before.

Successive 'rounds' of the simulation were carried out assuming the influence on diffusion of each of three ranges of mean annual rainfall, irrigation over 20 per cent of total area, population density over and under 200 per square kilometre, and tribal population as just noted. Data problems caused the abandonment of 'rounds' on the influence of tribal migrants (likely to be much more to the point than *proportions* of tribal to total population); on the possible influence of the main seasonal winds of the summer and winter monsoon (wind-blown infected black-flies are known to be significant for river blindness, see chapter 12 and Pedgley (1982)); on wet years in dry areas which seemed quite a possible influence on cartographic visual correlation (dry years in wet areas can be important, as in the epidemic in Sri Lanka in 1935, but did not seem to be relevant in our data set). Figure 10.12 is the simulation for 1975 for areas with over 20 per cent irrigated; regarded as the 'expected' map it may be compared with figure 10.10 of actual rates.

The findings were, as noted earlier, quite modest. Population density as such seems to be a negative or inhibiting factor; despite the increase in urban malaria, it remains overwhelmingly a rural disease. High proportions irrigated are also, and surprisingly to many people, an overall negative influence on malaria; this is despite the fact that locally, for instance, in the Rajasthan canal tract of new irrigation, it is very hard to believe that irrigation accompanied by over-watering and perhaps poor drainage, plays no part in the generally high API rates, characterized by Akhtar as 'stable malaria'. (For an African example of irrigated rice causing mosquito breeding, see Snow (1983).) From a general practice in New South Wales comes a confident report that the Ross River virus disease carried by culicine mosquitoes has increased with the introduction of flooded rice-paddies (Byrne 1984). Rainfall as such does not produce a simulation close to the actual rates, nor does tribal population as such produce a good simulation.

What of the failure to obtain data on wind influence, on wet years in dry areas, on local areas where irrigation *does* seem to be a factor, on tribal migration streams as possible influences on diffusion? Perhaps these

Figure 10.11 Simulated APIs by grid-square assuming only 'distance decay' from residual endemic foci of 1965
Source: Learmonth and Akhtar (1984)

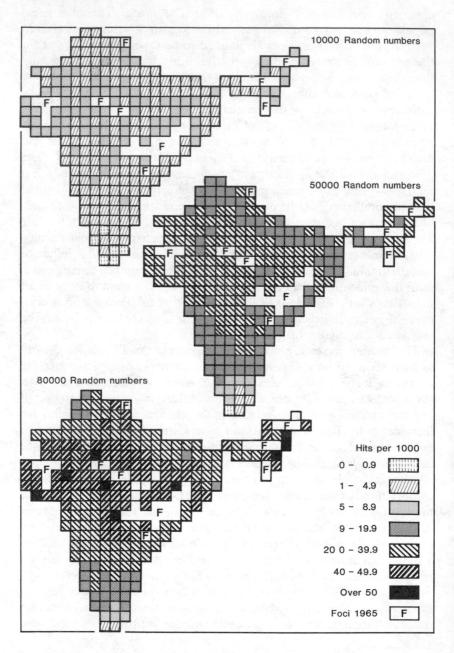

Figure 10.12 Simulated APIs by grid-square, assuming distance decay modified for areas with over or under 20 per cent irrigated to total area
Source: Learmonth and Akhtar (1984)

may point the way to future studies. It is significant that two recent Soviet studies of malaria in India stress the high rates of population mobility as affecting, for instance, the agewise incidence (Kondrashin 1983; Orlov et al. 1984). And from the All-India scale we very much hope that microscale studies of mosquito and human behaviour affecting contacts between people and mosquitoes will illume our meso-scale study.

Postscript: Malaria and Other Mosquito-borne Diseases

One of the local studies in India referred to earlier concerns the command area of a major irrigation dam at Sathanur on the Ponnaiyar river southwest of Madras (Hyma and Ramesh 1980). The present author and his collaborator in the studies of the malaria resurgence just cited were able to make a short trip to this already researched area in November 1981, with two colleagues. What follows is a summary of a paper flowing from that experience (Learmonth and Akhtar, in press).

We knew in advance that *falciparum* malaria would probably be encountered, and possibly in its chloroquine-resistant form; naturally we took appropriate precautions. Our main aim was to sharpen our ideas on possible collaborative and interdisciplinary research on contacts between people and mosquitoes, perhaps using a system of nested samples in order to link micro-scale studies with those at meso- and even macro-scale – a hope that so far has not materialized! A community of fisherfolk, the men fishing mainly at night in the reservoir above the dam were particularly severely affected, but agricultural villages and Harijan hamlets (of the formerly 'untouchable' people) were also affected. The malaria control authorities were active and reacting positively, and where appropriate attacking at more than one point. For instance systematic anti-larval treatment of the river below the dam was being done. We met with descriptions of people who seemed to have suffered from the cerebral form of *falciparum* malaria and met one young man recurrently affected by violent symptoms. I should add that all four in the party were geographers and we had no medically qualified researcher with us. As we visited four or five village communities and talked over glasses of buttermilk or tea, we heard of many cases of fever with violent cerebral symptoms, with a high death rate and more than a few young people left paralysed. On returning to Madras and consulting with geographical and medical colleagues we learned that what we had been hearing about was in all probability mainly Japanese encephalitis. (For a review of Japanese B encephalitis stimulated by a fatal case in an air traveller from Hong Kong to London see Gatus and Rose (1983).)

This is a mosquito-borne virus that is indeed commonly met and causes illness in Japan, mainly slight but sometimes severe; great efforts to control it have been made there, and an inoculation is available for which considerable protection is claimed. Its use in a cantonment in south-eastern Nepal is described in Henderson (1984); on the cycle in Japan, see Yamamoto (1981). The virus is primarily zoonotic, the main hosts in India being the fox and the pig – more intimately linked with human settlements, especially in South India the Harijan hamlets. On the role of pigs as 'amplifiers' of Japanese encephalitis, see Yoshida et al. (1981): this opens the possibility of immunization of pigs, not undertaken in Japan since the human disease is now rare (Sasaki et al. 1982). Birds are suspect as possible carriers of the virus across country. Its presence in India is thought to go back for only a decade or so; its progress across the country has been analysed from the biological viewpoint (Daschaudhuri 1980a) and the main vector identified as *Culex fatigans* (Latin, 'exhausting gnat'!), though certain *Aëdes* and the urban malaria vector *Anopheles stephensi* are capable of transmission. An epidemic in Raipur, Madhya Pradesh was focused on slums, on pig-keeping, and on urban ponds (Mathur et al. 1981); in Kolar district in southeastern Karnataka rice paddies are suspected; in an outbreak in Goa (Choudhury et al. 1983) the vector was *Culex tritaeniorhynchus* (roughly, 'three-tape-nosed'). See also, on Bihar, Kalimuddin et al. (1982a,b), Prasad et al. (1982) on Kolar in Karnataka, Khan et al. (1981) on a focus in Bangladesh.

Now *Aëdes* especially *A. aegypti* are the principal vectors of the dengue virus (and in Africa and the Americas of the urban yellow fever cycle), as noted briefly in chapter 9. As compared with *Anopheles* these culicine mosquitoes like *Culex* and *Aëdes* are able to use much more polluted water for egg-laying and the larval stage; at least organic pollution, even quite heavy, is tolerated, whereas *Anopheles* prefer clean even if still and perhaps stagnant water. Moreover *C. fatigans* is the main vector in India of the filariasis caused by *Wuchereria bancrofti*, one of the main causes of elephantiasis in India, locally a serious public health problem. A survey of over 2000 people twice yearly for four years in the Godavari delta area revealed 35 per cent infected and 21 per cent with acute or chronic disease (83 per cent in the lower extremities, 23 in the male genitals (Narasimham et al. 1983)). (The other is the similar *Brugia malayi*, named from Brug, a parasitologist, carried by *Mansonia* mosquitoes.) The filariases are also briefly noted in chapter 9; a recent estimate is that 220 million rural and 80 million urban people in India are at risk, with 16 million overt cases (Sharma et al. 1983). For a view of the spread of filariasis in Sri Lanka by an eminent German biogeographer, see Schweinfurth (1984).

It is now clear that if *Anopheles* are eradicated, their ecological niche is filled. Sometimes other species of *Anopheles* appear from unsprayed sites, as in Sardinia following the apparently total eradication of *Anopheles*. Sometimes another vector species becomes dominant, as in our Cameroon example, or as noted earlier for Assam. One possible biological control is deliberately to fill the ecological niche with *Anopheles* species that are known not to carry malaria. (A comparable technique to the release of large numbers of male mosquitoes sterilized by irradiation or by chemicals, sufficient to swamp the natural, fertile males. For a recent Soviet review of this topic see Zakharova (1983).) Some studies of the changing proportions of different genera and species of mosquito in India are available, including one on Calcutta (Daschaudhuri 1978, 1980a,b).

The present author has suggested with some support from a biomedical scientist (Diesfeld 1978) that one reason why the classic regional pattern of malaria in India has *not* been re-established, notably in West Bengal, may be that culicine mosquitoes have occupied many of the ecological niches formerly occupied by malaria vectors like *A. philippinenses*. Similarly it may be that in many of the densely peopled parts of India organic pollution of water-bodies favours the areal spread of dominance by the culicines, especially if *Anopheles* have been drastically reduced by the anti-malaria operations. Another possibility, of course, is the return of some species of *Anopheles* after an interval: to take a parallel case, the *Leishmaniasis* (Kala-azar) cycle involving sandflies (see chapter 9), *Phlebotomus argentipes*, having retreated under the impact of the DDT campaigns against malaria, returned in the 1970s to West Bengal and Bihar, causing a quite severe epidemic (ICMR 1983). Thus the considerable complex of diseases associated with the culicines and *Mansonia*, Japanese encephalitis, dengue and certain filariases, may tend to extend and perhaps become proportionately more important over much of the country. Already national bodies concerned with research and prevention of mosquito-borne disease have responded to the problem to a limited extent, but not so far with the confident and crusading zeal of the anti-malaria programme of the heady days of the mid-1950s (Raghavan 1955, 1957). Accepting malaria as the chief problem, some leading authorities put all their faith in the perfection of a malaria vaccine suitable for mass prophylaxis, and this indeed is devoutly to be hoped for. For reviews see WHO (1984c); Hope et al. (1984). The conquest of malaria by a vaccine need *not* of course leave vacant ecological niches for mosquitoes other than *Anopheles* to occupy. However, this lies in the future, and even if an effective vaccine becomes available the role of mosquito-borne diseases is likely to remain great. Biological and ecological methods of arthropod control are by no means dead or necessarily out-dated (see

Laird and Miles 1983; on the possibilities of a microbial larvicide such as *Bacillus sphaericus*, see WHO (1985)). There seems to remain a major role for biogeographical research on interlocking scales, perhaps by a system of nested samples, including both the biogeography of several mosquito genera and the patterns of human activities that expose them to risks of providing blood-meals to stimulate oviposition in gravid female mosquitoes. Ultimately the defeat of malaria and other arthropod-borne diseases will come from holistic or society-wide strategies or from changes in the society that make the people much more able to control their environment for themselves. It is interesting that the first in an important series of papers from USSR on malaria in South Asia concentrates on an account of societal elements, some of which are certainly direct factors in the resurgence, such as the effect of the 'Green Revolution' on increasing landless labour in some areas, population migration and mobility, including rapid urbanization, and their effects on the agewise incidence, deforestation and so on (Kondrashin 1983; Orlov et al. 1984). On neighbouring countries, see de Zulueta et al. (1980) on Pakistan; on Nepal Gramiccia (1981) and Sakya (1981); on Sri Lanka Dutt and Dutta (1985), Wickramasinghe (1981).

Conclusion

Looking back over this chapter, the sources drawn on are particularly selective from the vast literature dealing with malaria, and biased towards India and the author's own work. The interlocking cycles of mosquitoes, malaria parasites, and people involve complex and innumerable permutations, inviting geographical work on both the biogeographical and the social geography of the whole disease complex in its regional variations. A privileged few, but too few, geographers have been involved in team work on problems of malaria control. The chapter may have pointed to some pathways for future work, ideally of course action research, and opened some doors to the rich stores of knowledge – yet with yawning gaps – that should inform both the seeker after, say, a perspective on the population geography of a malarious area, or the committed researcher on the geography of malaria. It may well prove, however, that the anecdotal final paragraphs about interactions between the malaria cycle and other mosquito-borne diseases are a main growth point in the coming decades. If, as some authorities expect, an effective malaria vaccine is perfected in the next few years, then any spadework on the ecological geography of mosquito vectors and host populations will remain of continuing value, if only in relation to other mosquito-borne diseases.

11 The Schistosomiases

Introductory

The schistosomiasis group of fluke infections have been outlined in chapter 9 as a three-factor complex of world importance as a cause of debility, chronic illness and loss of efficiency and production (on the loss of well-being and physical output, see Awad el Karim et al. (1981); on the impact of development, see Prescott (1979)): there is the pathogen *Schistosoma* spp., the alternate host in aquatic or amphibious snails of several genera, and people wading, bathing or working in water polluted with urine (for *S. haematobium*) or faeces (*for S.mansoni, S.japonica* and *S.intercalatum*). (For a major treatise on snail-transmitted diseases in general, see Malek (1980), and for a bench-mark bibliography series, Hoffman and Warren (1978).) As two more 'One World' reminders, the skin eruption called 'swimmers' itch' in North America is a schistosomiasis, and the subject of a classic piece of medical geography (Jarcho and van Burkalow 1952); it also has water-snails as alternate hosts, but the main hosts are waterfowl and possibly muskrats. So it is an example of a zoonosis, with human infection as an accident – and a dead end for the life cycle of the particular schistosome. And in a broad survey of schistosomes in the countries around the Mediterranean, McCullough and Combes (1982) interestingly link the human and bovine cycles – the bovine found farther north than the human. A major treatise is in Jordan and Webb (1982a). Iarotski and Davis (1981) suggest 1–2 per cent are treated of 500 million cases (excluding China).

The Rich Literature

In the main human diseases, contacts between human excreta and water, and between the human skin and polluted water, clearly involve patterns of daily living – working in water, including wading to fill water-pots, washing clothes, bathing and swimming and so on. Irrigation and its extension in ways that offer new habitats to the snail hosts have a large literature on their own, mainly from Sudan and Egypt, and in recent years from the Lake Volta area (see for instance Coates and Redding-Coates (1981); F.D. Miller et al. (1981) and comment by Sturrock (1982d); Mansour et al. (1981); Fenwick et al. (1981); and on labour and labour migration as a factor Bella et al. (1980); Cheesmond (1980), Fenwick et al. (1982).

A major monograph on the management of schistosomiasis from a WHO scientist is in Rosenfield (1979): a model was evolved for St Lucia in the West Indies for selection of a cost-effective and practicable strategy from the options available, taking into account environmental changes accompanying economic development and the behavioural aspect of people's contacts with the cercariae in snail-infested water. This model was then applied to an irrigation project in Iran, with appropriate modifications for a different environment, where the recommended strategy was for a combination of engineering controls and chemotherapy, using mainly mollusciciding for maintenance. See also Rosenfield et al. (1977). The management technique is then applied to the Volta Lake development in Ghana where it is estimated that its adoption would not add excessively to the project costs while adding considerably to the people's well-being. WHO Technical Report 643 (1980) is also germane. Targetted mass chemotherapy, along with other measures against the disease cycle, is regarded as a main control: an apparent failure reported from Lubile, Zaïre, has been disputed as evidence that the approach is an ineffective control measure (Polderman and Manshande 1981; Jordan 1981). Integration of the various ways of breaking the disease cycle is also stressed in several recent publications, though some workers also stress that mass chemotherapy *after* examination is often cost-effective, as against blanket chemotherapy of total population. Mott and Cline (1980) review advances in quantitative epidemiology, and Davis (1984) stresses that planning control projects should be area-specific and calls for knowledge of five aspects of the local disease ecology: human prevalence, incidence and intensity rates, parasite strains, intermediate hosts, ecological backgrounds and human behavioural factors. Cross et al. (1984) use an example from the Leyte/Samar area of the Philippines to show how a probability map for schistosomiasis uses weather data and Landsat images. A review of biological control methods of the snail intermediate hosts is in McCullough (1981); see also Nasir (1981) and Combes (1982).

A symposium on schistosomiasis in the Sudan was largely concerned with *S.bovis* in cattle (*Trans. Roy. Soc. Trop. Med. and Hyg.* 1980):

however it is important in demonstrating that cattle can acquire resistance to the infection; possibilities of vaccines were also discussed. See also Hillyer (1981). The French literature includes some environmentally sensitive papers, among geographers, for instance, Doumenge et al. (1983) and a series of papers on Africa and the Caribbean in the same publication; by biomedical workers like Foba-Pagou et al. (1980), Nozais et al. (1980, 1981) on forest–savannah contrasts, and White et al. (1982) on swamp rice in Sierra Leone – its exoneration being queried by Sturrock (1982b). See also Petit et al. (1982) for a regional ecology of bilharzia in Madagascar.

Cost-effectiveness of chemotherapy as against mollusciciding is thought to vary with the local ecology: see Polderman (1984) on experience, on the whole favouring chemotherapy, among tin-mining labourers and their families in eastern Zaïre. Thus the whole disease complex is one that cries out for analysis using, amongst other approaches, the perspective that in this book is termed ecological medical geography and on several scales (Rée 1982). Zhao (1981) writes of arcal correspondence and a possible link between *S.japonica* and colon cancer in China.

Geographical Dimensions

The scale of the world problem is so vast as to demand international as well as interdisciplinary research, or, better, action research, rather than individual academic studies, and there are indeed WHO projects. Some include geographers in project teams, but nearly all the major reports include some geoecological insights of interest to geographers. I shall try to indicate some of these insights from macro-scale projects before citing some examples of geographical research, usually on meso- or micro-scale. A recent review article by two geographers (Weil and Kvale 1985), however, is so comprehensive that I shall quote comparatively few complementary biomedical references especially since it is in the widely available *Geographical Review*: it is clearly required reading for any student interested in the schistosomiases. See also Kloos and Thompson (1979); Kloos et al. (1982).

Figure 11.1 is a world map of the several forms of schistosomiasis taken from a study on that scale (Rée 1977; Doumenge 1984). As Rée points out, bilharzia has been traced in an Egyptian mummy before 1000 BC; and while the cause was established by Bilharz in 1851, the cycle of the disease clarified in 1915, and an effective treatment introduced in 1918, this is one of the few communicable diseases increasing in prevalence throughout the tropical and sub-tropical world. From the tartar emetic injections of 1918 onwards the search for a therapeutic or

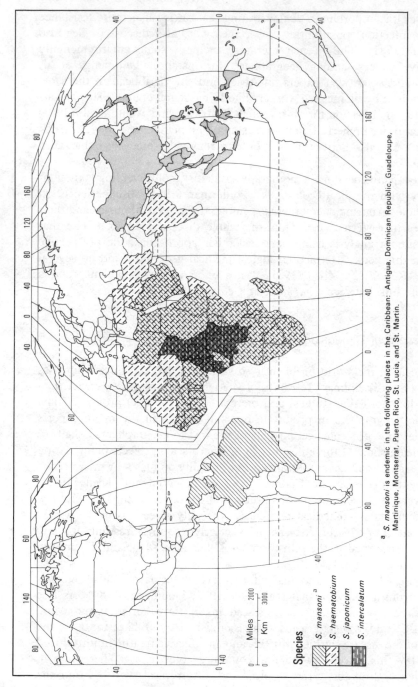

Figure 11.1 World map of the three important forms of schistosomiasis
Source: Rée (1977); Well and Kuale (1985)

a *S. mansoni* is endemic in the following places in the Caribbean: Antigua, Dominican Republic, Guadeloupe, Martinique, Montserrat, Puerto Rico, St. Lucia, and St. Martin.

Species

S. mansoni [a]
S. haematobium
S. japonicum
S. intercalatum

Miles 0 __ 2000
Km 0 140 __ 3000

prophylactic drug suitable for mass use has met with many difficulties and setbacks (Rée 1977). It has been regarded as neglected by geographers (Kvale 1981), and yet in many ways it calls for geographical analysis. There are climatic controls on the snail: thus for *Bulinus* for instance optimum water temperature is between 20°C and 33°C while below and above that range both snail and schistosome development are restricted. Relatively permanent and slow-moving water favours the snail, as does organic pollution (as near human settlements). On the other hand salinity of even as low as 0.16 per cent inhibits the snail population. Temperature – given suitable water – is discussed in relation to different species of schistosome in Pitchford (1981). Snails are believed to be susceptible to local strains of the schistosome but resistant to non-local strains, perhaps through antibody development. In humans, the disease has a predilection for children and young adults. While the cycles are clearly linked with poor disposal of faeces and urine, for the intestinal and bladder diseases respectively, their behavioural links are much more complex: irrigation and man-made lakes often encourage snail breeding, and also movement of people carrying the pathogens, while sparsely peopled areas and natural water-courses seem to be associated with less severe disease, probably owing to less intense transmission (Davey and Lightbody 1956).

Man-made Lakes

Several world surveys complement that of Rée already cited, particularly in emphasizing the role of man-made lakes and man-made disease including schistosomiasis. Two WHO workers offered a timely if too little regarded warning as long ago as 1971, when the effects were already becoming obvious of large water impoundments such as Lake Kariba on the Zambezi, Kainji on the Niger, Nasser on the Nile, and Volta in Ghana, while even in Africa alone others were in prospect such as those behind the Kossou Dam in the Ivory Coast, the Cabora Dassa Dam in Mozambique and the Tafilalet Dam in Morocco (Brown and Deom 1973). In south-western Iran the dam on the Dez river is near a known focus of bilharzia, and plans were envisaged to prevent its spread to the irrigation system below the dam. In Latin America dams planned for the São Francisco valley in Brazil were regarded as carrying risks of snail-borne (and mosquito-borne) disease and in Asia the great Mekong project, since disrupted by war. The section on schistosomiasis is worth quoting in part here:

> Schistosomiasis is essentially a 'water-based' disease, since it is dependent on an aquatic organism, namely, the snail intermediate

host, for a part of its transmission cycle. This serious debilitating disease affects over 200 million people. The prevalence of the infection is nearly always enhanced by the impoundment of water in made-made lakes and by the irrigation systems frequently associated with them. Irrigation systems have long been known as areas of schistosomiasis insofar as they increase the availability of water and consequent human contact with it; it is now becoming apparent that the man-made lakes themselves produce similar deleterious effects.

It is important to emphasize that the definitive host, man, is responsible for the dissemination of schistosomiasis by contaminating the aquatic environment, where he in turn becomes infected. The snail is only a passive intermediate host. Therefore, for the epidemiology and control of schistosomiasis, consideration must necessarily be given to the ecology of the human as well as to that of the snail hosts.

Where schistosomiasis is prevalent, a man-made lake is likely to present a considerable hazard for lake users, including the increasing numbers of fishermen and lakeside settlers who may come from schistosomiasis-free regions. It may also seriously jeopardize the health of the resettled population displaced by the impoundment. In Lake Kariba, transmission of both urinary and intestinal schistosomiasis has been demonstrated in limited foci, where the respective snail intermediate hosts *Bulinus (Physopsis) africanus* and *Biomphalaria pfeifferi* are associated with mats of the water fern *Salvinia auriculata*. In 1968, a decade after completion of the dam, the prevalence of *Schistosoma mansoni* was observed to be 16% among all age groups, whereas that of *S. haematobium* among children reached a mean of 69%. It is therefore vitally important that the presently focal transmission of schistosomiasis be contained.

In the vast Volta drainage area some 20 years ago the prevalence of schistosomiasis was low, the aquatic ecological conditions being generally unfavorable for the snail intermediate hosts. It was, however, predicted that on the west side of the future lake a number of areas might become ideal breeding grounds for *Bulinus* and *Biomphalaria* snails. In 1967–1968 a sharp rise in the transmission of *S. haematobium* occurred in lakeside communities because of enormous densities of *Bulinus truncatus rohlfsi*, developing principally in association with the weed *Ceratophyllum*. Specimens of *B. (Physopsis) globosus* have been found only recently in one location on the lake, although this species is the most numerous and widely distributed intermediate host of *S. haematobium* throughout west Africa, including Ghana. *Biomphalaria pfeifferi* has not been collected from Volta Lake, but it is expected that the species may be found, particularly in the northern part of the lake. Although one authority has stated that the prevalence rates of *S. haematobium* will drop in conjunction with an observed decline in the number of bulinid snails in certain places, a recent limited survey indicated that transmission of the parasite by *B. truncatus rohlfsi* is focally intense and may become more widespread with the possible development of even more favorable aquatic vegetation for snails, such as that that would be afforded by *Potamogeton* or *Nymphaea*, both of which occur in Ghana. This apparent conflict of opinion regarding transmission may only be a reflection of the seasonal fluctuation in snail densities and concomitant infections and certainly underlines the need for careful longitudinal epidemiologic studies in the area as a whole.

In Kainji Lake, the snail intermediate hosts of both *S. haematobium* and *S. mansoni* are now in evidence, and transmission of the parasites in settled areas is taking place, the mean prevalence rates of the two schistosome infections in 1970 being 31 and 1.8%. These observations, made 2 years after closure of the dam, also established that the snails were still confined to scattered foci.

In Lake Nasser, transmission of *S. haematobium* takes place around the entire perimeter as a consequence of the large colonies of *B. truncatus* present on algae-covered rock surfaces. No species of *Biomphalaria* have been found in the lake. An inevitable increase in transmission of *S. haematobium* and perhaps *S. mansoni* is predictable in relation to the development of irrigated area supplied from the lake.

Available evidence from the major man-made impoundments in Africa therefore clearly indicates that transmission of schistosomiasis is taking place in the main body of every lake as well as in the existing irrigation works. Despite the attempts to provide alternative water supplies in some resettlement villages, contamination of the environment through domestic, occupational, and recreational contacts by the new settlement and resettlement populations has resulted in new and increased transmission patterns in Africa.

Thus the containment and abatement of schistosomiasis calls for management of the impounded water by means of shoreline sanitation, education of the human population to improve its habits in disposing wastes and excreta, and sanitary engineering to minimize the contacts between man and lake water. These measures are particularly important in view of the impossibility of applying molluscicides over an entire lake to control the snail populations chemically.

(Brown and Deom 1973, pp. 757–8)

This paper has down-to-earth qualities remarkable in view of its wide coverage, and includes sections on resettlement of population displaced by man-made lakes, health protection during dam construction, administrative desiderata for public health in such projects, and of course covers many other diseases associated with water.

Hunter (1981a) also points out that the story of schistosomiasis in Upper Ghana may have been related to dam construction in the early 1960s, and that history is probably about to repeat itself with a new wave of agricultural dam building, again without built-in anti-bilharzia measures. On possible monitoring techniques, see Oomen (1981).

The long-term health survey in the Malumfashi area of Nigeria has produced a number of geographically useful papers on schistosomiasis, including a survey covering the disease (Pugh et al. 1981), a study of the effect of water conservation measures in increasing transmission (Pugh et al. 1980a, b), and one on water-contact activities in new small reservoirs – fishing, bathing, swimming and playing in water, being main contacts especially by boys and in the afternoon at a peak time for cercarial activity (Tayo et al. 1980).

A recent paper on policy issues concerning man-made lakes is by authors from geography, parasitology and project management on behalf of the United Nations/WHO project on schistosomiasis (J.M. Hunter et al. 1982). They make the point that schistosomiasis can act as a marker or indicator for a group of diseases including malaria and filariases, indeed that in a more or less predictable sequence a much larger group of infections including vector-borne and social diseases from venereal diseases to child diarrhoeas and malnutrition can follow large development projects, desirable as these may be. In Latin America these authors see the Parana–Paraquay basin projects as carrying considerable risks of increased malaria, leishmaniasis and yellow fever, but also increased schistosomiasis since endemic foci already exist in the region. In the São Francisco basin in Brazil schistosomiasis is a high risk, followed by yellow fever and kala-azar – and possibly plague which is still present in the area. The coming Amazon basin impoundment projects carry risks of increase in yellow fever, malaria, leishmaniasis, filariases, onchocerciasis and hookworm and bowel worm parasitism, and no doubt schistosomiasis also; the Tucurui dam project already demonstrates the likely trends. The pressures of population increase and rising expectations too, particularly in the Third World, imply inexorable pressure towards increased water impoundment mainly for irrigation, and data, admittedly imperfect, are assembled to show the extent of the 'future shock' and the need for holistic ecological assessment of what must rank as one of the major problems of Planet Earth in the next few decades.

Is India almost Bilharzia-free?

On the meso-scale a review of the evidence for bilharzia endemicity in India by a biomedical worker is challenging (Anantaraman 1984). There are reports of *S. haematobium* infection from Gimvi in coastal Maharashtra over the past 65 years – with a different indigenous vector *Ferrissia tenuis* – and the author regards this as the best-established record from India. The 30-year old report from Gimvi has been re-investigated (Sathe et al. 1981): water supplies had been improved in the hope of eliminating the problem, but low levels of prevalence seemed to persist and still with *Ferrissia tenuis* as alternate host – a freshwater limpet, also in the *Gasteropoda*, several species of snails (and possible animal hosts too) proving negative. There are reports from elsewhere – Delhi, Madurai in the south-east, Raipur in middle India, and a suggestion that *S. japonicum* may exist in eastern parts of the country. The infection seems to have come in from Africa and the Middle East, perhaps from early Persian settlers on the coast, more likely from Indian troops returning from campaigns in Africa and the Middle East in the two world wars, or from West African troops in the later years of the 1939–45 war. There are thought to be at least four snails suitable as alternate hosts of the schistosomes. The traditional ways of washing and bathing, laundering clothes etc. clearly favour the disease cycle, on evidence from Gimvi, and both detailed studies and action there seem to be justified. If the reasons for the comparative freedom of India from the disease can be established, they may well prove crucial in understanding the disease in ways useful in other areas, and for India, if any of the forms of it show signs of invading and spreading in the country.

Studies in Puerto Rico and the Caribbean

Still on the meso-scale, though for a smaller country, a study of Puerto Rico concerns the disease cycle of *S. mansoni*, the snail *Biomphalaria glabrata* (Latin *glaber*, 'smooth-skinned') (Haddock 1981). It is commoner in the more humid east of the island, and in the alluvial lowlands of the north and south coast, preferred by people and snails, rather than in the interior limestone and oldland (ancient rocks) plateaus. The route of excreted eggs from people to water is through defaecation on stream-banks, the placing of latrines within seeping distance of streams, and in extreme cases the use of streams as open sewers; the contact of the mobile larvae after maturing in the snail from water to and through human skin is through activities like swimming and bathing, wading and – quite important – washing clothes. *S.mansoni* was discovered on the island in 1904, and after various surveys a Bilharzia Control Unit established in the Department of Health in 1953. During the 1960s the useful but limited method of sampling using specimens of faeces was replaced by the intradermal skin test using schistosome antigen, and prevalence has declined from 12 per cent in 1963 to 5 per cent in 1976: figures 11.2 (a), (b) and (c) show – by catchment areas rather than by isopleths of prevalence – the retreat from 1963 to 1969 to 1976, in fact to a position regarded as on the brink of control. So far snail control has played a major role in the campaign against the disease, concurrently with encouragement of better sanitation and discouragement of insanitary practices. Chemotherapy in the human hosts, and molluscicides too, have been used in only a limited way, largely because they are expensive, and two 'biological' methods of control have achieved considerable success. 'Biological' methods, by convention, involve devices like drainage of snail habitats – avoiding the creation of fresh ones for this or some other vector! – or various other ways of tilting the ecological equilibrium against the snail population including introducing other animals preying on some stage of the snail. First, a carnivorous snail introduced from South America in the 1950s, *Marisa cornuarietis*, has proved able to control the

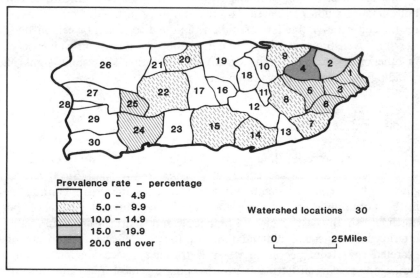

Figure 11.2 (a)   Schistosomiasis in Puerto Rico, 1963
Source: Haddock (1981)

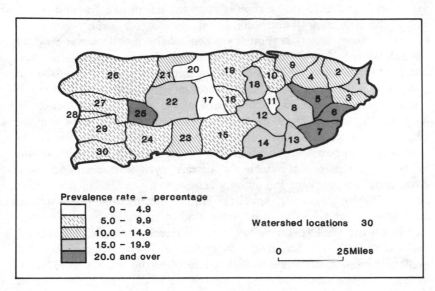

Figure 11.2 (b)   Schistosomiasis in Puerto Rico, 1969
Source: Haddock (1981)

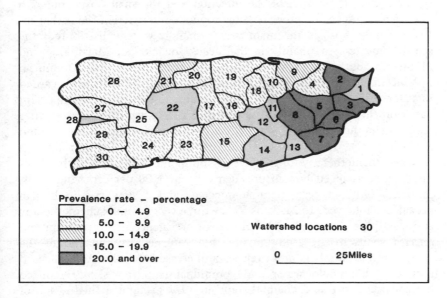

Figure 11.2 (c)   Schistosomiasis in Puerto Rico, 1976
Source: Haddock (1981)

vector snail in the 16 major reservoirs of the island at a fraction of the cost of chemical control; and second, a guppy minnow, *Lebistes reticulatus* (Latin *reticulum*, a net) is thought to control the mobile larval stage of the schistosome – and also to eat mosquito larvae. An abstract and critique by Sturrock (1982c) adds that a competitor snail *Tarebio (Thiara) granifera* was introduced, deliberately or accidentally, in the last 30 years. (*Marisa cornuarietus* has been introduced into a dam on a sisal estate in northern Tanzania (Nguma et al. 1982), rather against scientific opinion that the ecological consequences had not been adequately explored). As total control appears within grasp, the future strategy raises important issues on the points at which the disease cycle can best and most economically be broken: the authors believe that the human population affected is now sufficiently small that the campaign can now switch to chemotherapy at a cost of only one-seventh of that involved in further attacks on the snail adequate to attain nationwide control. A historical study of the South Coast irrigation system in Puerto Rico shows that small overnight storage reservoirs used early in the project were major harbours for the snail host and the prevalence in children in the town of Guyama soon rose to 25 per cent. Later parts of the project did not use these night stores, had better drainage and avoided the problem. Control measures from 1954 reduced child prevalence to nil by 1966 (Jobin 1978). A general review of *S.mansoni* in the Caribbean is in Bundy (1984), covering the distribution of the infection and the snail hosts, but also discussing primate and other possible zoonotic reservoirs of the pathogen. In the lesser Antilles the main vector snail is widely distributed, the schistosome less so, mainly in St Lucia, Guadeloupe, Martinique and Montserrat but with high potential for spread to Antigua, Dominica, St Vincent and Grenada. Barbados, St Maarten and St Kitts are regarded as at low risk because of factors unfavourable to the snail. An important paper on three areas in St Lucia concerns the return of *S.mansoni* after mass chemotherapy even with effective modern drugs (Prentice and Barnish 1981). The areas had different regimes. In Sulphur Springs repeated chemotherapy for three years and mollusciciding until the snails disappeared reduced human prevalence by over 90 per cent, but snails returned within a year, became infected, and a slow rise in human prevalence followed. In Marquis Valley three years' annual chemotherapy and standpipes for water reduced human prevalence by 70 per cent and *infected* snails disappeared initially, but returned by the end of the campaign and numbers and prevalence increased sharply. At Blanchard individual household water and communal laundries slowly reduced human prevalence and chemotherapy in 1977 brought a further fall of 60 per cent; there was a sharp fall in infected snails but an increase to pre-chemotherapy levels within two years but with steady human prevalence rates. Repeated and integrated measures are still essential. Improved domestic water supplies are thought crucial in maintaining schistosomiasis control, though vigilance against child infections will be needed (Jordan et al. 1982b; Jordan 1985).

Micro-scale Studies in Ethiopia

A paper on the Awash valley east of Addis Abbaba combines meso-scale studies of the valley (about 700 by 150–450 km) with micro-scale work on individual irrigated farms (Kloos 1985). The valley was formerly sparsely peopled by five semi-nomadic pastoralist groups, the Jile, Arsi, Kercyu and Ittu Oromo, and also the Afar who in addition had some irrigated agriculture based on simple basin flooding. Figure 11.3 (a) shows the valley divided, following the author, into the upper, middle and lower valley, the high dams Koka I (1960) and Koka II (1966), and the main irrigated farms.

Before the irrigation projects, the nomads of the middle valley were known to suffer from *S. haematobium*, as one of only three endemic foci of that cycle in Ethiopia; the valley is believed to have been free of *S. mansoni*, since even now its alternative host *B. pfeifferi* is absent from natural streams, swamps and stock ponds, and it seems to have come into the area with migrant labour from highland areas endemic for *Mansoni* to specific irrigation farms. Indeed *Mansoni* has spread from such farms to nomads in contact with them in new patterns of stock-watering following irrigation. Figure 11.3 (b) shows the recent picture of *B. pfeifferi*, the *Mansoni* vector, while figure 11.3 (c) shows the prevalence rates in migrant labour and indigenous pastoralists. Figure 11.3 (d) and (e) show the position in two commercial irrigation farms, one for bananas and one for cotton. In contrast, the map of *S. haematobium*, not reproduced here, still shows the main concentration in the middle valley. Mapping of other species of snail was carried out and risks assessed of the introduction of strains of schistosome compatible with some of these, and surveys made of water-plants congenial to the snails, and age and sex division of labour among the people in relation to risks of infection. Thus women and children gathering food plants were more at risk then men and boys engaged in cattle-herding.

Control schemes are envisaged as multi-pronged or integrated, necessarily so in view of the complexities in a catchment now dominated by irrigation, and involving local communities including health officials, engineers, farmers and pastoralists. This development is seen as entirely compatible with the emphasis on primary health care and devolution of health services under the socialist government's first ten-year plan. The

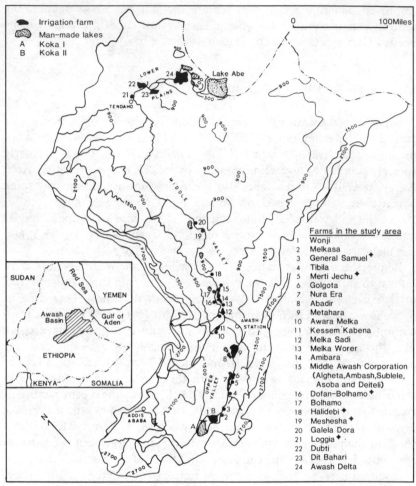

Figure 11.3 (a)   Schistosomiasis in the Awash valley, Ethiopia
Source: Kloos (1985)

emphasis varies in different parts of a large catchment, here by drying out irrigation canals between waterings, there by molluscicides (some from local plants, some synthetic compounds), and where appropriate by chemotherapy, by biological control (as in the Puerto Rico study cited above), and by improved water supplies and sanitation. Health education is seen as limited in value, simply because both forms of schistosomiasis are largely occupational diseases, and particular problems are encountered

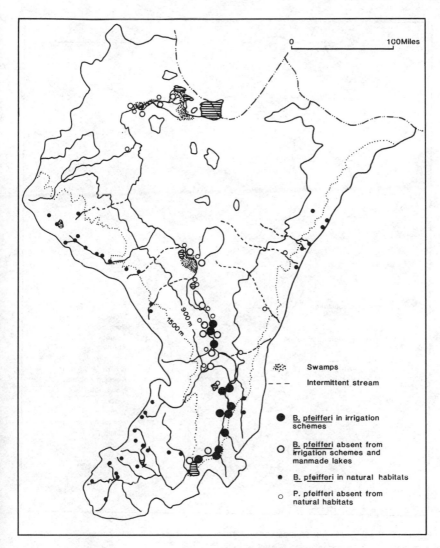

Figure 11.3 (b)   Snail vectors in the Awash valley, Ethiopia
Source: Kloos (1985)

with nomadic groups, especially the Afar, in establishing contact at all, and in maintaining it, e.g. for chemotherapy, where it has been achieved.

Kloos pleads the imperative need for such detailed ecological insights to complement broader mapping exercises, and his paper lends strong support to his plea.

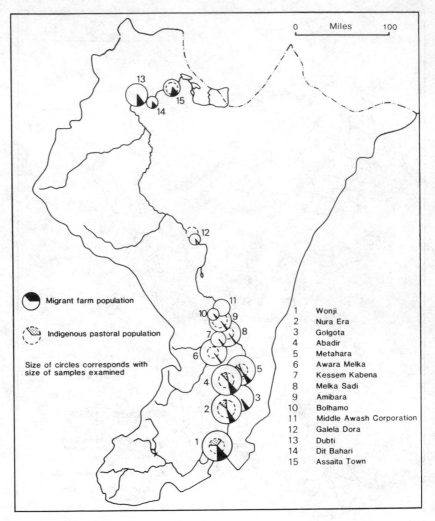

Figure 11.3 (c) Schistosomiasis prevalence in the Awash valley, Ethiopia, in relation to migrant labour and nomadic pastoralists
Source: Kloos (1985)

A Small Town in Brazil

A study from Brazil is primarily a micro-scale study of a new focus in a small but rapidly growing town, Pentecoste, in the north-east of the country and north-west of Recife (Kvale 1981): however it also links up

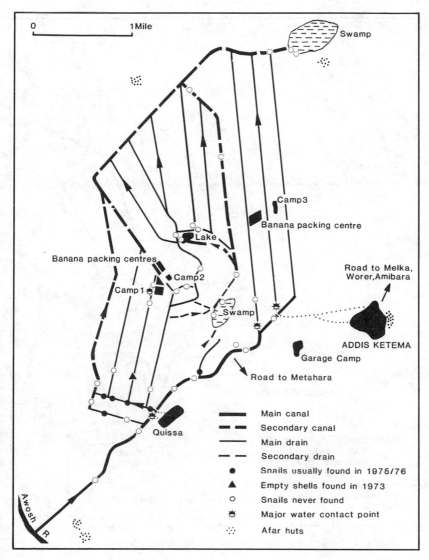

Figure 11.3 (d)   Schistosomiasis on a banana farm, Awash valley, Ethiopia
Source: Kloos (1985)

with much broader meso-scale material, even macro-scale in view of Brazil's sub-continental proportions and problems.

Figure 11.4 (a) shows patterns of diffusion of schistosomiasis in Brazil over the last 65 years. The endemic focus in the eastern shoulder of the country is at least some centuries old: it is believed to have been

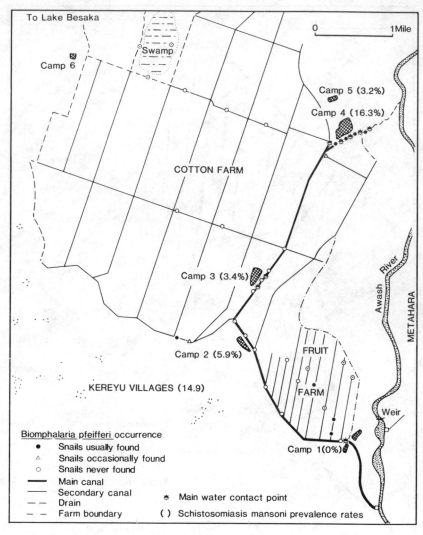

Figure 11.3 (e) Schistosomiasis on a cotton farm, Awash valley, Ethiopia
Source: Kloos (1985)

introduced along with slaves from Africa, finding an alternate host in local snail populations, and a congenial social environment in plantations for sugar and poor slave, then labour, housing. On migration and schistosomiasis, including its move from Africa to the Americas, see Brooks and Colley (1976) and Bousfield (1979). Slow expansion from Pernambuco and Bahia from, say, 1600 to 1800 with migrating people,

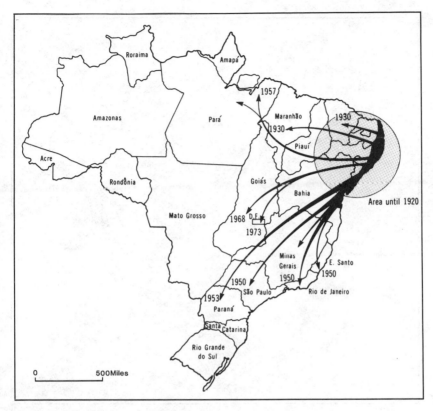

Figure 11.4 (a)   Diffusion of schistosomiasis in Brazil
Source: Kvale (1981)

was followed by the more rapid diffusion indicated as the *nordestinos* moved across the country in search of better living conditions. A 1977 map shows areas of high and low endemicity, and isolated foci (figure 11.4 (b), and figure 11.4 (c) the distribution of the three main *Biomphalaria* species of alternate hosts for the schistosomes, each with slightly differing ecological preferences. A locally important irrigation project is centred 4 km north of the town while the dam and reservoir lie on its south-western outskirts, and much of the population growth, from under 1000 in 1950 to almost 10000 in 1970, is due to employment on the project and its multiplier effects in the local agricultural and service economy.

Figure 11.4 (d) shows the town plan, along with several crucial factors: the reservoir and canal, the river and its associated creeks, and stagnant puddles found in housing areas near the creeks, are all congenial to the local snail alternate host *B. straminea* but of varying importance in the

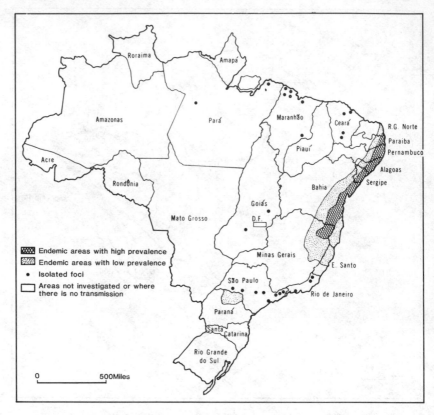

Figure 11.4 (b)   Schistosomiastis endemicity in Brazil
Source: Kvale (1981)

disease cycle, along with socioeconomic factors studied by sample survey. Sanitation is generally poor, and patches of ground along all these water-bodies are commonly used for defaecation, and near houses for dumping night-soil. Prevalence rates rose through childhood to over 30 per cent in older boys and young men, and to over 16 per cent in older girls and young women, tailing off in older age groups in both sexes. The young men bathe and swim for recreation in the reservoir, river and canal more than the young women and girls, and are also liable to prolonged exposure to infected water during agricultural work. The mobile larvae are more active between 10 a.m. and 4 p.m., and bathing or work then carries high risks: this includes a major source of infection in females, washing clothes in the river, creeks or the stagnant pools. Households with septic tank sewerage are less, but not significantly less, infected than people

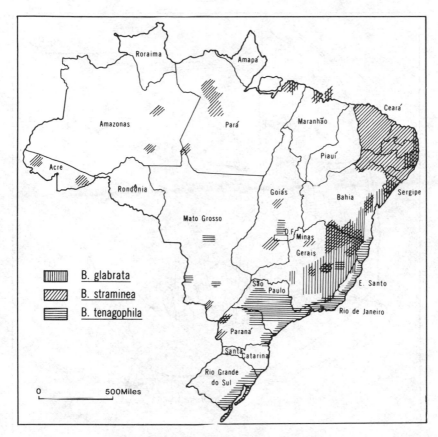

Figure 11.4 (c)   Snail vectors in Brazil
Source: Kvale (1981) (after W.L. Paraense)

without facilities, and the whole picture is one of a town where the changes brought by irrigation and mushroom growth with very poor hygiene, have brought a new focus of the disease, though the author is properly cautious about blaming the irrigation project in the absence of comparative studies with other settlements.

Other recent papers on schistosomiasis in Brazil include: a general review with maps by Barata (1981); an account of mollusciciding five sugar farms near Pernambuco, with two untreated as controls, leading to a conclusion that mollusciciding alone would be too costly as a strategy for north-east Brazil as a whole (Barbosa and Costa 1981); and a study of reinfection among poor people in the Belo Horizonte area north of Rio de Janeiro suggesting contacts with poor hygiene and the general

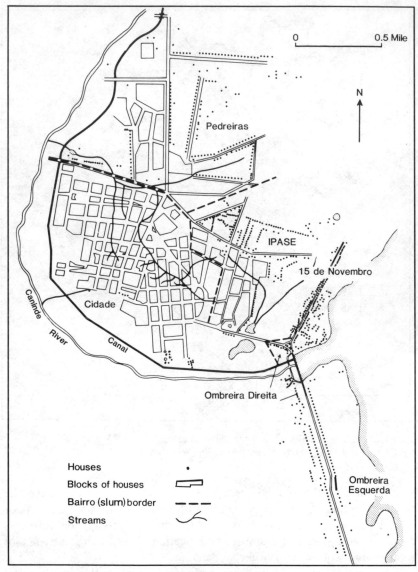

Figure 11.4 (d)   Town plan of Pentecosta
Source: Kvale (1981)

environment rather than that in or immediately around the home (Costa et al. 1980), chemotherapy having been avoided. A molluscicide campaign in a relatively prosperous and cooperative community at Boqueron brought a rapid fall in prevalence, incidence and intensity, then stability.

New Foci in Rwanda

An example of two recently developed foci apparently in retreat in high lakes in Rwanda's volcanic terrain is discussed by Gotanègre (1984): Lake Bulera lies at 1862 m above sea-level, lake Ruhondo at 1764 m, and endemicity is concentrated near the lakes, rapid and stony streams on the volcanic slopes being unfavourable to the water-snail and a campaign against the disease is producing a reduction in prevalence. The cycle is thought to have been introduced by migrant labourers from Zaïre working on a hydroelectric project, bringing in S. Mansoni (*Biomphalaria pfeifferi* being already present in the lakes); migrant Rwandese labourers returning from mines in Zaïre or plantations in Uganda are thought a less likely source in relation to the apparently recent growth of the disease. The author shows how pressure of population has led to more lakeside settlement, and brings out the significance of different economic activities: fishing, turf-cutting for pyrethrum-drying, cutting willow and papyrus for thatch and grain-drying platforms, and obtaining lake water for commercial manufacture of banana cider and cereal beer. While the health authorities have been pressing for widespread use of hygienic privies, that campaign meets with difficulties from old habits, particularly among the older people, and mass education and chemotherapy are thought to have achieved the significant reduction in prevalence from 6.5 per cent in 1980 to 2.9 per cent in late 1982. As with malaria, also a problem in the area, the altitude is not sufficient here to protect the people from a disease of the tropical rain-forests.

Water Behaviour in an Egyptian Village

A micro-scale and micro-spatial study of the *S. haematobium–Bulinus truncatus* cycle in a Nile and canal-side village in Upper Egypt sets new standards, though it should be stressed that the published report is but part of a longer-term study (Kloos et al. (1983), and see also Kloos et al. (1982) with critical comment by Forsyth (1983)). Ethnographic techniques like participant observation (as against questionnaire surveys) were combined with behavioural epidemiology observations of a quantitative nature such as using observers who knew most of the boys in the village and their home addresses to record bathing places, times, duration of swimming, proportion of body immersed during play in the water and so on. Observations were concentrated on boys in various age-groups, because of the importance of the build-up of infection rates and the light that may be thrown on the possibility of acquired immunity in humankind, and perhaps genetically based resistance or susceptibility; young girls were excluded for cultural and ethical reasons, but studies of adults of both sexes, and their behaviour patterns of likely relevance to bilharzia were also included. Twelve activity patterns were recorded in the main studies by observers of the boys: swimming, playing or walking in water, bathing, washing, washing animals, laundering, urination, irrigation, fishing, fetching water in jars for home use, ritual washing before prayer, and 'others' usually consisting of drinking and washing utensils. Relevant ecological observations included factors like the relative freedom from snails in the swifter water preferred for swimming by older boys, the movement down the Nile of water plants with a snail population, and so into snail populations in canals of various sizes, in fields during agricultural operations, and so on. Swimming was overwhelmingly the most likely source of exposure to the disease cycle, along with playing in the water; irrigation was probably not a high risk, and drinking water and fishing were low risk activities for these age-groups. It is difficult to do more in this book than suggest the flavour of this paper, but figure 11.5 (a) shows the egg-count for one of the 'cohorts' of boys, and figures 11.5 (b) and 11.5 (c) show contrasted patterns of water contact in boys of 5–7 years and the much more Nile-orientated pattern of those of 14–16.

Despite formidable problems of comprehending and analysing masses of such detailed data, this study seems to me to point the way for research on points of contact with disease cycles over a wide spectrum of diseases, not least man–mosquito contact in malaria. However, a somewhat similar study of urination, defaecation and subsequent washing habits, from the Gezira area of Sudan, has been criticised on ethical grounds, with the suggestion that a suitable questionnaire would cause less alienation in the community (Cheesmond and Fenwick (1981) and comment by Forsyth (1982)). Results were germane: most excretions were far from water, privacy being more sought, and the 31 per cent who washed were not particularly those who had excreted near water.

Technological Change in Japan and Eastern Asia

Last in this series is a micro-scale case-study of the Kofu basin north of Mt Fuji and southwest of Tokyo (Nihei et al. 1981). The basin is mapped as the remaining one of a series of main endemic foci of the *S. Japonica–Oncomelania* cycle in Honshu and Kyushu. Even in the Kofu basin it seems that no fresh cases are being reported, but that the snail population is still being treated seriously. While various control measures have been enforced by national laws, the authors point out that social and economic forces have also contributed to the retreat of the disease

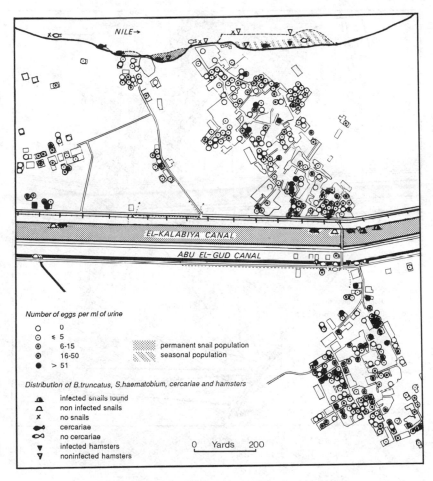

Figure 11.5 (a)   El Ayaisha village, Upper Egypt, schistosome egg count
Source: Kloos et al (1983)

from most of the endemic catchments: a fall in the agricultural population, or in rice-farming, changes in methods of farming and irrigation systems, part-time rather than full-time farming, a decrease in the use of draught animals, improved rural housing, hygiene and living standards, the construction of concrete ditches, and the extension of urban and periurban patterns of land-use and drainage. The authors map the landforms as lower deltaic plains, lower alluvial fans and one area of upper alluvial fans. Soil preferences of the snail, both as food and for placing around

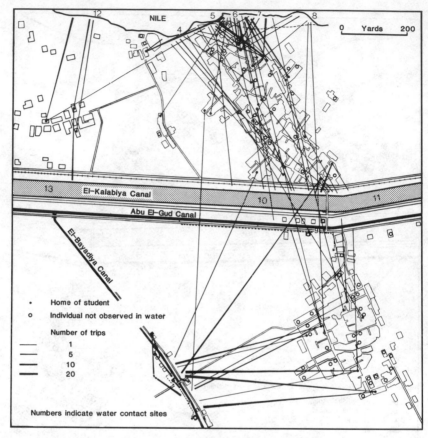

Figure 11.5 (b) Water contact map, boys 5–7 years
Source: Kloos et al (1983)

the eggs on oviposition, were studied in the field and in the laboratory, and landform, soil types and land use mapped as in figure 11.6; in province 1 the snail will probably keep on breeding in undulating land of mixed farming and widely distributed rice fields; in provinces 2 and 3, in similar terrain, urbanization is ousting farming and the snail habitat may vanish; in province 4 the water table is shallow and rice fields widely distributed, but the snail densities are low and decreasing because the rice fields are being moved to upland fields, and housing areas are spreading; in provinces 5, 6 and 7, formerly endemic areas with rice fields have been transformed for orchard development; and province 8 is an upland area, never endemic; though pasture is decreasing, orchards,

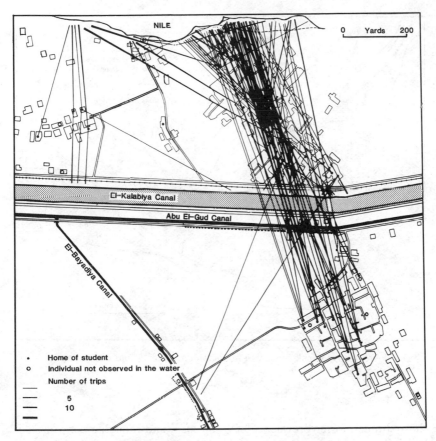

Figure 11.5 (c) Water contact map, boys 14–16 years
Source: Kloos et al. (1983)

greenhouses, etc. are coming in rather than rice cultivation so it remains free of the snail.

The emphasis on land-use change and improved standards of living, housing and drainage is reminiscent of the retreat of malaria from England, attributed mainly to changes in agricultural technology and housing (see chapters 8 and 10). For a complementary view of schistosomiasis control in Japan, see Hunter et al. (1982, 1984): the infection is seen as shifted from a human disease to a zoonosis only – of course with some risks of resurgence in people. The *S.japonica* remains important in parts of China and the Philippines, for instance (Olveda et al. 1983).

In the Philippines, a survey in northern Bohol island after 20 years

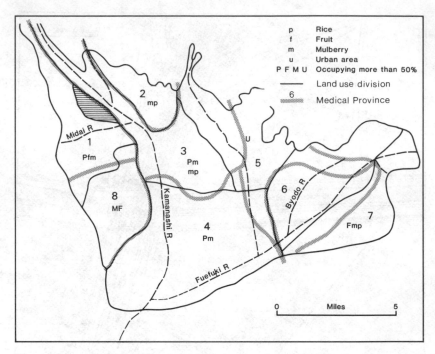

Figure 11.6   Schistosomiasis (japonica) 'provinces', Kofu basin, Japan
Source: Nihei et al. (1981)

showed much lower prevalence of *S.japonica*, and though a control team had been at work it was thought that the decrease was mainly because of an increase in intensive rice cultivation inhibiting to the snail vector (Carney et al. 1980). In China, campaigns against the snail vector are combined with community involvement in better sanitation (Yue et al. 1983; He et al. 1983). As with so many aspects of China, the massive action research programmes produce almost astronomical figures of manpower, areas cleared of snails, millions of people treated and so on (see Hillier and Jewell 1983). See also Lu Zhong-xian et al. (1983) on sewerage control in Shanghai partly because of schistosomiasis.

Relations of *S.Japonica* with cancers have been suspected: with liver cancer (Inaba et al. (1984), possibly as a multiplicative factor to the hepatitis B virus); with colo-rectal cancer (Xu and Su (1984) and several earlier papers) though Zhang et al. (1980) report only benign polyps as linked with the schistosomes. (And elsewhere *S. haematobium* has been linked with bladder cancer, for instance in Schwartz (1981).)

Conclusion

There is a certain paradox about this chapter: assuming as given the mainly descriptive outline of chapter 9, it opens with world perspectives not necessarily drawn from geographers, indeed it explicitly calls for interdisciplinary studies of a major cause of debility and social and economic depression in the Third World. Yet it goes on to present meso-scale studies of India, Puerto Rico and the Awash valley of Ethiopia, both of these latter linked with micro-scale work, and explicitly micro-scale studies from Brazil, Rwanda, Egypt and Japan. Some at least of these involve interdisciplinary studies, but I have tried to present the geographical viewpoint and as far as possible point up the geographical contribution. There is of course a concurrent literature of group research by biomedical disciplines, one example of which is the important series of papers on the dynamics of the disease cycle in 14 villages in Gambia (Wilkins et al. 1984); on Ethiopia, see Goll (1982). This book, however, is aimed primarily at students of geography, and this chapter may encourage them to see how quite traditional methods such as those mainly deployed in the papers cited, can contribute to the interdisciplinary studies that are so patently needed, as indeed Professor Hunter and his colleagues proclaim in the paper cited (J.M. Hunter et al. 1982). Even the interweaving of different scales can be a contribution, as indeed we have seen from developed world studies cited in chapter 7; I would add a special plea for geographers to be ready to integrate the spatial holism attainable through mapping with the studies, often individual and ethnographic like those in the Upper Egypt paper by Kloos et al. (1982) which will go far towards an integrated understanding of pattern and process.

12 Onchocerciasis or River Blindness

Introductory

River blindness has already been noted in chapter 9 as one of the main causes of eye disease and blindness in parts of tropical Africa and Latin America. The technical name is from *Onchocerca volvulus* (Greek *onkos* 'tumour', *kerkos* 'tail', Latin 'knot-like'); this is a worm parasitic on man, and also on some primates though the zoonotic element mentioned in chapter 9 is thought not to be important in the present world picture. See Brinkmann (1982) for a general survey of the disease in West Africa before major effects of the WHO campaign were apparent, and for a major symposium on onchocerciasis and other filariases, Institut de Médicine Tropical Prince Leopold (1981). Most long thread-like females and shorter and thinner males (see flow diagram, figure 12.1) live in an interlocked mass surrounded by fibrous tissue, forming distinctive nodules from pea to golfball size beneath the skin, though there may be some free adult filariae in the skin tissue. Egg-bearing females hatch out the microfilariae which spread through the skin as noted in the diagram, awaiting the chance of being picked up by the vector fly, a few particular tropical species of the almost worldwide genus of bloodsucking blackflies or gnats, *Simulium*. Species important in the main regions of river blindness are noted in figure 12.1. This is perhaps one of the comparatively few genuinely tropical diseases – though many a traveller in northern Canada will testify with oaths that the bloodthirsty biting black fly, or a close relative, is well-nigh worldwide. The microfilariae cause thickening of the skin, and if this affects the eye, damage and possibly blindness follow. However, some people seem able to generate immunity to the possible effects, while a diet rich in vitamin A, found in palm oil, offers some protection from blinding lesions, hence at least one cause of the contrast between serious infections and more and earlier blindness in the savannah belt as compared with the wetter coastal oil palm tracts of West

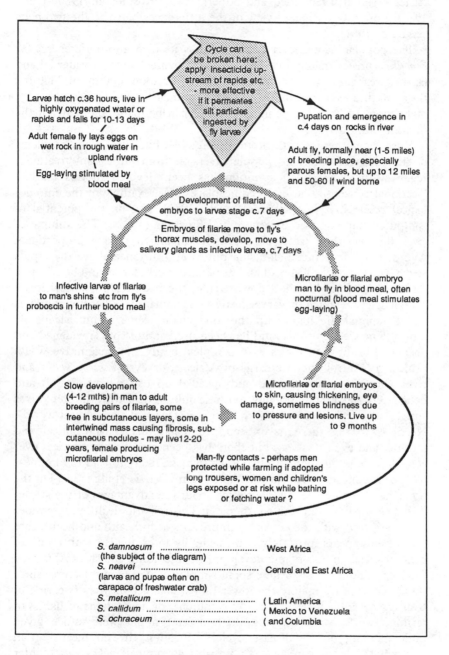

Figure 12.1 River blindness cycle
Source: Learmonth (1978)

Africa (Hunter 1966; Picq and Albert 1979; Prost et al. 1980; Duke 1981). For an evolutionary view of the differences between the two belts see Bain (1981).

The popular name, river blindness, has its own appropriateness, for *Simulium* breeds mainly in the oxygen-rich 'white water' of waterfall and cataract reaches of rivers, and on uplands over about 600 m (or 2000 ft); the adult flies feed voraciously on various animals including people within flight-range of breeding points – and this can be many kilometres if the flies are wind-driven.

Mass chemotherapy is theoretically possible, but raises many problems of skilled supervision and popular aversion from unpleasant treatment regimes, therefore much attention has been devoted to this marked locational concentration of breeding places. (An example of the entomological research is in Quillévéré et al. (1981), and on the potential of computer mapping, see Bickmore and Stocking (1982).) The volume of river flow at white water sites can be calculated, and a proportional volume of an insecticide emulsion put in at a distance above the rapids so designed that it will spread and disperse by turbulence, and be effective for up to 64 km (40 miles) downstream; the insecticide is absorbed by silt particles on which the larvae feed, while damage to other invertebrates and to animal life higher up the food chain seems within acceptable limits. Knowledge of this kind has been used and of course widened and deepened in the course of a vast, complex, costly and imaginitive WHO project to control onchocerciasis in Africa. Surveys of white water and river volumes were extended and speeded up using light aircraft and helicopters (hovercraft proving too inflexible to deal with different river sizes, widths of gorges etc. over such a vast part of the tropical world). Needless to say there have been problems, financial, technical and logistic, and even political, but there has been remarkable progress over considerable populations: in five years damage likely to lead to blindness has been reduced by half in the Volta basin (Dadzie et al. 1984). On the other hand the debate still continues about the advantages of the single-disease campaign – a recurrent theme in Third World health programmes – as compared with the all-round improvement in health and health care that often appears intimately and inevitably intermingled with issues of general social and economic development, including education. To stick to river blindness but to take some simple socioeconomic factors: since the black fly bites mainly the lower limbs, changes in dress (wearing of trousers by adult males is already common), or adaptations of habits of farming work, water-carrying, bathing etc. might well suffice given understanding of the disease cycle. Education, by no means at an unattainable level, can have an impact; already 20 years ago Hunter found that the people of northern Ghana were beginning to link the disease with the fly. Some of the simple elements of life style might equally well apply to breaking other disease cycles, such as malaria or sleeping sickness. Geographical studies over the last two decades are highly relevant to seeing this debate in perspective, and here I lean particularly on J.M. Hunter (1966 and later papers) and on Bradley (1972, 1981), though there are other valuable sources, notably Picq (1983), a modern synthesis based on the concept of the pathogenic complex.

Hunter on Ghana

Figure 12.2 is Hunter's map of black fly breeding sites in northern Ghana, extending north into Upper Volta, mainly south of 12°N. The fly is not seen for six months during the dry season, yet appears within hours of the first rains, and on Hunter's daring and now substantially verified geographical hypothesis of 1966 these adult flies are in fact immigrants moving north with the tropical maritime air mass that brings the wet season, warm, humid and congenial to insect life. Although the depressions of the early rains move east to west, and the east is an unlikely source of black fly, he suggested that the depressions are waves or troughs in the advancing front of tropical maritime air, and that adult flies might be wind-borne from more humid zones farther south rather than based on easterly air. However, Hunter's main contribution came with another hypothesis from human rather than physical geography – that river blindness is a main factor in a kind of cyclic advance and retreat of a settlement frontier.

Abandoned thatched and mud-walled villages are soon almost untraceable on the ground, but radial paths, poorer secondary vegetation on eroded former fields, and thick and varied vegetation on well-manured sites round former house plinths, are all relatively easily identified from air photographs. Figure 12.3 shows the result of patient sifting of the evidence and consideration of other possible explanations round Sakoti, a settlement about 5 km west of a focus of *Simulium* breeding on the Red Volta river, and as the caption says, Hunter now claims it as an instance of the retreat of a settlement frontier largely because of onchocerciasis, still continuing in the 1960s: thirty-six houses were abandoned from 1949 to 1963, yet the village elders said that settlement was *advancing* on the river as late as 1918, dating from memorable events. So Hunter reckoned on a retreat of villages and farms of almost 2 km every seven years in one area, about every 12–14 years in another. Chiefs' houses, once central, were now on the eastern edge of a retreating frontier, marked by neglected land and houses, much of the labour force

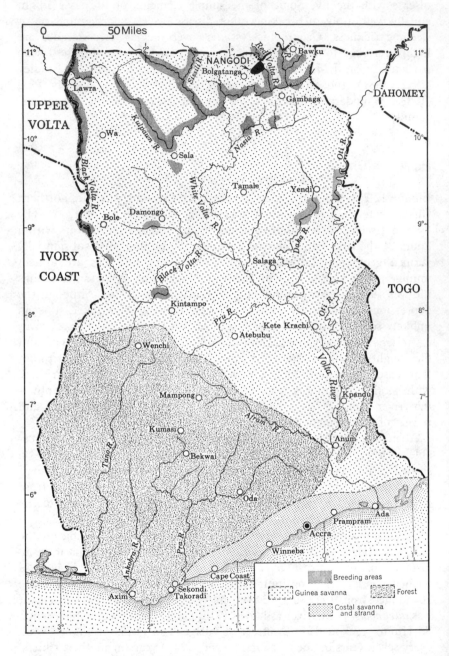

Figure 12.2   Foci of river blindness in Ghana
Source: Hunter (1966)

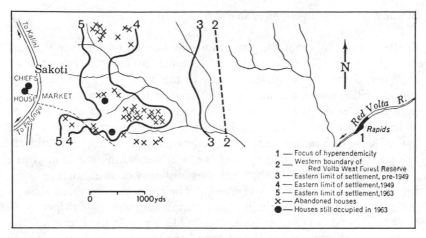

Figure 12.3 Retreat of human settlements attributed to river blindness, Nangodi, Ghana
Source: Hunter (1966)

being blind, by poor nutrition, much prevalence of minor ailments such as skin sores, and marked apathy compared with vigour and energy of the areas farther west. Hunter then came to his hypothesis of cyclic advance and retreat of the frontier of settlement, in earlier generations allowing for factors like the slave trade, sifting oral tradition with written history so far as relevant to such a question, comparing Forest Department records with air photographs and so on. He found evidence from diverse and scattered sources of an advance of settlements activated by widespread dearth into empty riverside terrain in the late nineteenth century, prospering from about the early 1890s to about the end of the 1914–18 war. Then disease began to take control, wiping out some communities, weakening others and initiating a vicious circle so that abandonment or retreat began, continuing into the 1960s. While other diseases including sleeping sickness may be partly involved, Hunter offers river blindness as the main cause with some confidence.

This work contributed towards solving the mystery of the sudden appearance of the black fly with the first rains, and also to the deeper understanding of the role of the disease cycle in the whole life and adjustment of African farming to the environment over time. It is a good example of the way that good human geography can contribute to knowledge of health and disease even where the mechanics of the disease cycle have been discovered.

Bradley on the Hawal valley in Nigeria

Bradley's work at about the same time was focused on the Hawal valley in east central Nigeria, carefully designed to compare prevalence, economy, demography, understanding of the disease etc. in a sample of affected villages and a matched set of control villages on uplands, free from the disease apart from returned temporary migrants after work in fly-infested lowlands. Relatively lower rates in men seemed to be related to the spread of wearing trousers, as compared with women and children, though risks in water-collection, clothes-washing, bathing etc. might be lessened by a possibility that the flies dislike wet skin (or are more vulnerable to a slap from a wet hand?). The links with impaired sight of lessened efficiency in farming, and simple indexes of prosperity in household goods were clear: even totally blind people tried to farm, but could travel shorter distances and were handicapped. Communal help to the handicapped does operate, but obviously with decreasing effectiveness in badly afflicted communities. The people understood the disease, its manifestations and progress very well, but at that time attributed it to spirits, witchcraft and the like, and the western concept of transmission was unknown. Data on age structure and migration history complemented Hunter's hypothesis well. In lowland villages only 7 per cent of the adults were still living in their birthplace, in upland ones 26 per cent; the average age in the lowlands was 29, in the uplands 40. Advance into the 'population low pressure areas' of the lowlands from the relatively densely peopled uplands was followed by a retreat back to the uplands after 10–15 years. There was marriage movement of brides from the uplands to the lowlands, but increasing reluctance to marry lowland men – suggestive of Daniel Defoe's comment about the numbers of young brides (non-immunes in our terms?) moving from the uplands to marry fen-men, well seasoned to ague (malaria?) (Defoe, 1724, pp. 11–15) (cf. chapter 8!).

Desertion of villages does occur, and while other diseases are also involved – including smallpox at the time of Bradley's work and the dusty dry-season meningitis epidemics (see chapter 9) – fear of spirits overlapping with fear of disease recognized as such, and actual attrition through death and loss of production (as in Hunter's study) were all largely attributable to onchocerciasis. Yet some people with years of contact with black fly did not become ill, so, as often, some individual immunity factor seemed to be at work that might point the way to control other than by attack on the vector – perhaps genetic, perhaps dietetic (differential use of oil palm?) or is it a matter of individual metabolism?

The study is a remarkable example of how much can be accomplished by a single worker in the course of a doctoral thesis – and was followed by some 20 years of fruitful interdisciplinary team research on tropical diseases. See also Melville (1979) and Prescott (1979) on implications for economic development.

The WHO/World Bank Project

Returning to Hunter's later work on this disease complex, since he wrote in 1966 he has become involved as consultant in further studies connected with a huge WHO/World Bank project to combat river blindness, and now almost twenty years later writes, still as geographer, but as generalist, even statesman (Hunter 1980, 1981b): these papers include more ecological details than can be included here, but are essential reading for in-depth study.

The project is sub-continental in scale: the east–west extent of the area covered is some 1350 km (comparable to the distance from Paris to Warsaw) and north–south is 500–600 km (cf. Paris–Marseilles or Warsaw–Budapest). Apart from the international agencies involved, several ex-colonial territories are included and political difficulties between agencies and between nations occasionally surface, despite all the goodwill toward a crusade against a major cause of blindness. Figure 12.4 shows the project area, with sub-areas numbered according to the phasing inevitable in such a large and complex project. Enormous investment is involved, and very great logistic problems, resolutely tackled. (On the economics, see Prescott and Jancloes (1984a) and Prescott et al. (1984b) debating cost-effectiveness as against the more complex concept of cost-benefit analysis, and taking measles immunization as an example for comparison with onchocerciasis in terms of cost-effectiveness.) Earlier, small projects had shown the potential of DDT against the larval stage of the filariae, and later insecticides, biodegradable and less environmentally damaging, had become available. The strategy adopted was for anti-larval spraying at distances upstream calculated to allow spread of the insecticide across the different streams, with modifications according to weather conditions – information being diffused by a special radio network. Light aircraft are used for more open white water sites, and the slower and more expensive helicopters for gorge and closely forested sites. The project is brilliantly imaginative, even audacious, and has been rewarded by equally remarkable success on all three accepted criteria for evaluation: (1) many transmission sites saw the cessation of black-fly breeding, others 75 to 95 per cent reduction; (2) infectivity in

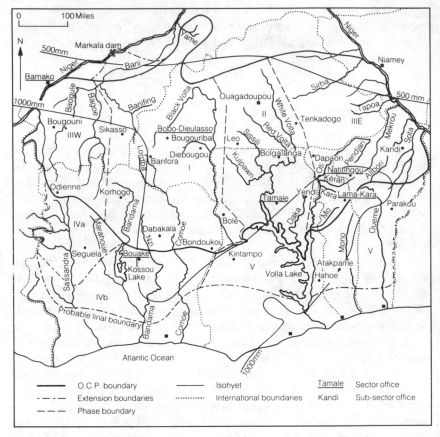

Figure 12.4   Onchocerciasis control areas, West Africa
Source: Hunter (1981b)

the female fly's head capsule leading to effective bites fell by some 95 per cent, and total bites by over 99 per cent; (3) in many villages no infections are found in children under five and few in children under ten. (Short of effective mass therapy becoming possible in future, adult populations will remain a potential source of resurgence of the disease for some 16 years after active transmission ceases.)

Major problems have, however, been encountered, some ecological and some economic and ultimately political. The fertile valley lands from which population had retreated because of the disease were mapped in terms of land quality and potential, and World Bank cost-benefit analysis to justify investment in the project was based on assumed resettlement of these lands, and consequent economic gains. Though by common consent the disease-free uplands are now overpopulated and subject to much severe accelerated soil erosion, resettlement of the valleys as these are cleared of river blindness has been slow. This may be a question of the time lag common in development of fresh or reclaimed land resources, or it may be that more government provision of infrastructure is required – possibly on a modest scale such as providing wells and agricultural extension services, possibly on a wider and costlier scale of provision including also roads, schools, clinics and perhaps the provision of measured plots, the allocation of crop quotas and the like. The overcrowded uplands are subject to increasing malnutrition and undernutrition, amongst other problems, increasing the vulnerability to other diseases, so that this problem does not lack urgency.

The ecological problems include the re-invasion of cleared areas, especially towards their windward margins, by large numbers of already infective black flies. Hunter's 1966 hypothesis of movement with change of air mass has largely been corroborated, though with important modifications: the movement is predominantly with the west-south-west to east-north-east monsoon rather than south to north and it seems to come mainly with the monsoon winds following the passage northwards of the intertropical convergence, rather than with that convergence zone itself as Hunter hypothesized. Black fly have been shown to move downwind for very long distances indeed, often for 100 km and up to 500 km. Concurrently the vector fly *Simulium damnosum* has been shown to have several different strains, and indeed several distinct sub-species have now been recognized. The disease cycle seems to be much more effective in parts of the savannah lands near white water than near breeding sites in the rain-forest belt; it is not clear whether this is due to differences in vector or pathogen, or because people, pathogens and vectors (or alternate hosts) are all drawn to water in a seasonally arid environment, cf. M.P. Hutchinson on trypanosomiasis in Gambia cited in Learmonth (1959). Inevitably the effect of these re-invasions is that the project managers have continually to consider extending the work into up-wind source areas of infective flies, sometimes involving negotiations with national governments not so far involved in the project, and concurrently to maintain vigilance in areas already worked over, and this to a much greater extent and at much greater cost than originally planned.

Lessons from the Project

At this point Hunter consciously goes beyond policies with which he has been involved as a worker with WHO, in two steps, one to consider other points at which this particular disease cycle may be broken, and two to question if this disease cycle is in fact best attacked using the single-disease programme so successful for smallpox eradication.

He reviews in turn a number of different points of attack. Could breeding places, that is waterfalls and cataracts, be eliminated by changes in river profiles, usually by damming – of course avoiding increased risks of schistosomiasis? Could the biological approach be used – that is, by introducing organisms known to be predatory or parasitic on *Simulium*? Could non-vector species of *Simulium* be induced to crowd vector species out of breeding sites? Could modern genetics be deployed, for instance by release of large populations of artificially reared male flies (possibly females) sterilized by low-level radiation? (Both of these have also been considered to eradicate *Anopheles* vector species – or to keep a particular ecological 'niche' that had been cleared of vectors, free from re-invasion.) Could the chemical composition of the water be altered at breeding sites without harmful effects on their ecology? It is worth noting that modern biodegradable insecticides as used in the project cause only slight loss of other non-vertebrates in the water and do not seem to cause fish losses or major alteration of ecological equilibrium. Can further studies of *Simulium* of different vector species reveal other points at which they can be attacked, such as emerging adults in their initial resting places? Can the filariae be attacked, in the human body by nodulectomy or by drugs? (The surgical removal of nodules is surprisingly popular where it has been tried, but is unlikely to be effective because some nodules are inaccessible to diagnosis in large buttock muscles. And existing drugs have such severe side effects that they are not practicable for mass chemotherapy.) Can a vaccine be evolved? Can people apparently immune to the disease yield clues as to why their immune system resists the filariae – and if so how to extend this to people without this immunity?

At this point Hunter moves to plead that, as with many other diseases, many victims are found to be subject to several parasitic diseases, and that a broader approach than the single-disease approach may be justified. In this case regional medical and health services may be envisaged as grading into regional and even quite local studies of behaviour patterns, so that, for instance, agricultural operations which put people at hazard may be at times of day or at seasons of the year (given modified cropping patterns) when risks are minimal, and tracts near white water at particularly high risk may be avoided altogether. Patterns of clothing may be changed, particularly that of the lower limbs, and colours of reflective surfaces disliked by the flies may be used, with additional precautions, change of occupation, or precise occupational pattern for very high-risk groups such as fishermen or honey-hunters. The provision of alternative blood meals in the shape of domestic or game animals might be tried – there is a precedent in malaria prevention in South-east

Asia. Design of houses and location of settlements might be altered to reduce contact between people and the fly. Nutritional patterns can be altered more rapidly than is sometimes thought (the use of Coca-Cola and of white bread in Africa show this), and higher consumption of vitamin A from palm oil may be encouraged at the expense of shea butter in the more severely affected savannah belt – it is already a staple in forest zone diets. Other foods rich in vitamin A may be encouraged in the savannah. Behavioural pattern 'cells' of people's movements at work, recreation and play may be identified, and those involving high risks of transmission pin-pointed and in time modified – the study of schistosomiasis in Upper Egypt in chapter 11 perhaps shows the way. And findings about crucial variables for an area may be modelled in order to identify how a combination of alterations of environment and lifestyle might break the cycle. Given studies in depth of particular local communities and the total disease burden, the approach can be extended towards holism and ideally to a fresh ecological adjustment to the local environment and resources. Above all, this approach, whether for a single disease or for a spectrum of the main scourges affecting a local community, demands participation by local people on quite a different scale from the *deus ex machina* of the aircraft or helicopter spraying of white water areas, attacking a single point of the arthropod vector's life cycle, with little or no action by the people themselves. Parallels with house spraying against malaria are close.

Conclusion

This part of the book has deliberately spanned twenty years of geographers' interest in the disease. Initial research of good quality, with imaginative leaps in formation of a hypothesis later shown to be valid with qualifications, was followed by contributions to a huge international crusade. The crusade's fine achievements were muted by re-invasion of the disease, involving extension in area and continuation in time beyond the original plans. And a leading geographical researcher has been led to plead for a multiple-disease approach rather than a single-disease attack, and moreover to plead for a holism that extends to consider community health as a whole, ultimately to put health and disease into a community and societal context, always – ideally at least – with respect for and conservation of the ecological balance of people, plants and animals in a particular setting.

13 Some Third World Cancers

Introductory

Chapter 9 concentrated on 'tropical' diseases, meaning mainly infectious vector-borne ones, including the universal diseases like measles and influenza. Apart from the 'western diseases' that are tending to increase in urban elites in the Third World, certain cancers, for instance, are proportionately more important in many parts of the Third World. Parkin et al. (1984) and Parkin (1986) point out that the *numbers* of cancer cases in the Third World now exceed those in the developed countries – though of course their proportion of total mortality is much less. A world survey that includes Third World material is in Krastev (1979). An Indian surgeon interested in geography has published a book entitled *Surgical Diseases in the Tropics* (Joshi 1982), a valuable pioneering viewpoint – though subject to criticism from his surgeon colleagues mainly as to definitions of what constitutes a 'surgical disease' (arguing that there are simply diseases in which sometimes, say, chemotherapy may be indicated, sometimes surgery), and also that tropical areas outside India are under-represented. About half the book concerns a wide range of degenerative diseases including cancers, in which surgery is commonly deployed; the other half concerns surgical aspects of infectious and vectored diseases like those discussed earlier – surgery for onchocerciasis nodules is an example of this, mentioned in chapter 12. Considering cancers by site, liver and oesophagus cancers are important in many parts of the Third World, while Burkitt's lymphoma, a mainly child cancer affecting lymph nodes in the neck and common in East Africa has been the subject of geographical studies for reasons outlined later in this chapter. Of course there are regional variations in such a vast area. A recent report based on a cancer registry in Iraq stresses bladder cancer associated with schistosomiasis, lung cancer and lymphomas, but low incidence of cancer of the cervix in women (Al Fouadi and Parkin 1984). Mouth and liver cancers seem to be commoner in the Solomon Islands than in Australia, and colon and lung cancer less so (Taylor et al. 1983). Asian immigrants in the Trent regional health authority area in England had higher than expected rates for cancer of the tongue, mouth, oesophagus and pharynx, and lower than expected for stomach, skin and testis (Donaldson and Clayton 1984). And geographers studying the high incidence of nasopharyngeal cancer in the Chinese in Malaysia tentatively point to the high consumption of salted fish in childhood and youth as compared with Malay and Indian populations (Armstrong and Armstrong 1983a) – though the almost universal Epstein-Barr (or 'glandular fever') virus is somehow involved, as noted later. Professor Armstrong's many linked papers with various collaborators are perhaps best followed up from the references in this paper or in Armstrong and Eng (1983c); however, it is important to note that his researches have led him to important contributions to geographical methodology such as his idea of 'self-specific environments' that may be related to this cancer (1973, 1976). And note his (1984) paper on exposure to air pollution in a tropical city.

Some Literature Surveyed

For cancers as a group Waterhouse et al. (1982) present data from five continents, and see also the special issue of *Médicine Tropicale* (1983). B. Armstrong on China (1980) draws attention to the importance of stomach cancers in the east of the country already noted in chapter 3, linked at least suggestively with regional diets high in salted and pickled vegetables and sweet potatoes; he notes too that liver cancer is common in the warm south-east coastal belt, possible links including hepatitis B, aflatoxins (discussed a little further presently) and nitrosamines (again see below), and perhaps water contamination. The remarkable regional concentration of cancer of the oesophagus in certain hilly northern tracts is discussed in relation to possible factors – low riboflavin (vitamin B2) and ascorbic acid (vitamin C), possible carcinogens in pickled vegetables and perhaps *Aspergillus* fungi, or alcohol, or very hot tea (as has been suggested for Soviet central Asian groups also). Nasopharyngeal cancers are high in southern Quangdong province with high rates in women. Expatriate populations are discussed (cf. the Malaysian Chinese referred to earlier in this chapter in the Armstrong and Armstrong study of 1983): suspected causes include the Epstein-Barr virus (causing glandular fever or infectious mononucleosis), salted fish, cigarettes and exposure to fumes at work (see Yu et al. (1981); also Haynes (1984) conducting statistical analyses based on the great atlas of cancers in China, and finding four cancer sites to be significantly associated with urbanization – 'western diseases'?).

Marks (1981) edits an important symposium comparing cancers in China and in the USA. See also Lam (1986).

McGlashan (1981, 1982a,b) analyses main causes of mortality between ten Caribbean island states, including cancers: Barbados and Antigua were high for oesophageal cancer for males and almost comparably so for females, but Grenada low; Jamaica and Barbados were high for male stomach cancer, Antigua and Dominica low and so on.

A geographical pathology view of cancers, strong on Third World illustrations, is in Hutt (1979) and see also Hutt and Burkitt (1986). There are a number of regional studies of cancers as a whole. Habibi (1982), makes a countrywise review of the Near East. Habibi (1979) on Iran finds several cancers including cervix and skin, but not lymphomas, to be related to socioeconomic group. Akhtar (1983) maps the regional combination by site in India. Hazra (1984a) looks at West Bengal in more detail with some suggested environmental correlates. Jayant et al. (1971) comment briefly on differential incidence in endogamous caste groups in western India, and McGlashan and Mathur (1984) map regions within Rajasthan. All of these were trying to give a geographical view allowing for imperfect data, while Armstrong (1980) similarly gives a broad view of South-east Asia, stressing the importance of cervical cancer over most of the macro-region. Chin (1979) gives a broad geography of cancers in Africa, Cook and Burkitt (1970) an epidemiology of seven cancers in East Africa including an atlas and commentary, Mbalawa (1981) reports on cancers in Congo, and Kasili (1983) on those in sub-Saharan Africa but mainly in Kenya. And McGlashan of Hobart and his colleagues in South Africa continue the series of revealing analyses of cancers in black goldminers from different areas already noted in chapter 5 as methodology (on the 'isomell' or contour of equal risk concept); see McGlashan and Harington (1976), McGlashan and Bradshaw (1982); Bradshaw et al. (1985). Roy (1982) reviews breast cancer in developing countries.

Taking Chile as having some developing-country characteristics, Haynes' (1983) analysis of mortality as a whole includes sections on cancers: high rates seem to have some relationship with nitrate use in the main farming areas, rather than with the nitrate mining areas of the north. His survey is complemented from the medical side by that of Armijo et al. (1981a,b).

Lung Cancers and Smoking

Third World lung cancers have a considerable literature. Examples include Jindal et al. (1982) on data from Chandigarh, and using migrant data in comparative studies and Hinds et al. (1981) on rates in Japanese,

Chinese and Hawaiian women in Hawaii where the smoking risk was highest in Hawaiians, followed by Japanese, and comparatively low in Chinese. In Chandigarh, India, nearly all women patients and one-third of the men had never smoked; smokers and ex-smokers comprised 48 per cent who had smoked only cigarettes, 28 per cent only *bidis* (of naturally cured tobacco in the leaf of a jungle tree – these have been referred to as 'cigarette-like things'!; the leaf is from the *temburni* tree, *Diospyros melanoxylon*, and 3 per cent hookahs. (There is probably a class bias, with hookahs upper and *bidis* lower class.) A study mainly on oral cancers in Ernakulam in the south-western state, Kerala, shows male patients as linked with smoking and mixed use of tobacco, women more with chewing (Mehta et al. 1982; Gupta et al. 1984). In a ten-year study 10 per cent of the respondents gave up smoking and 5 per cent started! This study has now been extended to several regions, as action research including propaganda against tobacco and research on pre-cancerous lesions; and compare the various smoking and chewing patterns, the latter including tea leaves, in northern Thailand (Mougne et al. 1982). Chewing of 'betel nut' or *pān* (actually ground areca nut wrapped with various condiments in a leaf from the betel vine) is linked with oral cancer, but with increased risk if the wad includes lime, as it commonly does, or tobacco (Wilson et al. 1983; WHO 1984a). For mapping and a geographical conspectus of regional smoking and chewing habits, see Akhtar (1983). On health policy and tobacco, Milio (1985) writes on Third World problems as well as on the USA.

Cancer of the Liver

Of the cancer sites here selected as Third World cancers, the liver is perhaps the one most widespread as a serious public health problem, responsible for large numbers of premature deaths, economic loss, orphaning, suffering and distress. Table 13.1 represents some estimates of incidence in tabular form, rates increasing from left to right. The left hand column is entirely of developed countries, the next includes western and central Europe, black and Latin American people in the USA, coloured and Indian populations in South Africa, while the third includes northern Japan (Hokkaido), Maori New Zealanders and southern Europe. The three right hand columns include only developing countries, some of them of course very rapidly industrializing like Taiwan, Singapore and Hong Kong (Cook-Mozaffari and van Rensburg 1984). It seems certain that at least several, perhaps many environmental factors – broadly defined – play a part in this disease, world-wide even if proportionally more important in the Third World. Evidence from developed countries

Table 13.1 Approximate level of incidence for PLC in different parts of the world

Age-standardized incidence per 100 000 for men aged 35–64

<4	4–	12–	25–	50–	100–
Canada	USA (blacks)	Southern Uganda[a]	Southern Nigeria	Dakar, Senegal[b]	Maputo, Mozambique
USA (whites)	USA (Latin)	North-west Tanzania[a]	Southern Ivory Coast[a]	Northern Ivory Coast[a]	Bulawayo, Zimbabwe
Northern Europe	Caribbean[a]	Botswana	Most of East Africa[a]	North-west Uganda[a]	Taiwan
UK	South America	Lesotho	Most of Malawi and Zambia[a]	Southern Malawi[a]	
South Africa (whites)	Western Europe	Swaziland (High veld)	Most of South Africa	Natal, South Africa	
New Zealand (non-Maori)	Central Europe	Singapore (Indian)	Swaziland (Middle veld)	Swaziland (Low veld)	
Australia	South Africa (coloured)	Southern Europe	Singapore (Malayan)	Inhambane, Mozambique	
	South Africa (Indian)	Northern Japan (Hokkaido)[a]	Southern Japan (Kyushu)[a]	Singapore (Chinese)	
	Bombay, India	New Zealand (Maori)	Hawaii (Hawaiians)	Hong Kong[b]	
		West-central China[c]	North-eastern China[c]	Shanghai, China[b]	
			East-central China[c]	Coastal China south of Shanghai[c]	

[a] Estimates of incidence include liver tumours of unspecified origin (WHO International Classification of Diseases 7th Edition, Code 156 and 8th Edition, Code 197.8)
[b] Liver tumours of unspecified origin not included; true incidence of PLC may be higher
[c] Not clear whether liver tumours of unspecified origin are included; true incidence of PLC may be higher
Source: Cook-Mozaffari and van Rensburg 1984

suggests the importance of alcohol, cigarettes and, locally, chemical industries; the higher male rates may be related to hormonal factors, as also the suggestions of higher risks in women taking oral contraceptives.

In the Third World countries with the highest rates, such as Mozambique, two factors seem to be crucial, probably acting synergistically – working together to have a more than a simple additive effect. The first is aflatoxin, a toxin derived from certain moulds of the genus *Aspergillus* (allied to that sometimes seen on the top of jars of home-made jam!) and especially species of the mould found on badly stored groundnuts (peanuts) and maize (for a general review of the mycotoxins including the aflatoxins, see *WHO Environmental Health Criteria* (1979)). The aflatoxins have long been known to cause toxaemia and deaths in poultry and other domestic animals, and the association with human liver cancer from epidemiology is now regarded as very strong though apparently lacking laboratory confirmation. (See for instance Patten (1981); Van Rensburg et al. (1985) on Mozambique and Transkei, pleading that aflatoxin–hepatitis B interaction demands more action than just vaccination against the virus; and Casadei et al. (1982) on a government survey of aflatoxins in food in Mozambique.) See also Bulatao-Jayme et al. (1982) for a case-control study in the Philippines, Shah et al. (1981) for data on aflatoxins in food and fodder in Pakistan, and Ngindu et al. (1982) for a report of *acute* symptoms – epidemics are by no means unknown. (See chapter 14 for a possible relationship of aflatoxins with Kwashiorkor.)

The second synergistic factor, then, is the hepatitis B virus. African populations have long been known to have high rates of various serological markers of past hepatitis B infection and of carriers of the virus, so that over the last 15 years or so causal links with liver cancer have been suspected. (See for instance the important retrospective survey by Maupas and a group of workers from Tours and Dakar (1981), 25 years after the link was first suggested by M. Payet and his team; also Zuckermann (1982), *Médicine d'Afrique Noire* (1982), and regional studies by McGlashan (1982c) on Swaziland, Zhuang et al. (1982) on Indian–Fijian contrasts in Fiji, Ying et al. (1984) reporting on 1000 autopsies in different parts of China, and Hann et al. (1982) on Korea.)

However, high rates of carriers of the virus in Greenland, Lesotho, Botswana and New Zealand are associated with low rates of the cancer – and with rare occurrence of mouldy groundnuts or maize in the diet – and some researchers believe that on present evidence the aflatoxin must be accepted as the necessary and sufficient factor leading to this Third World cancer. Low to moderate rates are found in south-eastern USA where much maize is consumed by both black and white groups (as 'grits' or coarsely ground corn meal), and economically disastrous epidemics of aflatoxin toxaemia in poultry etc. are on record. The apparent anomaly as compared with African experience may be related to the relative preponderance of contaminated groundnut or maize in the diet? McGlashan (1982c) points out that in the high risk areas of Mozambique rates have been tending to fall, perhaps with changes in life style. And again that policies to modify agricultural practices to reduce the risks of *Aspergillus* contamination in Swaziland have led to better preparation of crops for storage, and to groundnut supplies that are much more acceptable for export – a health measure has here proved economically advantageous. From China, climate is seen as influencing the formation of the mould, though the aflatoxin is thought to be synergistic with hepatitis B (Wang Yaobin et al. 1983). Aflatoxin contamination has been under suspicion in the Kazakh republic in the USSR (Kulmanov 1985).

Cancer of the Oesophagus

Cancer of the oesophagus has been ranked seventh in the world in frequency of occurrence and, given the data problems, may well rank equally with liver cancer so far as Third World incidence is concerned; its regional variations are so marked that it is 'the malignancy *par excellence*' where geographical pathology should illumine the aetiology (Day 1984). Day points out the much higher rates in men than women in most groups (the exceptions, as we shall see, may be challenging), the high rates in male blacks in South Africa and North America, medium to high rates in the Caribbean and Latin America, high rates in the Indian sub-continent and high rates in China (though regionally concentrated) and in emigrants from China.

Day's 1984 survey already cited pulls together available knowledge of the distribution pattern of cancer of the oesophagus in central Asia. There is a suggestive relationship with various groups of Turkic origin, Turkoman, Uzbek and Kazakh, and the former kingdoms of Uleg Beg and Timur, with Samarkand as the old capital: major concentrations are in the Soviet republics of Kazakhstan and Uzbekistan, in Kazakh areas of north-west China, in Afghanistan and in north-east Iran, while China has another major concentration in Henan province in east-central China (peaking with extraordinarily high rates in Linxian county, as pointed out in Marks (1981)). The rates for men in China are roughly twice those for women, a much smaller difference than recorded in many countries, while there is high incidence in women in north-east Iran as noted presently. The Samarkand area of the Uzbek SSR, noted for high rates of oral and oesophageal cancers, has many men especially who chew *nass*, a mixture of tobacco, ash, cotton oil and lime (quite reminiscent of Indian chewing of tobacco with areca nut, betel leaf and lime), and rates are slightly higher in smokers and drinkers (Zaridze et al. 1985). See also Rahu (1986) on the high rates in Kazakhstan and Turkmeniz. It has been suggested that silica fragments in millet bran may play a part in cancer of the oesophagus in people, and also in poultry (O'Neill et al. 1980); millet is a staple cereal in many other parts of the world that do not have high rates of the cancer, on present knowledge. Lu et al. (1981) discuss mutagenicity of pickled vegetables in the high-incidence area of Linhsien county in China; a possible role for opium has been suggested (Ghadirian et al. 1985) including contaminants in the pipes used (see also Dowlatshahi and Miller 1985). In all these central Asian concentrations, and in that in east central China, tobacco and alcohol consumption are generally regarded as playing a negligible role. Opium may formerly have been important, and perhaps residually still.

Nitrates rather than nitrites were found in Thai salted fish and other foods, and in the rock-salt commonly used in the north-east of Thailand (Migasena et al. 1980). Do the regional patterns of concentration in Europe offer any hints, granting that the disease is generally less common? Tobacco and alcohol are suspected in Brittany and Normandy, as noted presently, and in north-east Italy, but the high rates of northern Scandinavia have been linked with poor diets, along with the inflammation of throat tissues that may be prodromal to this cancer (and known as the Plummer-Vinson syndrome). So micro-nutritional imbalance or deficiencies may be crucial, and it may be that alcohol (possibly even tobacco and opium?) is operating as in other problems through its detrimental effect on nutrition? Current action research in China is aimed at intervention by dietary improvement when precursor symptoms are found in community surveys. On Scotland, see Blythe (1986).

An important and wide-ranging review is in van Rensburg (1985): he attributes a limited role to alcohol and tobacco, and interestingly goes right back to the poor and unreliable rain and water supplies, poor soils, stressed plants, bad food storage especially mycotoxins, and possibly trace element deficiencies (zinc, molybdenum, selenium, magnesium) and vitamins too (riboflavin, also in the vitamin B complex) seen as enhancing risks from carcinogens. Excess energy foods and Vitamin A may also add to risks. But probably mycotoxins are basic.

McGlashan (1968, 1972) was the first to draw the attention of geographers to this problem: figures 13.1 and 13.2 bring out a possible relationship between cancer of the oesophagus and certain types of locally distilled alcoholic spirits, though it should be stressed that full allowance was made for the admittedly crude nature of the data (as well as of the alcohol!) and that cartography was accompanied by statistical analyses. Types of still vary locally, from kettles to petrol drums to arrangements

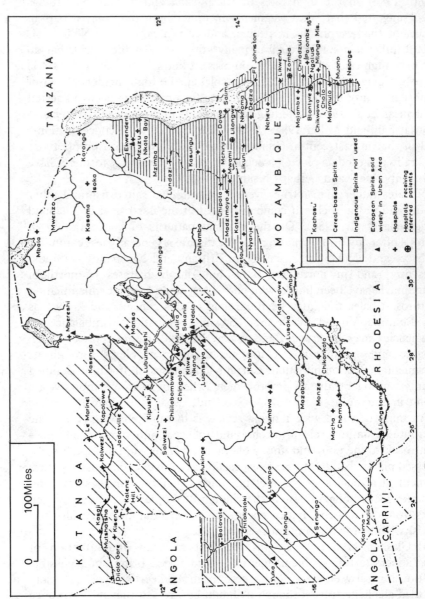

Figure 13.1   Indigenous distilled spirits in parts of central Africa
Source: McGlashan (1972)

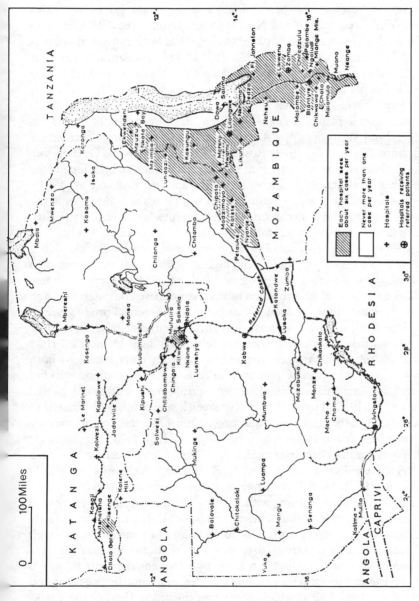

Figure 13.2 Cancer of the oesophagus in parts of central Africa
Source McGlashan (1972)

of earthenware pots. First, metal contamination was suspected, then a constituent of certain types of fermentation, nitrosamine, found in a very wide range of foods, some used commonly in the west, where there is a fermentation stage in the processing. (For a general survey of health aspects of nitrates, nitrites and N-nitroso compounds, see *WHO Environmental Health Criteria 5* 1978; carcinogenesis has been proved in animals but not in humans, see O'Neill et al. (1985).) The correlation seems clear enough and it is possible that repeated insult to throat and gullet tissues by crude alcohol might be a cause but that alone does not seem sufficient. Concurrent smoking has been suggested (Bradshaw and Schonland 1974) and carcinogenic plants, *Solanum incanum*, used to sour milk quickly in Transkei, and Mexican poppy *Argemone mexicana* which may contaminate grain crops (Rose 1976, 1979; Rose and Fellingham 1981). Overlapping with McGlashan's work came a report whose authors included the geographer Paula Cook (Cook et al. 1971, and see Collis et al. 1971), who was to follow that up with the atlas and analysis done with the surgeon Denis Burkitt already noted as covering seven cancers (1970). Similar factors are suspected for Ivory Coast (Cornet et al. 1983).

In western countries alcohol and tobacco may well be suspected but difficult to pin down. In France, the high incidence in the Calvados area (Picheral 1976) makes it tempting to think of crudely prepared home distillation of the well-known spirit of that name, based on cider – though as with Scotch whisky the carefully monitored commercial product seems to be free from suspicion at least as a direct source of carcinogens like the nitrosamines. In western societies tobacco is held to increase risks five-fold, alcohol much more and increasing with daily intake in both sexes – thus the high male rate in France is ascribed to higher alcohol consumption in men; and smokers who drink are at additional hazard (Tuyns et al. 1982; Tuyns 1983). Moreover heavy drinking is known to cause vitamin deficiency, and lack of vitamin C in the system may be involved in upper alimentary tract cancers (Yanai et al. 1979). McGlashan's work on Australia encountered the problem of small sample size in a relatively rare disease, with beer and laundry detergents as faintly suspicious (1976). Both McGlashan and Cook were able to visit the area south of the Caspian in Iran, with high rates that increase from west to east (and actually extend into Turkey and Soviet Asia). Incidence is fairly even between the sexes, especially in the east, in contrast to the high male rates in many countries that may link with alcohol and tobacco. McGlashan suggested further work on two fermented products, one a local vinegar and the other a preparation used as a tonic by pregnant and lactating women. The research team that included Cook (now Cook-Mozaffari) formed a cancer registry and tested these and many other foods, soils in case trace elements could be implicated, and life-style elements, but unfortunately the work was interrupted in 1978 by the Iranian revolution. The reports by Cook-Mozaffari et al. (1979) and by Mahboub et al. (1973) suggested links with low intake of protein, vitamins A and C and riboflavin, lack of green vegetables and high intake of opium (see 'also Ghadirian et al. 1985); nitrosamines, nitrates or nitrites, polycyclic aromatic hydrocarbons, and mycotoxins on food, stored grain and flour, all seemed to be excluded. A link has been suggested with a fine fibrous contaminant of flour (O'Neill et al. 1980). On eastern Anatolia, see Memik 1979.

Burkitt's Lymphoma

Burkitt's lymphoma was mapped, rather simplistically (1962) by Burkitt himself, along with his suggestion that since the distribution pattern seemed to exclude high-altitude areas, free from many of the disease-carrying arthropods, the cancer might be caused by an arbovirus. The over-simplified presentation was criticized, and soon the mapping was complemented by the Burkitt–Cook atlas and commentary on cancers of seven sites for East Africa already mentioned (Cook and Burkitt 1970). Perhaps the 1962 paper should be treated as one putting forward a hunch with some sketch-maps? If so it makes the case for the hunch that flows from experience at the grassroots, for a stream of exciting research has followed. After a good deal of work on time-space clustering – negative in the economically developed area of high population mobility round Kampala (Brubaker et al. 1973) – and on relations with blood-groups, it began to emerge that there was a sort of wave movement across this part of the continent that seemed to relate to movements of malaria. However, the tumours in such areas yield numbers of the Epstein-Barr (glandular fever) virus already mentioned in connection with nasopharyngeal cancer. A recent hypothesis that would link the observations on the lymphoma with both malaria and the Epstein-Barr virus is that malaria may impair the immune system's reaction to the virus and thus act as a synergistic factor in tumour activity (Moss et al. 1983; Whittle et al. 1984); see Williams et al. (1985) for a review of several cancers associated with viruses in Africa. It may be significant that a somewhat similar lymphoma, though occurring mainly in older males, and less benign than Burkitt's, is common in AIDS patients where the immune system is also impaired. Geser et al. (1980) argue that since the Epstein-Barr virus occurs at both high and low altitudes, malaria must be regarded as synergistic with it, but from West African evidence Biggar et al. (1981) think that if *Plasmodium* and the E-B virus are both involved, they must operate separately – malaria is mainly a rural disease, the E-B virus both rural and urban (and presumably the lymphoma occurs in children in both groups). The debate continues, and clearly its resolution lies beyond the competence of all but the rarest individual geographers; however, this probably applies almost as much to people in individual branches of biomedicine, and team-work will probably be needed to crack the problem – important in itself and for understanding of tumour formation in general. The West African evidence just cited suggests that this story that began with a hunch and some crude mapping has still a role for good cartography – given data! – and good geographical analysis.

Conclusion

The great relative importance of certain cancers in Third World countries is an important phenomenon in itself, and amongst other things probably supports the view that a major part of the total burden of the cancer group of diseases on humankind has causes lying in the environment, broadly defined. That liver cancer should have, on existing evidence, a likely cause in mouldy groundnuts and maize, with the virus hepatitis B as a synergistic factor, can lead to preventive action, already in train in several quite different parts of the world. The geographical techniques used so far are quite basic ones, and further research can usefully go on to bring out quite local patterns of risk where again simple action may have important preventive effects. Mapping either of liver cancer incidence or of mouldy groundnuts or maize seems likely to be equally effective, though as often biomedical or agricultural science collaboration would be ideal. A recent study aimed at correlating life style with age-standardized cancer ratios in Liberia, Cameroon and part of Tanzania raises promising possibilities for geographical studies (Sobo 1984).

On cancer of the oesophagus the story so far shows how a challenging hypothesis can come from a single worker struggling with a very imperfect data base. The subsequent more detailed research, happily with a geographer involved with biomedical scientists in field work in Iran, demonstrates the scientific value of eliminating certain possible causal relations, directing attention rather to micro-nutritional hypotheses and diet surveys. Only a little further progress is needed in this detective work before areally directed health education may take over – indeed precursor systems are already being linked with diet modification programmes in China.

In the work on Burkitt's lymphoma the story started with the eminent tropical surgeon turning amateur cartographer and geographer, with a plausible hypothesis based on very simple visual inspection of dot maps of children affected compared with climate and relief maps. After criticism, more refined mapping was done with geographer-surgeon teamwork, and meantime links between the tumours and arboviruses and other vector-borne diseases followed more biomedical lines, with a tentative link now widely accepted between the lymphoma and malaria. How much time could be saved if geographical analyses were employed as soon as a spatial pattern and environmental relations are suspected?

Lastly, the work of Bradshaw, Harington, van Rensburg and McGlashan on the different cancers found in different groups of immigrant gold-miners in South Africa shows how good data and imaginative use of opportunities can yield results of potential benefit far beyond the immigrant labour force. Like the research on acute pancreatitis by Giggs and others cited in chapter 8, this is an example of geographical opportunism in its best sense.

As with cardiovascular diseases, however, the Third World picture is changing, in some places very rapidly. There is disquieting evidence that populations at risk of lung cancer, for instance, are not only or necessarily urban elites. A study of 1000 rural people in Bangladesh – where 130 000 acres of useful land are used for tobacco in a country with an annual food-grain deficit of 1.5 million tons – reveals that 71 per cent of men smoke (only one per cent of women), of whom a fifth began smoking at under ten years. The local tobacco is higher in carcinogens than is imported tobacco, advertising is widespread, and without any government health warning. As with western men a generation ago, and women at present, an epidemic of lung cancer and other diseases induced by tobacco now seems inevitable (Cohen et al. 1983). Lung cancer in Cuba is known to be higher than in neighbouring countries, and smoking patterns have been incriminated with high risks to smokers of dark tobacco, while inhaling cigar smoke carries a four-fold increase of risk (Joly et al. 1983).

Equally impressive in looking back over this chapter, I believe, are the roles attributed to the hepatitis B virus and to the Epstein-Barr virus in modern thinking about carcinogenesis, and perhaps also to loss of efficiency in the immune system. Infections seem to be more involved in what were thought of as degenerative diseases only a few years ago; but it now seems reasonable to speculate that loss of efficiency in the immune system with ageing may be the link with the physical degeneration of the ageing process?

As this book goes to press, another quarry of data has become available in Parkin (1986).

14   Is there a Geography of Hunger?

Introductory

Geographers, I sometimes used to tell my students, should never be surprised – well, hardly ever! Certainly few geographers can have been surprised at the parts of the world involved in recent famines, particularly those in the Sahel belt stretching across Africa south of the Sahara and into the Sudan, northern Ethiopia and southern Somalia. Figure 14.1 is a sketch map of the world belts of moderately low rainfall, marginal for production of several of the cereals of semi-arid zones, which are also belts of high variability of rainfall from year to year. In the world as a whole there is a general tendency for drier climates to be associated with high variability – with high risks of crop failures: even if there is not a total failure of the rains, the timing through a growing season may not accord with the moisture requirements of, say, eleusine millet (*Eleusine coracana*) at different phases of its growth. Several of the shaded regions have been known as famine tracts almost throughout history – regions in which there will be an expectation along the lines of the saying in parts of India: one lean year in three, one famine year in seven. Of course there were devastating famines in many different climates and societies historically: for instance in 1695–7 Finland lost 25–33 per cent of her population, Estonia 20 per cent, much worse than contemporary famines in France, Italy and Scotland (Neumann and Lindgren 1979). Readers in the British Isles looking back to the mid-nineteenth century and the potato famine in Ireland and north-western Scotland (not shaded on the map) will not need to be reminded that it is the poor, the women and children, the aged too who suffer most in a famine – for in many cultures the tradition is strong that the lion's share goes to the male head of household. (For geographical work on Ireland, see Cousens (1960a,b).) So already it begins to be clear that human arrangements as well as natural vagaries are involved in famine deaths. And this is strengthened

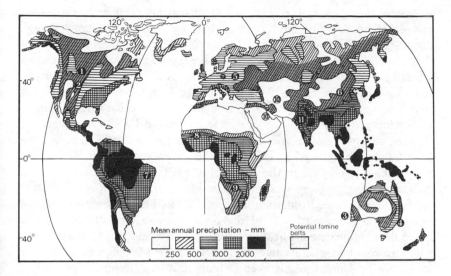

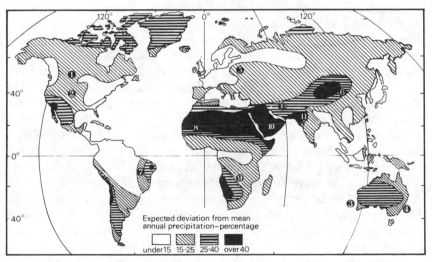

Figure 14.1 Famine belts (numbered regions mentioned in text)
Source: compiled

if one compares various regions within the shaded famine tracts, numbered in figure 14.1.

Famines and Famine Tracts

In North America regions 1 and 2 are areas of cereal production in a capitalist mixed economy, mainly prosperous, and drought years, or even a series of them, are marked by economic hardship, perhaps bankruptcies and enforced sales of land, rather than by famine deaths – though documentary or feature films, or Steinbeck's *Grapes of Wrath*, remind us that at worst conditions approached famine levels. Similarly in Australia's wheat and barley or wheat and sheep areas (regions 3 and 4). Region 5 stretching from the fertile black soils of the Ukraine east across Russia into Siberia is now comparable, granting that the mechanisms of coping with widespread crop failures are different in the USSR; however, the western part of region 5 had a very severe famine, accompanied, like the Irish famine, by typhus, in 1921–2, within a few years of the Revolution and owing a good deal to the chaos of war. (This was perhaps the first occasion on which there was a considerable *international* effort at famine (and epidemic) relief, from nations acceptable to the still new and insecure Soviet government and led by the Norwegian explorer Nansen.) For much detail and some illustrations of Russian famines, see Dando (1980), who stresses their mainly man-made character, including one in 1946–7 attributed by Dando to mistaken farming and food shipment policies of the Stalin government. Edmondson (1977) is also relevant. Dando gives much detailed information about the terrible famines of the nineteenth century in region 6, in inland China, and up to 1921; again modern droughts are met by relief measures by the communist government but see Ashton et al. (1984) on famine in 1958–61. Region 7 is the variable rainfall region of north-east Brazil, where the economically vulnerable share-croppers are still at or near famine levels every few years; government measures are taken, including some movement of population to the new settlements in Amazonia, but where radical restructuring of landholding has evaded successive governments and the poorest remain extremely vulnerable. Region 8 is the Sahel belt of Africa already referred to briefly, and region 9 the corresponding area in southern Africa: the position in Africa is so crucial to the world geography of famine today that it will be discussed separately later in the chapter. Region 10 is the variable region area covering much of the Middle East, in which of course the oil-rich states can now protect their people from famine by food imports. In a sense this region extends to region 11 in the north and west of the Indian sub-continent, in Pakistan and adjacent parts of India but extending south into the Deccan. In this region there arose many, though by no means all, of the famines of India in recent centuries for which Dando (1980) is again a convenient source of detail; the extension of irrigation has ensured that the Punjab canal tracts in both countries, and Sind in Pakistan, more than cover food requirements for the intermediate area and beyond, though, reaching ahead to later paragraphs, the question of entitlement (or command of cash-flow) must arise locally and in economically vulnerable groups. The Deccan area is a more difficult one in that only parts are irrigable; since Independence in 1947 there has been no widespread famine, though the only village I have visited during really severe local food shortage was in the south of this belt in 1957. South India has known some devastating famines. (See McAlpin (1979) for the period 1870–1920, with an attempt to weigh the benefits of the colonial economy and famine relief system.) Bengal had a terrible famine that cost at least two million lives in 1943–4 and the eastern part of the Bengal delta, now Bangladesh, has had at least one famine, very severe locally, in 1974–5 and several local outbreaks of severe food shortage. The other areas of the Indian sub-continent outside region 11 illustrate two important points. One is that rainfall variability can be devastating in a wetter area that nevertheless has an average rainfall, the one the optimistic farmer looks for, that is marginal for the local staple food-crop – at least as catastrophic as in the semi-arid famine belts of figure 14.1, maybe more so if population densities are very high. Thus the Ganga plains in northern Bihar, with mean annual precipitation of about 40 inches (100 cm) have rainfall marginal for rice in the flood-plains and maize on the slightly higher interfluves; shortage of rain and bad timing in relation to the needs of rice and maize at different stages of growth, including interruptions to the monsoon, have both caused very severe famines in this area. The second point requires a new paragraph.

The Bihar famine of 1966–7, twenty years after Independence, showed the advantages of the Famine Codes evolved under the British Raj almost a century before. Its evolution over two or three decades up to the 1880s was by no means without opposition from *laissez-faire* and post-Malthus economists arguing that famine relief would merely result in population increase without any matching increase in food production, as Brennan (1984) notes in a fascinating review of issues and personalities using many contemporary sources (see also Passmore (1951)). Following the heavy financial costs of relief in the Bengal and Bihar famine of 1873–4, there was sufficient opposition to the principle to delay relief measures in the severe and very widespread famines in South India in 1876–8 until several hundred thousand lives had been lost. After that tragic experience there was no real argument about the principle, right to the end of colonial rule: thus in 1939 a relatively local famine occurred in Hissar and Rohtak districts (now in Haryana and largely irrigated from canals), and relief measures proved very effective. The catastrophic famine in Bengal in 1943–4 was another matter, the most terrible blemish on the closing years of colonial rule, discussed briefly later in another context. Meantime it is sufficient to note some virtues in the Famine Codes, which were adopted province by province rather than agreed for the whole of India, or for even the old British India that excluded the 'native states' of the rajahs and nawabs; they must be classed as lasting virtues, for they endured until the 1970s. Thus the Bengal Famine Code, apart from indicating action to be taken once famine was identified, used a number of 'early warning' signs of approaching crisis: a contraction of the private charity normal in village life, indicated by the movements of paupers; a contraction of credit, normally a complex and changing web; feverish activity in the grain trade (probably including hoarding or 'bullish' buying for an anticipated price rise, perhaps astronomical if famine develops); restiveness and an increase in crime, like a kind of bubbling cauldron; unusual wandering of people, either unattached males in search of livelihood for the family back home, or at worst, whole families moving out in search of wages but ultimately of food (Currey 1986).

Sen's Entitlement Theory

From the end of the introduction of this chapter onwards it has been clear that even if there is a natural disaster, like a drought, involved in a famine, there is nevertheless a more or less strong man-made element in it too. This may be very general, perhaps the world trading patterns in tropical products against imports from developed countries, or relatively local, such as, say, population increase following epidemic control, or again storage irrigation that does not have sufficient capacity to provide water over a *run* of drought years. Or a hurricane or crop disease in a small area may start a price rise that develops into hoarding for higher prices, as already mentioned. (For the 1972–3 period a valuable compilation of world climate and famine statistics is in Garcia and Escudero (1982); the analytical element of this work has been criticized as naïve.)

There is, then, a geography of famine, but it has moved a long way from reductionist physical determinism. The argument that famine is *not* caused by climatic change, progressive desiccation of the desert margins, drought, flood etc. has been very prominent in recent years, and one focus has been the elegant economic analyses of A.K. Sen (1981), who himself remembers the Bengal famine of 1943 as a child. Sen's argument is that famine is primarily a failure of entitlement. To quote:

> Some of the relations are simple (e.g. the peasant's entitlement to the food grown by him), while others are more complex (e.g. the nomad's entitlement to grain through exchange of animals, leading to a net gain in calories). Some involve the use of the market mechanism (e.g. selling craft products to buy food), while others depend on public policy (e.g. employment benefits, or relief in destitution camps). Some are affected by macro-economic

developments (e.g. demand-pull inflation), while others deal with local calamities (e.g. regional slump), or with micro-economic failures (e.g. denial of fishing rights to a particular community in a particular region). Some are much influenced by speculative activities, while others are not.

For a similar argument couched in somewhat different terms see Timmer (1977).

Sen justifies his stress on entitlement by wide historical references. Food was actually exported from famine areas in Wollo, Ethiopia in 1973, in Bangladesh in 1974, in the Irish famine of the 1840s. He points out that the Bengal famine of 1943 took place when there was no widespread failure of the rice crops and in conditions of economic boom, not slump. Locally, south of Calcutta, there had been cyclone damage in the autumn of 1942, and locally some crop damage from disease. The war had brought a wholly exceptional complex of circumstances: the seizure of food stocks by the military in order to deny them to the Japanese should seaborne invasion come, and for the same reason the seizure of many of the 'country boats' essential for communication in the semi-aquatic environment of the delta, and perhaps as crucial as any, the censorship and secrecy that kept news of the gathering disaster from parliament and the public in still imperial Britain and even – rumours apart – from the wider Indian public. Maybe the fact that the tide of war had not yet turned against the Japanese made for panic buying and hoarding, but it was largely for profit from rising famine prices rather than for personal stocks – there were appalling malpractices by some trading groups and the small but important import of rice from Burma was of course prevented by the Japanese occupation there. An epidemic followed in this 'world endemic home' of cholera, in the wake of enormous refugee movement from the country to the cities. Once the appalling death-rates were 'leaked' and then officially admitted, government procurement of rice improved (including using prominent merchants for the task) and military resources deployed in famine relief, the situation improved – but too late to avoid 2 to 3 million deaths. Of course it is no surprise that the famine struck mainly at the poor, or that enforced sale of lands etc. by small landowners added permanently to the total of landless labourers after the famine. Sen's childhood memories were at least one stimulus for his later analyses of famines across the world, and it is the common thread of failed entitlement in different societies and economies that gives a fresh view of the need for short-term and long-term change in the entitlement of the economically vulnerable in future famines. After reviewing both the Sahel and the 1974 Bangladesh famine in an account aimed at geography students, Crow (1985) stresses that

Sen's work above all prevents any serious student of recent famines from regarding them as anything but man-made, even if there was a trigger in some natural disaster like flood or drought.

Currey's Concatenation Process Model

There is much convergence of thought along these lines, see for instance Glantz (1977a,b); Currey (1984); and it is surely significant that a Conservative ex-Prime Minister, addressing the Royal Geographical Society (a generally conservative rather than notably radical body), should have referred to starvation in the 'poverty belts of Africa and of Asia' rather than to drought belts (Heath 1981). For a critical view of Sen's work, however, see Currey (1984) on 'concatenation process models':

> Sen's 'entitlement' approach does not, however, explain the causes of famine. The work is in fact an elegant description using economic terminology of concepts similar to those of Greenough (1975) and other historians (e.g. Bhatia 1975), of the reasons why some groups suffer more than others during famines. To date the policy analyst, Sanderson (1975) at the international level, the economist Alamgir (1980) at the national level and the anthropologist Firth (1959) at the community level have probably come closest to an exposition of the complex concatenation processes which explain the causes of famine.

(Currey's sources here are included in the references for this book.) To an extent Currey's own approach is idiographic and deals with the unique rather than nomothetic and law-seeking – or at least the law is to search for the concatenation; he illustrates this from two recent food crises in Bangladesh:

> *The 1974–75 food crisis*: in the wake of the independence war, the administration was inexperienced: relations with aid donors were strained; government personnel in rural areas were left unpaid. Annual flooding was severely out of phase with the agricultural calendar both in 1973 and 1974. The dumping of sterile sand and the ponding of flood waters on the fields lessened the need for agricultural labour. The Government's initial response was minimal amidst widespread speculation, hoarding and smuggling by certain people.

> *The 1978–79 food crisis*: population numbers had grown beyond the previously estimated needs for stocks of food. The worst drought in Rangpur District's meteorological history affected internal production, particularly in the northern region. Anxiety arose after

difficulties with food aid negotiations. The Government released large amounts of food stocks (already low) to urban elites because of an impending election. The cash crop, jute, was poor in quality and gave little remuneration to poorer groups so that they were then unable to purchase back supplies of rice for subsistence.

So on this reading the 1943 Bengal famine was, as older accounts had always thought, a concatenation: this does not excuse the appalling blot on the closing years of the British Raj, but it does suggest that the lack of free communication was crucial, and this may be important for the future. How do the Sahel famines of recent years appear in the light of this argument?

The Sahel Famines

The Sahel belt, stretching right across Africa south of the Sahara and north of the Ethiopian highlands into the Horn of Africa, has seen very widespread famine accompanied by considerable movement of people as refugees from the worst-hit areas, an accentuation of an age-old response to drought, stock losses, crop failures and hunger (Tymowski 1978; Miller 1982; Hill 1985). There is a climatic element in the pattern of recurrent drought – that is, a shortage of rain as compared with that expected or hoped for by pastoralist, farmer or in some contexts water authority supplying human needs or irrigation canals: this is best seen as a secular trend towards a drier climate in the Sahel, of course with annual fluctuations above and below the descending totals (Bryson and Murray 1977). Climatic change interacts with changing human impact on the environment: as elsewhere in Africa, population growth has increased with the extension of preventive medicine and economic development, and provision of boreholes to water stock can lead to changes in traditional nomadic patterns of land-use and overgrazing and loss of semi-desert vegetation within easy journeys to a borehole for cattle (for a general perspective see Grove (1977) in a United Nations conference report). This is an example of the 'desertification process' that has caused much concern in recent decades. Swift (1977) analyses loss of ecological equilibrium with increased pastoral and agricultural farming and gives some pointers to ways of attaining a new state of balance. Ibrahim (1978) points specifically to extension of millet cultivation in the western Sudan, to tree-felling for firewood and general degradation of vegetation by overgrazing. On Nigeria Apeldoorn (1981) opposes 'victim-blaming' of peasants as inefficient and shiftless; he traces the tradition of gifts of food and cash to the distressed by the feudal Emirs of the desert trade towns, through to the related but changed post-Independence policy of government redistribution in famine years – but with stocks inadequate and badly used. This author sees socioeconomic change as fundamental to the present problems: the increase in cash crop marketing has changed the structure of rural society; the poor depend greatly – too much? – on the rich, and on the south of the country, while the northern farmers do not have sufficient command over the surpluses they produce in good years as insurance against bad; thus he recommends more investment from such local surpluses, including food stores and reserves (see also Berry et al. (1977); Nicolas (1977)).

Migration of desert and desert margin groups as a response to drought has already been noted as normal and age-old, and Tuareg, for example, came to towns as far south in Nigeria as Zaria and took jobs as watchmen, caretakers and the like that fitted oddly with their proud bearing – and then vanished silently when the rains improved; Bein (1977) suggests that governments could provide more employment in receiving areas at the first signs of this type of migration. E.P. Scott's (1984) edited volume, *Life before the Drought*, concerns traditional coping strategies and makes a case for more consultation with the people before outsiders try to find remedies for famine; Grove (1978) offers an authoritative geographical introduction to the area; and Hill's (1985) edited book demonstrates the kind of sample surveys and statistics from Mali that could be carried out over wider areas with benefit, and makes the point that nomadic people can be adaptable, and can move in and out of agriculture. From the Sudan Awad El Karim et al. (1985) consider the question of availability of water in relation to water quality and disease potential, as well as the distances and time spent in fetching drinking water. In Mauritania, the pastoral nomads of the centre and east, retaining more of the traditional responses to drought, were less severely affected than those in the west who had moved further towards permanent settlements, attracted to the town of Nouakchott (Toupet 1977). Bernus (1977) further develops the theme of the plight of the nomadic herdsmen: he sees the deterioration of the vegetation as linked with the stress imposed on it by the technical services' encouragement of increased cattle populations, more demanding on fodder resources than other stock; and he brings out forcibly the enormous impact of complete loss of stock to a herder community – loss of animals and milk to barter for cereals, of religious symbols including animal sacrifice, or security for loans, and very disruptive breaking of social ties, exchanges and relations. See also Museur and Pirson (1976) on the Ahaggar area, and for bibliographies, Peterson and Newman (1977) and *Sahel Bibliographic Bulletin* (1977). A kind of spatial operational research approach to the problem of food distribution in the Sahel is in Gould and Rogier (1984).

It is rare to have actual nutritional data during the crisis-laden period of famine relief, but there is a study from the 1970s famine in the West African part of the Sahel, on rural communities: this suggests improvement between 1974 and 1975, apparently due to relief measures (Hogan et al. 1977). The degree to which the famine was an information crisis is dealt with by Baker (1977), and one looks back to the wartime censorship in Bengal in 1943, and also to the tremendous influence of a television report of the conditions in Ethiopia in 1984, especially film of dying children. The demographic implications of the 1970s drought in the Sahel are discussed by Caldwell (1975) and in a broader survey Hugo (1984) looks forward to the prognostic value of even quite small variations in, for instance, infant mortality – *if* the information flow is both good and heeded! Harriss (1985) looks back on recent African famines and asks 'Are there any solutions?'

While it may be too early for a full analysis of the course and causes of the Sudan–Ethiopia famine of 1984–5, Cutler's 1986 paper offers a wide interdisciplinary view of the crisis, including figures 14.2(a) and (b) of the dramatic fluctuations in price over short distances of a local staple food, a millet, *neff* (*Eragrostis neff* or *Eragrostis abyssinica*). It would be premature – and perhaps reductionist too? – to say that this is evidence supporting Sen's entitlement thesis, but it does illustrate the extent to which lack of income to pay the crisis prices (panic prices? hoarding prices? profiteering prices?) was crucial – as indeed some of the relief organizations made clear at the time. Cutler, however, adds in a personal communication (1986) that in many areas even the offer of high prices would not have brought food to the market; for such areas the prices quoted are notional.

Part of Currey's concatenation (literally 'a joining' like the links of a chain!) is too often war between nations or between a government and dissident groups or between warring tribes or factions. Once the television reports were coming through in the 1984–5 famine in north-east Africa, few family sitting-rooms in the west were free from the impact of the Ethiopia–Somalia war on the famine and the responses of the communist government in Addis Ababa to it; the Sudan government too is affected by warfare with dissident groups near the border with troubled Uganda. A regional famine in Karamoja, Uganda, was largely caused by a breakdown in civil order, cattle raiding and the like affecting semi-nomadic herders with some subsistence agriculture; very simple emergency foods included skim-milk powder, but happily lactose intolerance – an enemy of this simple form of western aid for protein-deficient babies in particular – was not a problem (Robinson et al. 1980; Biellik and Henderson 1981).

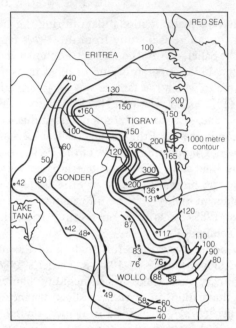

Figure 14.2 (a) Ethiopia, price fluctuations over short distances and short periods 1983
Source: Cutler (1986)

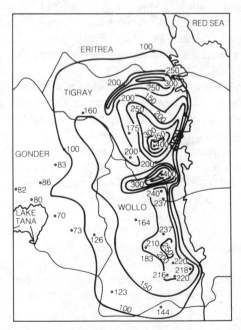

Figure 14.2 (b) Ethiopia, price fluctuations over short distances and short periods 1984
Source: Cutler (1986)

Food aid has its critics, often on the argument that the benefits may not reach those for whom it is intended, through corruption and the like – though there is a counter-argument that even so it does represent an injection of capital, often much-needed, into the developing economy (Dustin and Lavoipierre 1981). For a geography of food aid see Tarrant (1980) Currey (1980), familiar with famine in South Asia, looks at past famines and future prospects in the Pacific Islands, suggesting that food aid may delay the evolution of farming patterns appropriate to the local environments.

Geography and Famines

Among geographical contributions to famine studies the edited volume by Currey and Hugo (1984) occupies a unique place: it is strong in historical components yet in the end up-to-date except for the Sahel and Ethiopian famines of 1984–5 and not uncritical of geography's relatively small part in academic and practical work in recent decades. It culminates in Currey's essay on early warning and forecasting systems based on this concatenation process concept and of course linking back to the Indian Famine Codes noted earlier in this chapter. Currey (personal communication, 1986) warns that satellite imagery is by no means a panacea for all early warning problems. However, it does have some potential if indications of poor rains and vegetation development from satellite photographs are complemented by ground survey and, over large territories, by low-level air photography using light aircraft or helicopters (Gwynne 1985). See also O'Keefe and Wisner (1976) on early warning systems, and Currey (1986) on the need for these to be locally *specific*.

A television programme cited in the references of Crow (1985) emphasizes the mainly man-made nature of the 1974 Bangladesh famine, showing geographically how the peak weeks for 'street deaths' in Dhaka corresponded with the period of very high prices – rather than shortage – of rice. The area of greatest demand for famine relief in the north is shown in figure 14.3(a) as not corresponding with low *per capita* availability of rice (figure 14.3(b)) to those who could afford to buy it, but rather with very high prices in relation to the purchasing power of average wages (figure 14.3(c)).

From Famine or Epidemic Undernutrition to Chronic or Endemic Hunger

After the terrible Sahel famine of 1984–5 it seemed right to put catastrophic hunger first, but on the world scale there is at least as great

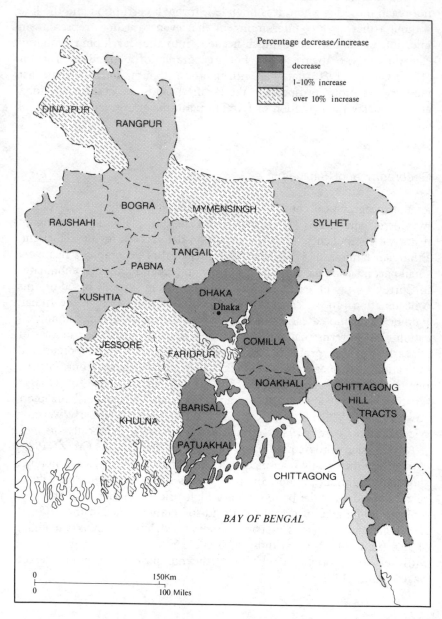

Figure 14.3 (a) Bangladesh 1974: rice available *per capita*
Source: Crow (1985), based on Sen 1981

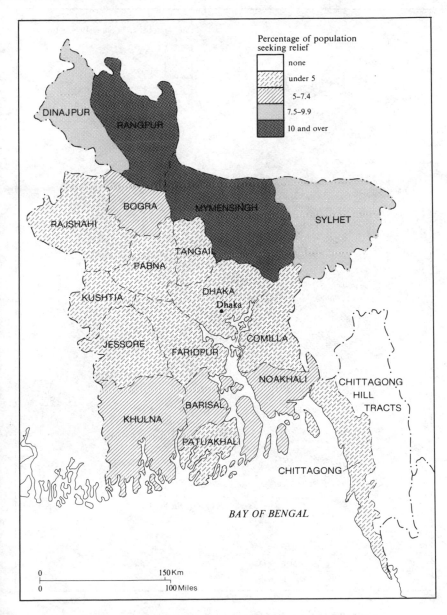

Figure 14.3 (b) Bangladesh 1974: demand for famine relief
Source: Crow (1985)

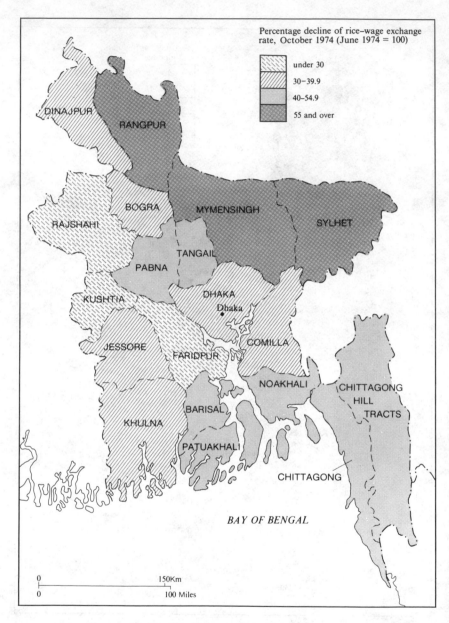

Percentage decline of rice–wage exchange
rate, October 1974 (June 1974 = 100)

under 30

30–39.9

40–54.9

55 and over

DINAJPUR

RANGPUR

BOGRA

MYMENSINGH

SYLHET

RAJSHAHI

TANGAIL

PABNA

KUSHTIA

DHAKA

• Dhaka

JESSORE

FARIDPUR

COMILLA

NOAKHALI

CHITTAGONG
HILL
TRACTS

BARISAL

KHULNA

PATUAKHALI

CHITTAGONG

BAY OF BENGAL

0   150Km
0   100 Miles

Figure 14.3 (c)   Bangladesh 1974: rice price/wage ratio
Source: Crow (1985)

a problem in chronic or endemic undernutrition, often coupled with malnutrition or lack of specific dietary components such as protein or vitamins, and also with seasonal hunger. This aspect is intimately bound up with questions of world food production, and these involve a minefield of political issues and values, yet there is an underlying geography. Fortunately there is a major geographical survey, perhaps as objective and value-free as any comparable work (Grigg 1985). That author looks back to the 1950s, at the fairly general gloom about the prospects for population growth and at least matching food production, at the doubling of the population of the Third World since the 1950s, but then turns to the remarkable increases in food productivity in much of the developed world and, with a different complex of resource utilization, in most of Latin America and Asia, exceeding the considerable to high rates of population growth in those parts of the Third World. This leaves Africa, in this context as for famines, as the major problem continent, with many very high rates of population growth while output of food remains static or shows inadequate and faltering growth. So, finding good cause for some thankfulness, if not optimism, he then adds the necessary qualifications, and here I quote from his concluding chapter:

In the 1950s, at the time that malnutrition was becoming a minor issue in the developed countries, the problems of hunger in Africa, Asia and Latin America were receiving a great deal of attention; the rapid growth of population led to fears of catastrophe. In the event, the world as a whole has increased its food output faster than population since 1950, as have all the major developing regions except Africa. But the record is not as satisfactory as this might suggest. First, it must be reiterated that there are countries – mainly in Africa but also in Latin America and parts of South Asia – where food output per caput has been in decline since the early 1960s. Second, in spite of the remarkable growth of food output, one-third of the population of the developing world live in countries where in 1977–80 available food supplies – output, stocks and imports – were insufficient to provide the population with an adequate diet even if it were distributed according to need rather than purchasing power. Third, even among those countries which had supplies in excess of national requirements, many were perilously balanced a percentage point or two above the minimum needs, and any major crises – such as the disruption in China during the Great Leap Forward or the failure of the Indian monsoon in 1964–6 – can lead to acute difficulties in feeding the population. Thus whereas it is unquestionably true that poverty is the principal cause of undernutrition and malnutrition, it does not follow that food production can be neglected. It is not only that in many countries food output is still insufficient to provide the minimum national diet; although there has been some slight decline in the rate of population growth in the last decade, rates of increase will remain high well into the next century in most countries in Africa, Asia and Latin America.

(Grigg 1985)

Figure 14.4, from a valuable series in Grigg's survey, is one of two maps based on the figure of 1.2 times the basal metabolic rate, that is the food intake is estimated as enough to cope with needs of the body at rest (at 1.0) plus a fairly arbitrary figure of 0.2 to allow for normal physical activities demanding more than the resting rate. In terms of calories, intakes are from under 1500 to over 1600 calories. This is much lower than earlier attempts to find out the proportions of undernourished people in different countries, some criticised as using criteria based on western overnourishment; as it is, these intakes probably allow excessively for the known adaptability of the chronically undernourished to make more efficient use of intake than better-nourished people while sustaining remarkable outputs of energy in work (Edmundson 1980a,b). As Grigg points out, on this basis, in 1978–80, 535 million people had diets inadequate in quantity,12 per cent of the world population and 17 per cent of that in the Third World, with the highest proportions in Africa and least in Latin America, but the greatest numbers in Asia. And as always and in all countries the economically vulnerable groups, castes or classes bore the heaviest burdens. Recent estimates of prevalence of protein–energy malnutrition include Keller and Fillmore (1983) and WER (1984b). Waterlow et al. (1980) also use a wide range of data from tropical countries to show that babies' weight tends to falter at 4–6 months unless suitable solid food is given to supplement milk. It is well to note that Burkitt's advocacy of increased dietary fibre in western diets is balanced by concern for the damaging role of high-fibre low-energy diets on Third World children, (Burkitt et al. 1980). Experience in the UK of severe diarrhoea in Asian children returning to Britain from visits to their ancestral homelands has stimulated a suggestion that damage to the mucous membrane of the small intestine may reduce assimilation of foodstuffs, and that this may give a clue to the diarrhoea–malnutrition cycle in the Third World (Hutchins et al. 1982).

The Protein/Energy Debate

At one time there was a heavy stress on protein malnutrition and on *kwashiorkor* (discussed in a later paragraph) which was then seen as a

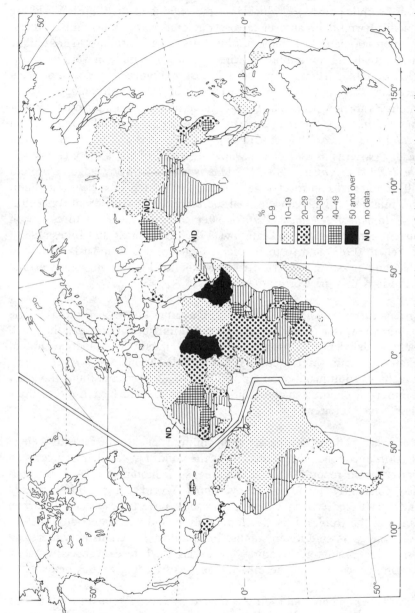

Figure 14.4 World map of areas with proportions of populations with under 1.2 times the basal metabolic rate expressed in terms of energy values of food intake
Source Grigg (1985)

protein malnutrition especially of weanlings: this led to what is now seen as over-emphasis on the protein problem and on wasteful food aid in the form of milk powders – which in some regions of the Third World are actually harmful because of lactose intolerance in babies and toddlers. (Human populations in much but by no means all of the world are unique in mammals in continuing to drink mammalian milk in various forms into adult life, having acquired a lactose tolerance that does not seem necessarily to be a built-in characteristic of human physiology.) These emphases are now part of such consensus as now exists among nutritionists: thus for instance the relevant part of the course for undergraduates on *Health and Disease* (Open University 1985) stresses the need to view dietary patterns as part of the whole structure of the society (Book III, *The Health of Nations*, 118–37). This is a field of knowledge at present full of internal controversy and perhaps in search of a new paradigm. One might start with conventional sources like the Ministry of Agriculture's *Manual of Nutrition* (1970 or later edition), move on to essays on current controversies like Waterlow (1982), Neuberger and Jukes (1982), or Pellett (1983) and so to problems of nutritional standards (Wretlind 1982) and measuring undernutrition (Sukhatme 1977). Still, some working definitions may be worth attempting.

Protein–energy malnutrition or PEM   Sometimes known as Protein–calorie malnutrition, this is now used to cover 'all nutritional disorders in which there is deficiency of protein and energy in any combination and of whatever origin' (McLaren (1981)). On global trends see *WER* (1984b). It includes adult inanition or starvation, and also two conditions tragically common in children in the Third World, and here I continue to draw mainly on McLaren.

Marasmus   This is wasting in young children, in extreme cases to skeletal or 'skin and bone' appearance. It is the condition familiar to television viewers from reports from famine areas of Ethiopia in 1984–5, but it is also constantly found in many Third World communities, mainly underprivileged economically. A disease of poverty, especially in urban slums in the tropics, it is also commonly linked with infections, such as fly-borne gastroenteritis in summer, respiratory infections in winter, and also with premature weaning on to artificial feeds especially using contaminated water in the mixture, or dirty feeding bottles or teats.

Kwashiorkor   This condition was named by Cicely Williams from the Ga dialect of Ghana in 1933 and the implications of the name were said to include 'red boy' and 'the deprived child'. The child is not skeletal but rather oedemic, and *very* miserable, and there is often reddish hair and skin in black babies as 'red boy' suggests. The 'deprived child' idea is from premature displacement from the mother's breast by a new baby and against the normal tradition of prolonged lactation in many African communities. Early workers related the syndrome – regarding it as a group of symptoms rather than a specific disease – with some confidence to sudden, especially premature weaning on to an excessively starchy and protein-deficient diet, particularly if the staple is starchy roots like cassava (tapioca) and yam, or in some areas bananas (Trowell et al. 1954). This is still held to be the main causal link in a general guide like McLaren's 'atlas' (of diagnostic photographs rather than maps!) and it is probably still the prevailing orthodoxy. Controversy has already been implied.

As long ago as 1968 Gopalan produced convincing case series from India widely accepted as evidence that from a population of babies on the same diet some would remain healthy, some develop marasmus and some kwashiorkor. Fifty years after Dame Cicely Williams identified and named the syndrome, a symposium was held in honour of her 90th birthday, and two papers reflect the continuing controversy since Gopalan's report. One view signals a return to the classical view that it is a protein malnutrition of children especially on weaning (Waterlow 1984a), and that individual physiological differences in the babies on similar diets may cause some to develop marasmus, some kwashiorkor. In contrast, Hendrickse (1984) argues that kwashiorkor occurs over quite a wide socioeconomic spectrum, whereas marasmus is always linked with poverty (see also Hendrickse et al. (1982) and Long (1982)) and that kwashiorkor does have a specific cause, that it is a specific disease, and that it is one of the diseases caused by aflatoxins arising from fungi living on ill-stored crops especially of maize or groundnuts. (See also chapter 13 on liver cancer; early workers like Brock (1954) suspected a link between kwashiorkor and liver cancer but knowledge of the aflatoxins as possible carcinogens lay in the future.) Hendrickse points to some evidence from animal experiments – an avenue that has never produced animal analogues to kwashiorkor by protein-deficient diets alone.

In the mid-1950s, along with Dr Hugh Trowell, I conducted a questionnaire to tropical doctors and paediatricians on kwashiorkor which produced a good deal of evidence of a relationship with rapid urbanization, social disruption and the like and evidence of this is still coming forward and of course need not exclude the aflatoxin theory: for instance Waterston (1982) stresses 'substitute mothers' as a possible factor. Incidentally the questionnaire was also the basis of a map which I showed to Cicely Williams, who said: 'Oh, Dr Learmonth, what a lovely map – of paediatricians!' Cartographic evidence has its perils and pitfalls! So what of the modern geography of these three linked conditions – protein–energy malnutrition, marasmus and kwashiorkor? I have not attempted to update maps like those used in my (1978) book, simply because the field is in such a turmoil – perhaps the spectators have invaded the pitch! The field is wide open for geographical input, preferably in contributions to team work; indeed these may well be overdue. May devoted his last years to the geography of nutrition, always appealing for the international geographical community to join in cooperative projects, but on any scale these have so far failed to materialize – see the review of what has been done in Currey and Hugo (1984) in their introduction to their edited volume and see May (1961–8) and May and McLellan (1970–4); also Newman (1980).

Seasonal Hunger

As for seasonal hunger, this can be thought of as pressing on vulnerable groups through the Third World, in the belt of semi-arid climate and variable rainfall in figure 14.1. The interface between nutrition studies, physiology and biology is explored in Haas and Harrison (1977), for instance in relation to climatic stress and behavioural responses in quantity and quality of food. The hungry season before the harvest, and the need also for high energy outputs during the hard work of harvest, are topics long familiar to geographers, lingering in folk memories from 'what is sown with tears is reaped with joy!' through to the 'hunger and a burst' attributed to the less provident members of the community in rural Scotland (or the more economically vulnerable?); how much more immanent is the problem to the landless labour of the Third World today (Geddes 1982; Currey 1984). This topic is something of a growing point in nutrition studies at present. And apart from the vulnerability of children and the old already mentioned there is also a gender difference: it is not only a matter of the tradition of the heaped plate or banana leaf for the male head of the household, but also of the additional stress on females at menarche, during pregnancy and during lactation. A valuable systems-based survey of nutrition in Tamil Nadu found that this stress occurred throughout the socioeconomic groupings they used, though naturally it was in the poorest that the nutritional stress brought real danger to health (Sidney M. Cantor Associates 1973). The relations with seasons and their fluctuations from year to year, with cropping patterns and with behavioural patterns cry out for this kind of holism that geography can offer (see Currey (1984), or the older study of seasonal graphs of climate and cropping in Geddes (1982), chapter 6 on the plains of Biharia).

Some Sequelae to Malnutrition

As chilling as anything from the Third World, to me at least, is Dugald Baird's confident attribution of excess congenital malformations including anencephaly in Aberdeen in the 1950s and 1960s to the slump years of the 1930s and – apparently – irreparable damage to the oöcytes of girl babies at or soon after birth (Baird 1973).

An introduction to the important topic of malnutrition as a possible impairing factor for brain growth and intellectual development is in Clugston (1981), though there are critical comments from R.J.C. Stewart in abstracting the paper for *Trop. Dis. Bull.* (1981, 78, p. 507): that some of the papers used by Clugston have been criticized as to documentation, and that more attention should be paid to longer-term studies by Richardson et al. (1978) in Jamaica and in Mexico by Cravioto and De Licardie (1976). Richardson et al. think that the effects may have a sharp impact above some threshold degree of malnutrition (rather than acting as a continuous variable so that increasing degrees of malnutrition cause increasing degrees of mental impairment). A local study in Guatemala concluded that cognitive development was probably improved by a regime of vitamin-fortified high-protein dietary supplement, ideally for the pregnant and lactating mothers and then carried through to the children (Freeman et al. 1980). A report from South Africa again supports the idea that medical supervision and food supplements can improve intellectual development as compared with three sibling groups – some who had recovered from kwashiorkor, some who had received medical supervision but no supplements, and those who had received neither (Evans et al. 1980). An important study from the West Indies took a different line from dietary supplementation: development quotients were recorded in malnourished groups receiving and not receiving 'psychosocial stimulation' (being played with!), and also in a well-nourished group receiving hospital treatment for other illnesses and *not* receiving the stimulating play (Grantham-McGregor et al. 1980). The abstracters for *Trop. Dis. Bull.* for these last two studies make the point that it is extraordinarily difficult to sift out the variables – the nutritional from the 'Hawthorne effects' (to borrow the sociologists' term for the stimulating effect of experiments on human subjects): these might include the stimulating effects, possibly both intellectual and emotional, of the studies on the children's mothers, siblings, and possibly fathers too. Interactions with infections have already been noted in chapter 9. A bench-mark survey is in Faulk et al. (1975).

The Geography of Overnutrition

Overnutrition is at least part of the problem of 'western diseases' discussed in chapter 2, and a reminder that this also has a geography may be justified at this point. The lack of geographical study of foods and food habits is quite remarkable, as Thouvenot (1978) points out in introducing a valuable paper on food geography in France, concerned not with calories, protein and vitamins but with patterns of combination of particular foods; see also Favier and Thouvenot (1980) for maps of food patterns in France. Returning to nutrition as such, Klatzmann (1979) attempts a three-fold world classification by countries, stressing internal divisions and disparities within countries: overnourished countries, mainly developed countries; those with just about enough food, like China; and those seriously deficient in food, like many Third World countries. Grigg (1985) is again essential reading in this context. Nutritional needs naturally vary somewhat in different climates and in relation to physical activity, see Waterlow (1982) and Evenson et al. (1979).

Overnutrition may be general, from excessive food intake in relation to climate, physical activity and individual metabolism – the more common problem in many, perhaps most, developed countries; or it may be specific, for malnutrition can occur from over-consumption of specific items. Too much vitamin D can cause excess calcium deposition in the kidneys, for instance; and alcoholism is commonly accompanied by vitamin deficiency, often of vitamin B_1 (Thiamin or aneurin) a substance needed for alcohol assimilation, but sometimes as a more general vitamin deficiency due to a poor and ill-balanced diet (WHO 1980, TRS 650, p. 44). (Alcoholics with low incomes will often spend money on alcohol to the neglect of food.) General, and some specific, overnutritions may contribute to, even cause, obesity and associated problems of heart disease and other disorders of the circulatory system. Many readers will have encountered official and commercial campaigns to persuade us to alter our eating (and exercise) habits, and their relevance is discussed briefly in chapter 4. Geographical studies of obesity are not numerous, but an exemplar is proffered by Thouez and Munan (1981b): they found the proportion of obese women in eastern Quebec province to rise very consistently with age as compared with obese men; obesity seemed a higher risk in rural areas and small industrial centres; and the problem seemed to have its root in adolescence, in a nutritionally vulnerable age-group. Comparative studies might be enlightening, even by countries with different policies: thus for instance the USA seem to have undergone something of a dietary revolution mainly on a free-market approach, whereas Norway seems to have moved away from that approach according to Ringen (1980), with a combination of subsidies, regulations and education. From the Third World comes a study of obesity in children in Abeokuta, capital of Ogun state in Nigeria (Akesode and Ajibode 1983): as in inner city USA, obesity was greater among children from poorer families, largely owing to socioeconomic factors including high consumption of cheap starchy foods, and more in girls (8 per cent overweight, 5 per cent obese) than in boys (9 and 3 per cent).

Vitamin Deficiency Diseases

Most readers will know that scurvy was common in 'scurvy knaves' in the Middle Ages, and important in sailing ships into last century, causing serious problems to the Royal Navy until lemons and later the less efficient limes were made part of the rations as a countermeasure. Fewer would know that, like so many useful practices, this lesson was forgotten in the first flush of post-Pasteur 'germ theory', so that scurvy was one cause of the loss of Captain R.F. Scott and his companions on their return trek from the South Pole in 1912 (Open University 1985, III, p. 120). The disease itself, if neglected, can be serious, the lack of the vitamin leading to a breakdown of connective tissue e.g. in gums, but also bone defects. It does occur in artificially fed babies who are not given a vitamin supplement, in old people living on poor diets, and in alcoholics whose vitamin C absorption is impaired. But it is not like so many of the diseases described in this part of the book particularly a Third World problem, except locally where urban slum populations have lost touch with traditional sources of the vitamin, and in some poor rural diets – see Farooqi et al. (1981) on diets in Orissa in north-eastern India, and Akhtar (1985b) on the Kumaon district and especially people in Himalayan villages.

Rickets has been a familiar deficiency disease in Britain and other western countries until the last two generations or so, for instance in sunless slum areas where children often had unbalanced diets, northern cities like Glasgow being notorious. And it has recently returned to similar areas in underprivileged immigrant groups, especially in Muslim groups practising purdah and where children, especially girls, may not be able to use the synthesizing power of the skin in sunshine to make vitamin D. (Some writers stress sunshine alone as a source, deprecating diet as a factor, see Loomis (1970); for some measurements of the surprisingly short and partial exposure of the skin needed to produce adequate amounts of the vitamin see Webb and Steven (1985).) The general problem in Britain is set out in DHSS (1980b); Goel et al. (1981)

report on the anti-rickets campaign in Glasgow. Stephens et al. (1982) report that Asian children in Manchester show improved vitamin D status (though still below that of a white control group) but adults manifest little improvement despite a health education campaign. The need for a balanced and not faddish approach to diet is urged in Robertson et al. (1981) suggesting that the re-emergence of rickets in Dublin is related to an excessive increase in dietary fibre in some diets, a factor long known to affect calcium absorption and so bone formation; rather similarly there is a report from the Netherlands of rickets not only in immigrant groups but also in strictly vegetarian households (Schulpen 1982). For a study from a rich country, Saudi Arabia, see Serenius et al. (1984) and while vitamin D levels in Pakistan are reported as generally within normal limits, *purdah* does provide exceptions (Rashid et al. (1983) – and the older literature at least gives evidence of the related adult bone malformations of osteomalacia, especially in pregnant women, see Learmonth (1958)). The problem of rickets in a sunny country, it is now suggested, may partly be that protein–energy malnutrition causes such lassitude and inactivity that exposure to the sun does not occur (Raghuramulu and Reddy 1982).

Vitamin A deficiency as a cause of eye disease and blindness has been briefly noted in chapter 9. In Asia alone some 5 million children develop xerophthalmia each year, and 250 000 of them go permanently blind: WHO's field guide for the detection and control of this preventible blindness (Sommer 1982b) is seen by a doyen among nutritionists as a call for action and 'the energies of angry men and women' (Passmore 1983). See also V. Ramalingaswami (1984) on the comparative ease of control by massive doses of vitamin A every six months. This again seems a field wide open for geographical work and preferably action research with an interdisciplinary team. An avenue of approach is in Perisse and Polacchi (1980) on the world distribution of sources of vitamin A, and changes therein, calculated from FAO data on national food supplies. A study of vitamin A deficiency in Upper Volta, south Mali and Senegal in 1977–9 showed proportions with inadequate intake from 37 per cent in the south (with more growing and tradition of use of palm oil, rich in the vitamin), but higher in the dry season, rising to 100 per cent in the north (Le François et al. 1980). Lechat et al. (1976) report on mass vitamin dosing, with needs greater in the host population than among nomadic refugees from drought, and plead for relevant health education. A campaign against this avitaminosis in Hyderabad City, India brought a fall of 80 per cent in hospital admissions, but the needs of 80 per cent of the total population of the city as a whole remained unmet, so a campaign targetted at the city's children is urgently needed (Vijayaraghavan et al. 1984). Solon et al. (1980) report on a survey in four ecologically different zones in the island of Cebu in the Philippines – densely peopled urban fringe *barrios* or squatter areas, rural coastal fishing communities, rural coastal farming areas, and upland hilly areas in the hinterland. There were deficiencies in 3 per cent of 1700 children of 1–16 years, but varying from nil to 8 per cent in different age groups and zones, and interestingly with high rates in adolescents in an area of high general intake of the vitamin. A cost–benefit study as part of this project found that strictly on xerophthalmia *either* vitamin capsules or food fortification (using monosodium glutamate as a vehicle) would be adequate without any health education campaign which might, however, well be justified on wider health grounds (Popkin et al. 1980). Assumptions are always difficult in such exercises; Erica F. Wheeler, the reviewer in the *Trop. Dis. Bull.* (1981), notes an assumption here that population not affected by xerophthalmia would have potential productivity increased by the mass vitamin dosage by about 1 per cent, because resistance to infections would be enhanced. Possibly, however, the assumption might be justified, even modest: in urban squatter and rural farming *barrios* the overt xerophthalmia rate was 4.5 per cent, but this was indeed the tip of the iceberg or the snout of the bathing water-buffalo, for 57 per cent of this group showed low or deficient vitamin A levels by international standards. From Indonesia Fritz (1980) records some of the problems met in aid programmes across cultural boundaries, using the example of a vitamin A and xerophthalmia project; in 5000 children between six months and five years the xerophthalmia rate was 7 per cent, while in Lombok island children of the same age group showed responses to vitamin dosage including reductions in night blindness, Bitot's spots (hardened conjunctival tissue), corneal xerosis and ulcers and keratomalacia (*WER* 1984a). On xerophthalmia in poor rural households in Bangladesh, see Cohen et al. (1985). In intriguing contrast, see Landy (1985) on a possible effect of excessive vitamin A in an Inuit (Eskimo) group.

For the vitamin deficiencies it seems justified to include a version of one of Dr May's maps from his *World Atlas of Disease*, dated as it is, to show the potential and as archival material (figure 14.5).

Goitre

Goitre and iodine deficiency has been selected for brief discussion because the topic has received some attention from geographers. Trace element deficiencies or excesses have a more general literature, and entry points are in a special issue of the *Journal of the Geological Society* (1980) or in the many papers of Professor H.V. Warren (1972, 1973). Bench-mark papers on the environment and thyroid disorders are in Greig et al. (1973)

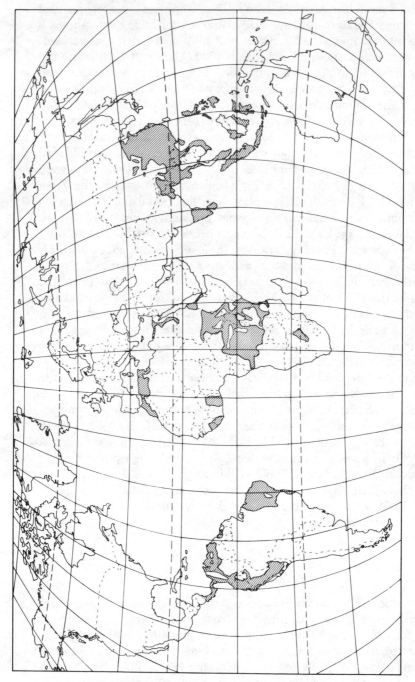

Figure 14.5 World map of vitamin deficiencies
Source: May (1977)

and a brief but important discussion in Hutt and Burkitt (1986).

Goitre (ultimately from the Latin for throat, *guttur*) is enlargement of the thyroid glands in the neck. From this swelling come terms like Derbyshire Neck, denoting a regional concentration of which only residuals happily are left; struma (Latin for scrofula); scrofula (Latin for 'brood sow' though that also applies to tuberculosis of the cervical lymph nodes) and king's evil from the notion that the king's touch could cure the disease. All these are popular terms from the past, but goitre rather unusually is both popular and scientific usage, implying that somewhat similar symptoms may arise from different specific causes. Simple endemic goitre responds best to geographical analysis, and this is confidently linked mainly with iodine deficiency in the diet, causing over-stimulation of the gland, and swelling in the neck sometimes large enough to interfere with the nearby gullet, windpipe, veins, nerves etc. Hormones from the thyroid gland and from the pituitary (also a ductless gland at the base of the brain), operate together in the normal individual to maintain homeostasis or balance in energy utilization from tissue glucose; this homeostatic mechanism is important, for while iodine deficiency in food and water intake seems to be the primary cause of simple endemic goitre, there are areas where goitrogens seem to be involved. One theory is that these produce goitre by reducing the thyroid gland's ability to use iodines in the bloodstream, and thus produce symptoms similar to those caused by iodine deficiency. Thus some years ago a minor epidemic of goitre in schoolchildren in Tasmania was attributed to the introduction of school milk from cows fed too predominantly on brassicas like kale in the cool Tasmanian winter, while, as often, lactation had a concentrating effect that in the particular circumstances included a goitrogen from the brassicas. On present knowledge this does not account for much of the world pattern of goitre as compiled from various sources in figure 14.6, but alert medical geographers may produce a change in this judgment, and the ailment is amply serious enough to make this a worth while field of research.

Apart from inconvenience and sometimes personality changes in individuals, there has long been noted some degree of association between goitre, deaf-mutism and cretinism, particularly in countries with very marked regional patterns such as India; at present the weight of opinion seems to be against the direct link that would exist if goitre were a proven cause of deaf-mutism and cretinism, but rather that similarities in spatial distribution patterns of the three conditions may arise from some third causal factor at present not known. However, on terminology, a recent paper suggests that for many purposes the term iodine deficiency disorders (IDD) should be substituted for goitre, the swollen glands being a symptom (though not an invariable one) of an underlying deficiency that

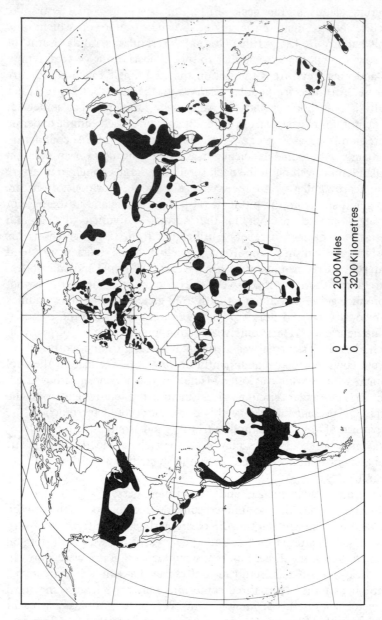

Figure 14.6 World map of goitre
Source: Learmonth (1978) after WHO (1960)

commonly affects intellectual ability including initiative and decision-making; its author believes that there may be 400 million people suffering from IDD in Asia alone, with millions more in Africa, Latin America and Oceania (Hetzel (1983) and see also Ramalingaswami (1984)).

The WHO monograph of 1960 from which figure 14.6 has been compiled stresses the influence of glaciation in removing mature soils from many temperate and high latitude areas: some 12–15 thousand years after the Quaternary glaciers retreated from many now inhabited and cultivated areas, there are many immature soils based on limited organic action on rock-flour, boulder-clay, outwash sands and the like, and these are often very deficient in iodine, affecting crops and drinking-water. (For a WHO report, see DeMaeyer et al. (1979).) Research on iodine content of soils suggests that this gradually builds up as soils mature by vegetative recycling from the parent material (Aston and Brazier 1979). One might add the considerable areas of periglacial action involving much solifluction, mass movement of superficial deposits and so on, and no doubt involving radical alteration of pre-glacial soil profiles. The world pattern forces one to hypothesize that rain-forest climates, with heavy leaching and very deep soil profiles, may have somewhat comparable effects on iodine content of the soils, crops and drinking water, and even more speculatively that seasonally heavy leaching during summer monsoons might be an influence. In some rain-forest areas where the root crop cassava (tapioca) is a staple food – and in many areas increasingly so – it is now accepted that iodine deficiency is aggravated by a goitrogen, linamarin, a glucoside from which cyanide is liberated in the gut (Delange and Ahluwalia 1983). In reviewing this book the eminent nutritionist Dr R. Passmore refers back to the pioneer work of Sir Robert McCarrison in India over 50 years ago – some of it referred to below – and how horrified McCarrison would be to know that as many infants are at risk today in a disease which, Passmore pleads, could be eliminated by AD 2000 given the international will (Passmore 1984). (Cassava inadequately cleared of its cyanide content is also one cause of disorders of the peripheral nervous system: see WHO TRS 654 (1980) for a general account, Osuntokun (1981) for a report from Nigeria.)

There remain puzzling anomalies, like the concentration in northern Chile, roughly in the nitrate mining area. Are nitrates an influence? – other diseases with suspected links with nitrates seem to be more serious in nitrate-using areas of Chile than in the mining areas (see chapter 13).

The old name of Derbyshire Neck is from a largely limestone terrain, and there is some popular association at least with limestone parts of the mountain arcs of the Old World from the Pyrenees through the Alps and the Balkan chains, through the mountains north of the fertile crescent in the Middle East to the Himalayas and into China and Burma and

Malaysia. McCarrison hypothesized that polluted calcium-rich water was a causal factor, and after experiments using trout he conducted some experiments using volunteers. This theory is almost forgotten, apparently, though the geographer Rais Akhtar found some support in his village surveys from the plains to the Himalayas in Kumaon (Akhtar 1978, 1980, 1985b), and recent studies in western Colombia of goitre persisting after iodization of dietary salt do point tentatively to water supplies downstream from organic-rich sediments (Gaitan 1983). Years ago Stott and Gupta (1930–1) found some links with calcium-rich alluvium in the plains, but fifty years afterwards Singh and Singh (1980) suggest a correlation with socioeconomic status rather than lime-rich alluvium. These workers are sure that calcium-rich soil and water cannot be an independent factor, though they may operate synergistically with iodine deficiency, poverty and poor diet and hygiene, perhaps contributing because of more locally based food in the poorer groups.

Seaweed was used as a treatment for goitre in China some four centuries ago (Langer 1960), and well into the age of western scientific medicine in 1915 David Marine, thinking of iodine additives in salt (bread is now found more effective), declared that 'simple goitre is the easiest of all known diseases to prevent . . . It may be excluded from the list of human diseases as soon as society decides to make the effort.' Passmore's comment quoted above may serve as a postscript – or prescript to action?

Iron Deficiency

A note on another avoidable mineral deficiency may be justified: in at least some Third World conditions mass addition of iron to diets is justified – as an additive to salt in villages near Calcutta and Hyderabad (and in Madras with less effect), and as tablets to school children in Varanasi (Working Group on Fortification of Salt with Iron 1982; Singla et al. 1980; see also Agarwal et al. (1980) on anaemia as a concomitant of protein–energy malnutrition in India; and Akinkugbe (1980) on the frequency of anaemia in village children near Ibadan).

Toxic Plants

Illnesses resulting from the consumption of toxic plants sometimes have strong geographical relations. Lathyrism, causing paralysis and crippling of various degrees, results from high proportions of a pulse in the diet, *Lathyrus sativa*, a vetch and relative of the garden sweet pea. This vetch grows in drought years in various parts of India, and too easily forms part, an excessively large part, of the diet of landless labourers and poor peasants. It appears to attack especially boys and young men, but this may be related to larger rations allocated to males. It is described in an early paper by the present author and his wife (Learmonth and Learmonth 1955) and more recently in a pamphlet from the Indian Council of Medical Research (ICMR 1974) and a paper by Hinz (1984). A more general source is in WHO (1980 TRS 654).

Any geographical reader interested in detective stories would be fascinated by the use of maps and plans of all scales by two Indian medical men (Lal and Roy 1937–8) tracking down the cause of epidemic dropsy in north-eastern India in the 1930s, eventually incriminating a toxic weed namely the prickly poppy *Argemone mexicana*, growing in crops of mustard, the source of the staple cooking oil in that part of the sub-continent.

Conclusion

Looking back over this chapter there is every reason to stress the One World element. Many readers with Irish or Scots surnames must have grandparents whose grandparents were able to tell them at first hand about the potato famine. What one might call the political economy viewpoint on famine and chronic hunger and malnutrition – not necessarily left-wing – urges that much of the world's hunger is part of the world economy and related to developed country use of Third World crops and to the terms of trade between North and South, between developed and developing. Broad surveys of this exist, like Grigg's (1985) book. Given appreciation of this, coloured, perhaps by individual political and even ethical values, there is nevertheless a whole world of regional problems on all scales, micro, meso and macro, with geographical dimensions. Grigg points out the change in perspective on the world food problem since the 1950s in his book and in a valuable paper (1981). This chapter reflects these changes and those following Amartya Sen's elegant economic presentations of the famine problem in particular. Geographers, too long absent or underrepresented in an interdisciplinary field of endeavour of enormous practical moment, now have guidance such as the edited volume from Currey and Hugo (1984). Over a decade after the tragic death in a car accident in Morocco of Jacques May and his wife Donna McLellan – at work in the field, both, to the very end – it may be that the pleas he made for geographical research will now be answered by the post-Ethiopia and post-Geldof, post Band-Aid generation. How Jacques May would have rejoiced at such an outcome!

Part III   Towards Synthesis

15 Approaches to Regional Synthesis

. . .from the waters the people get their food, also their cholera, their dysenteries, their typhoid fevers, their malaria; from the earth they get their hookworm; from the crowded villages they get their tuberculosis and their yaws; from the type of housing they have been forced to adopt they get their plague and typhus and from the food which the earth, temperature and rain produce, their protein deficiencies and their beri-beri.

J.M. May (1958) on the Song Koi (Red River) delta, Vietnam

Introductory

This quotation from a medical man turned geographer, or the one by Dr William Pickles quoted at the beginning of the book, might well serve as a text for micro-scale regional synthesis. Both of course are by medical doctors, and except for the very rare medically qualified geographer, or one having the almost as rare chance to engage in team-work of this type, a medical geographer interested in regional synthesis often has to take at second-hand a medical survey of all-round health (and such are also quite rare apart from routine public health reports) and try to complement the medical findings by geographical insights. Both May and Pickles were working on a micro-scale, studying a comparatively small area in depth, one in an underdeveloped country, the other in a still relatively isolated part of a developed one. So it seems appropriate to start with a micro-scale survey in India to which I have tried to add some geographical input, then go on to a meso-scale and macro-scale study from that country.

A West Bengal Village, *c.*1950

Figure 15.1 is a composite portrait of 'Kalipura' drawn from descriptions or experience in several villages in West Bengal (Learmonth and

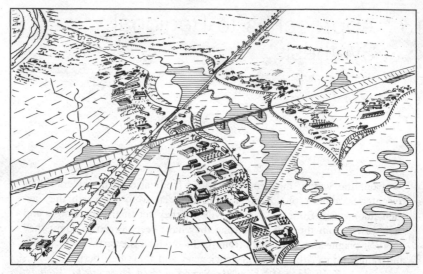

Figure 15.1   'Kalipura', a composite portrait of a West Bengal village
Source: Learmonth and Learmonth (1955)

Learmonth 1955); however the details of health conditions are drawn almost entirely from Lal and Seal (1949). Kalipura lies in the western 'dying' delta, shown as highly malarious in figure 1.2, as compared with the 'active' eastern part of the Ganga-Brahmaputra delta that was much less malarious at the time that map was drawn. Round Kalipura, river channels, chains of stagnant pools for much of the year, are linked with the local disease complex and – along with the land tenure system – with the poor physique of its inhabitants: the soils are no longer renewed by sheet-floods and in a mean annual rainfall of about 140 cm (50 in), mainly in the summer monsoon, leaching of nutrients is quite marked. There is stagnant water too, behind carelessly engineered or maintained rail and road embankments, in ponds behind small dams across the water-courses used for local irrigation, and in the rectangular excavated water 'tanks' – here used mainly for ceremonial ablution and clothes washing and often rather neglected. All these give harbourage to mosquito larvae – including the local malaria vector *Anopheles philippinensis* (see chapters 1 and 10). Many water-bodies are at least partially covered by the water hyacinth *Eichhornia crassipes* – the 'lilac devil' – which spreads into paddy fields and reduces yields. Seventy per cent of the inhabitants cultivate their own land, usually as rice-growing and rice-eating subsistence farmers, the rest including landless labourers and 'village menials' often of lower caste such as leather-workers and sweepers. The village economy and community (or set of factions!) have already been affected a great deal by the great industrial conurbation of Calcutta-Howrah, some 30 miles away. It adds to the cash income required to buy in additional rice to tide over the lean time before the main autumn rice harvest, in two ways: some of the people travel daily to the city to work, or migrate there for shorter or longer periods, some as pavement-dwellers, and send some of their earnings home to the village; and the huge urban market attracts much of the fruit, vegetables, milk and eggs from this countryside. Again there is a cash flow into the village economy, but at a cost, for all these foods of high nutritive value are much needed in the diet of the poorer peasant and landless families.

The sketch shows that the richer houses are in courtyard form, of course including cattle-sheds etc. The courtyard may be covered by a trellis with a pumpkin giving shade and food; there may be some hens, and by the tank some ducks, and date palms to be tapped for syrup or toddy. The health and status especially of the poorer people are unsatisfactory. Much disease is related in some way to the pools of more-or-less stagnant water. *Vivax* malaria is always present, depressing to adults even though they carry on working through the periodic rigors, men, say, ploughing with their oxen, women transplanting rice seedlings from nursery beds, soaked by the afternoon storms; and it takes a very heavy toll of the elderly, the young and the unborn. Few except widows – of low status at this time in poor but orthodox families – now drink habitually from tank or stream, and the virtues of deep tube-wells are becoming known; but ritual cleanliness demands bathing, invariably including washing out the mouth and complete submersion, and this is often done in such polluted places. Urination may occur in the water, and the search for privacy for defaecation often leads to fouling of the lower banks of tank or stream. The village lies near the world endemic home of cholera, and very near a notorious local focus, and water-, fly- and food-borne intestinal diseases include periodic epidemics of cholera, and much and severe endemic dysentery and typhoid, as well as hookworm from bare feet on polluted soil. Outdoor living is restricted during the rains and in the quite sharp cool season, poor people being ill-clad, and overcrowding spreads colds and coughs, influenza, often succeeded by pneumonia, tuberculosis – perhaps from the city with a returning migrant – and at that time smallpox too in occasional years. The poor farmer or farm labourer will be given preference at the hot evening meal, and the early cold breakfast of left-over rice – though that may be polluted by the eggs of the rat tape-worm *Hymenolepis nana* – so stress to pregnant or lactating women or girls at menarche is implied. For an attempt by the author to bring this account up to about 1980, see Open University (1985, III, chapter 4); many improvements are largely due to much greater urban influence but there is a return of malaria and a sharp impact of filariasis and Japanese encephalitis carried by culicine mosquitoes. Hazra and Banerjee (1979) give a statewide context for this micro-scale study; and for an urban micro-study of Sagar, Madhya Pradesh, see Choubey (1985). From the Middle East a micro-study of Kuwait is based on a different organizing principle, the quality of the statistical data available being judged suitable for multivariate analysis (Ffrench and Hill (1971), discussed in Learmonth (1978)).

The Meso-scale: Chandigarh Dun

A reconnaissance survey of the Chandigarh Dun, a comparatively isolated cul-de-sac of valley between the Lower Himalayan ranges and the outer foothills of the Siwalik range some 15 km north of the city, offers one of the rather few studies from India on the meso-scale. The valley is about 40 km north-west to south-east, and between 2 and 8 km across (Mukerji 1980). The north-western three-quarters of the valley are drained north-west to the Sutlej catchment, while the Ghaggar river breaks through the Siwaliks to flow south-west across the Punjab plains. The rivers flow quite close to the northern edge of the Siwaliks forced southwards by three major and several minor alluvial fans or alluvial cone-segments of coarse gravels resulting from erosion of the outer slopes of the Lower Himalaya: their southern fringes contain more clay, and the southern quarter of the longitudinal valley is dominated by the flood plains of three rivers (the third is the Jhajra) and a series of low terraces. The alluvial cones are very permeable, mainly calcareous and iodine-deficient. Apart from the summer monsoon season (with about 85 of the 120 cm (50 in) of mean annual rainfall) the radial streams across the alluvial fans are dry with occasional stagnant pools, rapidly becoming covered by green algae. There are springs where the water-table meets the surface, especially in limited patches of clay towards the southern edges of the cones, but these are very seasonal. Wells for human or animal use, or for small-scale irrigation, are usually quite deep – and so involving long hauls for buckets or hand-pumps – and yet in mainly coarse gravel they are very liable to pollution from surface flow; in the eastern part of the dun water tanks are common, fed by rainfall or springs, for human and animal use and described by Mukerji as very liable to pollution from human and animal washing, laundering and excretion near tanks. Winter wheat and summer maize are grown on the rather light and dry sands and sandy loams of the fans, with much poorish grazing also; the clay soils are hard to drain and liable to have pools of stagnant water for long periods. The sandy loams are mainly near settlements receiving more water (and human excreta).

The 90 per cent of various Hindu castes and groups, and the 10 per cent of Sikh Jats, live for preference in courtyard houses, regarded as encouraging the spread of non-vectored infections like measles and influenza, and especially so among one Hindu group, Gujars, whose houses usually are linked to linear courtyards. Woodsmoke in the houses may add to eye, skin and lung troubles.

Diet is largely vegetarian, with dairy products and in some groups a little animal protein – but the river fish are a neglected source of this. Mukerji found eating of many kinds of vegetables and fruits to be almost unknown, and the diet deficient in protein, vitamins, mineral salts and especially iodine. Disposal of excreta is often haphazard, and where sewers exist they are often open, with stagnant pools breeding culicine mosquitoes and flies that can act as mechanical vectors of intestinal diseases. There is one all-weather road along the dun, but apart from that, movement is difficult and limited, on tracks along streams including beds cut deep into the heads of the alluvial fans, and links between settlement by footpaths and cart and camel-tracks, mainly running parallel to the north-east–south-west streams on the fans. Mukerji sees this as making for quite local concentrations of disease – yet, as will appear shortly, even such a cul-de-sac and backwater has surprised him by the importance of 'new' diseases spreading by contact from the outside world to the south. Religious gatherings may spread disease through pollution of water and food, pilgrims diffuse infections along the dun, and cremations of say cholera victims by streams or ponds are sometimes a hazard.

Much of this is in common, perhaps surprisingly so, with the micro-scale study from West Bengal, some 1500 km (1000 m) away and in a humid delta; however, Mukerji's sampling – on an unstated sample design – gave him evidence of marked sub-regional contrasts within the dun. The general picture is of endemic goitre, venereal diseases from limited outside contacts and liability to invasion from influenza epidemics, and variable risk of influenza, trachoma, typhoid fever, syphilis, gonorrhoea, tuberculosis, leprosy, amoebiasis, malaria, hookworm, asthma, anaemia, pellagra and rickets. Within this he finds the regional complexes indicated in figure 15.2.

Area 1. The Southern Flood Plain Endemic Malaria Belt

There are many pools suitable for anopheline breeding (*Anopheles culicifacies?*) especially in autumn and winter after the monsoon rains,

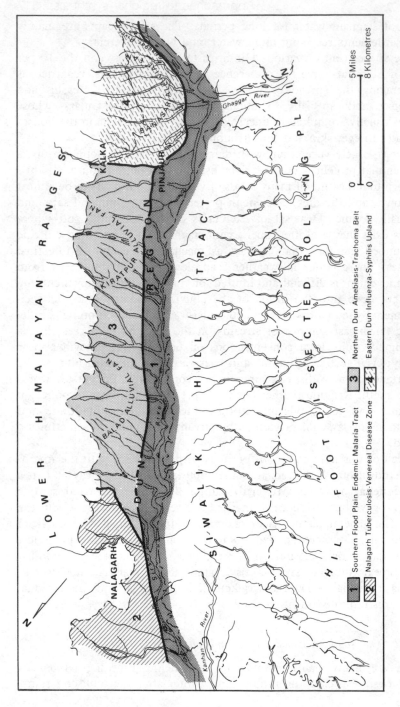

Figure 15.2 Chandigarh Dun, sub-regions
Source: Mukerji (1980)

1 Southern Flood Plain Endemic Malaria Tract

2 Nalagarh Tuberculosis-Venereal Disease Zone

3 Northern Dun Amebiasis-Trachoma Belt

4 Eastern Dun Influenza-Syphilis Upland

and malaria is overwhelmingly important in this tract, though hookworm is widespread and debilitating and typhoid troublesome. In the 20 years since the malaria resurgence in India (from near-eradication), some authorities class the whole dun as hyperendemic.

Area 2. The Nalagarh Tuberculosis–Venereal Disease Tract

In contrast with the post-monsoon waterlogging of region 1, this is an area of alluvial cones of sand and gravels, with *kuhl* irrigation (that is from leats led along a 'falling contour' from a stream, more or less incised into the cone). Water is calcium-rich and iodine-deficient, goitre widespread. This is an area of Rajput landlords and Kanet tenant-farmers or peasants: the Rajputs' greater interaction with the Punjab plains may be related to their greater prevalence of venereal diseases, the inadequate housing and nutrition of the peasants to their higher prevalence of tuberculosis.

Area 3. The Northern Amoebiasis–Trachoma Belt

This is the traditional area of Gujar culture, involving the linear courtyards common to a number of households, with sewage and sullage water of several households flowing in an open drain to some local sump: ponds are not used for drinking but for washing clothes and household utensils and bathing cattle, and commonly with defaecation and urination nearby. The depth of the wells, often draw-wells without even a hand-pump, is seen as a deterrent (perhaps quite sharp winter temperatures too?) to the thorough bathing and personal hygiene normal in India under the most unpromising conditions. There is high room-density, with children and adult family members often sharing bed and pillows, and this along with the poor personal hygiene in a hot dusty climate is linked with the high incidence of trachoma especially from May to September (see chapter 9). Amoebiasis is a complex problem, attributed by Mukerji to contamination of food and water under the conditions described above, and certainly intestinal infections in general must be favoured. Many Gujar farmers leave their fields as seasonal merchants in the towns: complex malnutritional problems are attributed to this movement. Anaemia is thought to be particularly prevalent in this belt.

Area 4. The Eastern Dun Influenza–Syphilis Upland

This is a tract partly covered by dense mixed jungles of tropical and sub-tropical vegetation, with outliers of Himalayan rocks on which clay soils have developed; there are many ponds and marshes, and a good deal of *kuhl* irrigation. Nearly all suitable areas are farmed, mainly by Sikh Jats. While malaria is prevalent, as elsewhere in the Dun, it is influenza and syphilis that stand out as higher in proportion here – gonorrhoea too, and asthma. Mukerji sees the venereal disease problem as controllable given treatment and education programmes, but that of influenza as more intractable because it is difficult to account for its greater relative importance in this sub-region of the Dun. He hints that wild or domestic mammals and fowl may somehow be involved, but clearly the answer lies beyond his reconnaissance scale of study.

Summing up, Mukerji points to the diversity within a small and rather backwater area, and to interactions between physiographic, biogeographical and cultural factors; he looks to better public health and medical treatment as improving a somewhat depressing picture, and for the 40 per cent of all hospitals' and private doctors' patients that present with malaria, he looks forward to the discovery of an effective vaccine as the only likely remedy for *community* health – a not uncommon reaction in Indian workers in the post-resurgence era (see chapter 10).

The Macro-scale: Late Colonial India

Turning to the macro-scale and to late colonial British India, excluding the then 'Native States' but still on a sub-continental scale, the present author attempted a regional synthesis from the series of maps based on the annual public health reports of the then British Provinces, which together gave data for some 400 districts – of doubtful and variable accuracy, but yielding some spatial patterns that seemed to make sense and to justify analysis. Figure 15.3 of a general index of health and well-being, infant mortality, and figure 15.4 of a notoriously epidemic disease, cholera, are examples of the mapping on which the synthetic map 15.5 was based, and their captions make some points about the patterns revealed in the first two figures. A synthesis based on a quantitative search for common patterns was attempted, but failed – given the flexibility of modern computer technology, a similar attempt today might well be successful. So, in the event, figure 15.5 was based on careful visual inspection of the series of eight maps resembling figures 15.3 and 15.4 and of course many other maps and a great deal of reading (Learmonth 1958).

The publication summed up the regional synthesis thus:

> On the broadest scale the 'chief zones' of mainland South Asia may be outlined thus from point of view of medical geography. First, a pluviose, tropical and rice-eating zone might be distinguished, associated with severe endemicity of several diseases. These are

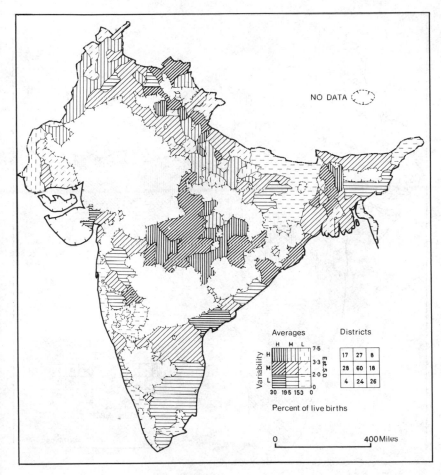

Figure 15.3 Infant mortality British India 1921–1940, showing average incidence and a measure of variability from year to year, thus reflecting epidemic as against endemic diseases
Source: Learmonth (1958)

partly mosquito-borne (malaria and filariasis), partly water-borne and fly-borne (cholera and other intestinal diseases). Chronic malnutrition among many of the people results from inadequate diets, based on rice, or on rice-and-tapioca in the south-west. Poverty and backwardness are linked to such diseases as leprosy and smallpox which are severe in this zone. Yaws seems to be widespread in humid South Asia, while syphilis and gonorrhoea, urban diseases of both zones, unfortunately extend their impact back into the villages with returning migrants.

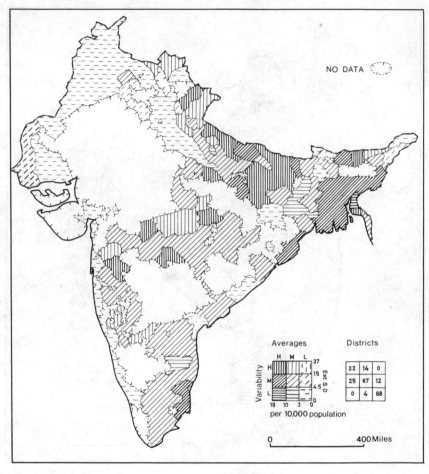

Figure 15.4 Cholera, British India, 1921–40, using the same conventions as in figure 15.3
Source: Learmonth (1958)

The semi-arid zone

In contrast, one might distinguish a zone of semi-arid conditions and variable rainfall. The northern half is somewhat continental in climate, with millet and wheat-eating; the southern half is mainly millet-eating. This great zone is associated above all with instability and fluctuations in its conditions of economy, health, nutrition and disease. Great variations occur in harvests, bringing alternations of relative plenty with lean years or actual famine, often accompanied

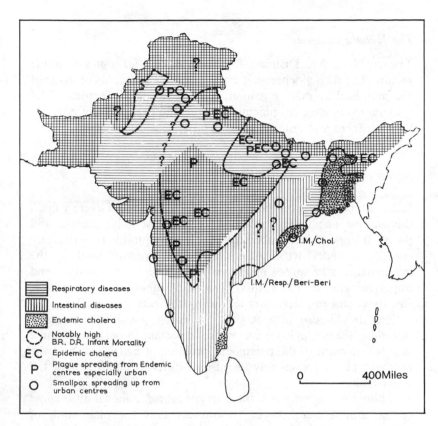

Figure 15.5 Regional synthesis based on a series of maps similar to figures 15.3 and 15.4
Source: Learmonth (1958)

by epidemics of disease spread by insects, water and man. Malaria, plague, intestinal disease and influenza may all strike in this fashion. These epidemics typically spread from endemic centres either outside the zone or within it. Plague spreads from urban centres or large villages within the zone, and beyond that from the enzootic of the marmots etc. in Central Asia, while malaria is maintained in wet and forested hill and hill-foot tracts within the zone. Cholera, however, usually spreads into the zone from its endemic homes in eastern deltaic India. In the northern half of this zone, universal diseases such as pneumonia, measles and influenza are probably more important in the cool season, especially during a famine.

The Himalayan zone

The few Himalayan Districts afford glimpses of a far from favourable picture, but with a depressing complex of low standards of material life and health, poor nutrition, liability to severe epidemics of cholera, to endemic or epidemic malaria, and to diseases of poverty, backwardness and ignorance like leprosy and osteomalacia.

Some Relevant Disease Aspects

Still conceptualizing on the broadest scale, one should overlay upon this outline one disease which is certainly of great present and potential importance – tuberculosis. The profoundly unsatisfactory conditions under which most townsfolk live are vital in the maintenance and spread of tuberculosis. They play a similar and important role in the natural history of other diseases such as smallpox, and in places plague, during the period studied.

One should also consider an interesting possibility, that the intestinal diseases may be even more important in peninsular India as a sub-stratum to the paramount problem of malaria than in the northern plain, presumably because of different conditions of the water-table.

Within these great zones, there are, of course, regional differences of the utmost significance. To consider only the plain-lands of north-eastern India, fundamentally different problems are found in the mature delta of West Bengal, whose population is in the state termed 'stagnation', in the active delta of East Bengal (now Bangladesh) with its high natural increase in population until 1943 and in the colonisation tract of the Assam valley . . . (see Geddes 1942).

Population Disequilibrium

Regional differences in health and demographic trends may be considered in ecological terms, as evidence of differing stages of adjustment of equilibrium between groups of men and their environment. In a sub-continent in which the greater proportion of the people still largely depend on the food they produce themselves from the land, there is still much justification for this point of view. One view of the unfavourable extremes of population stagnation and recurrent crises might be that they represent different varieties of Malthusian checks on population growth; and that they therefore represent a state of 'unstable equilibrium' or of oscillation, more or less violent according to climatic and biotic complexes involved. On this view, if disequilibrium has arisen, it is because of a number of new factors. Thus during the later British period major famines were prevented save during the stress of war, and many outbreaks of epidemic disease were checked which might have spread as pandemics. Craft workers were ousted by competition from large-scale manufacturing industries in Britain, India and elsewhere, and this had driven yet more people back to the land. Cash cropping has been increased.

All these new factors had operated with few major steps – except the great irrigation schemes – either to increase the amount and flow of food supplies through increase in cultivated areas or in yields, or to pave the way to a higher standard of living, a more even balance between agriculture and industry, and a new state of equilibrium, given the more or less limited natural resources of the land.

The present review of the medical literature and statistics leads the writer to lend some support to such a view. Western medicine, and its many devoted servants in India, both European and Indian, have accomplished great work especially by acquiring basic knowledge, notably of pathogens and nutritional diseases. They have prevented the spread of many epidemics and have saved many lives and much individual suffering. Yet though the literature has been written mainly by doctors trained in curative rather than in preventive medicine, it reiterates the theme of interlocking vicious circles – poverty, backward agriculture and malnutrition; ignorance, poor environmental hygiene and disease. Here it might be argued that from any practical point of view geographical studies of these problems must be futile, since man cannot alter the regional differences of climate. Conversely, social and economic elements are factors very largely common to the whole subcontinent.

(Learmonth 1958)

However, the logistics of remedial campaigns and targeting of health education can only benefit from regional studies: indeed all experience suggests that they are essential for rational planning of campaigns.

A fresh synthetic map, then is not yet available, though it may be just around the corner at least for India. However, some outstanding trends may be outlined, at severe risk of over-generalization. Economic development programmes in India and Pakistan – hardly as yet in Bangladesh? – have made the rich richer and the poor at least a little less

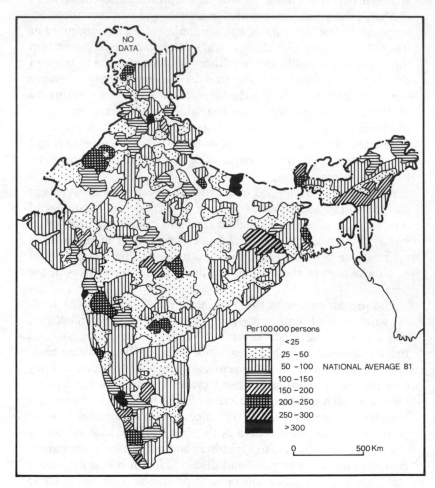

Figure 15.6 (a)   Ratio of hospital beds to population, India, 1975
Source: Akhtar and Izhar (1985)

poor. Falling death rates and rising population have brought rapid urbanization, some of it in 'shanty towns', and also major efforts in population control. Malaria eradication programmes were close to success in 1965, but then came the resurgence and re-diffusion over much but not all of the pre-1945 endemic areas: this was followed by fresh strategies aimed at control rather than eradication, with some success. Other major changes include the decline of plague, the eradication of smallpox, and the partially successful anti-cholera measures, the enormously difficult campaigns against tuberculosis and leprosy, and the obdurate problems

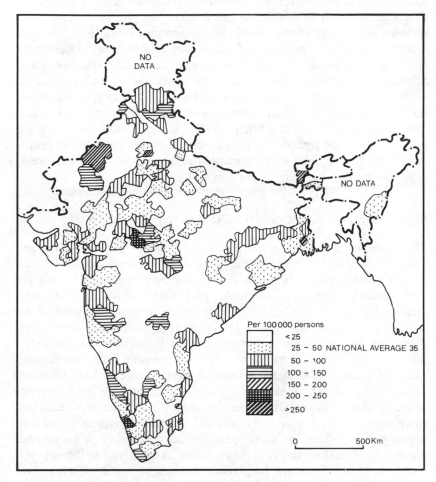

NO
DATA

NO DATA

Per 100 000 persons

< 25

25 - 50 NATIONAL AVERAGE 35

50 - 100

100 - 150

150 - 200

200 - 250

>250

0   500 Km

Figure 15.6 (b)   Ratio of hospital beds to population, India, 1957
Source: Akhtar and Izhar (1985)

of bronchial and intestinal diseases, including the dysenteries, until general living standards can be raised. Economic development and modern technologies in agriculture and manufacturing have brought prosperity to many, but still side-by-side with little-relieved poverty and squalor. There are still possibilities, perhaps slipping from grasp day by day, of avoiding some of the errors of the Industrial Revolution in the West, including further extension of the 'western diseases' already evident in urban middle-class groups.

On the state of the art in India, useful reviews are in Ramesh (1983),

Akhtar (1985a). And for an important complementary geographical viewpoint of India in a wider Asian context, see the joint paper by a surgeon and a geographer in Joshi and Deshpande (1972, 1985): they see – and map – a watershed across India between a South-east Asian and a South-west Asian or Middle East disease complex. And not least, Schweinfurth (1979) makes the case for geoecological and geomedical analysis and regional synthesis, with Sri Lanka as an example. Moreover India is a country for which there is a complementary study of health care facilities (Akhtar and Izhar 1985): figures 15.6(a) and (b), for instance, show the remarkable change in bed spaces per 100 000 people from 1957 to 1975, yet leaving marked disparities in backwater areas, including part of the Ganga plains in eastern Bihar.

Africa: Mainly on a Macro-scale Study of Kenya

The relevant literature on Africa is now rich – see the wide and discriminating review by Prothero (1983) and the special issues of *Social Science and Medicine* (1983a,b,c; 1986b) and *GeoJournal* (1981), and not least Akhtar's major edited volume of 1987. Only one macro-scale study, that on Kenya by Diesfeld and Hecklau (1978) has been selected for detailed discussion, but first it is important to stress that the three scales illustrated for India could easily be matched for Africa. On the micro-scale, from the medical viewpoint there is the very deep and detailed study by Gilles (1964) of the village of Akufo, some 20 km (12 miles) northwest of Ibadan, a million population city but one with perhaps uniquely close ties to villages in the area which even now maintain compounds in the city; the medical data from the years of living and working in the village, with environmental information that a geographer can re-sift, re-analyse and re-synthesize, are in one sense at the opposite pole from Mukerji's geographical reconnaissance of the Chandigarh Dun. Or there is the series of studies of the Malumfashi endemic disease project farther north, about 100 km (60 miles) north of Zaria, the first report having a geographer as first author (Bradley et al. 1977). Or Petit's (1984) geographical survey of needs and services in the service area of a dispensary at Batoumé in Togo. For an urban study see Herbert and Hijazi (1984) on Khartoum/Omdurman. On the meso-scale there is, for instance, a valuable edited volume on Rwanda (Meheus et al. 1982). And on the macro-scale there are two of the Heidelberg geomedical monographs earlier than Diesfeld and Hecklau, namely Kanter (1967) on Libya – used in my 1978 book, and Schaller and Kuls (1972) on Ethiopia. From the medical side, too, two decades after independence of the former French Africa territories, a remarkable synthesis includes a context in the physical and human environment for the epidemiological content

(Pène et al. 1980). A pioneer study by a geographer is Sharaf's (1968) paper on Sudan. The reason for concentrating on Diesfeld and Hecklau on Kenya is that their synthesis is based on a different organizing principle. The authors explain that compared to most earlier volumes in the geomedical monograph series their study concerns a well-studied area so that an encyclopaedic compilation of information would be inappropriate, and that they therefore propose to base their work on an analysis and eventually a synthesis of the relations between the ecological endowment, the social and economic structures and disease and health services viewed regionally within Kenya. On their methodology see Diesfeld and Hecklau (1976), Hecklau (1978). Their combination of skills makes for quite unusual analyses: in places there is a Christaller-like spatial analysis, elsewhere integrated description in the great *landschaft* tradition. A curious aspect is that urban issues are little discussed. After a 'systematic geography' of land, people, the economy, health services and diseases, the synthesis deals with the inter-relations, just as promised, the regionalization in the event being based on a map of what one might almost call life styles (figure 15.7). There is a broad distinction between 'African peasant and pastoral societies' and 'Class societies' (including Afro–Arabic ones); these are further classified according to key factors in their environment for health and disease; altitude as affecting temperature, rainfall, type of agriculture – for example, peasant rain-fed farming in 'marginal areas', or peasants using irrigation. Class societies are given this neutral term rather than say the White Highlands, or White Settlers with Large farms, in response to the fact that these areas are subject to rapid change in these first decades after independence from colonial rule. These range from Afro–European class societies of pastoral economy in arid areas, to those with large rain-fed farms, those with plantations for coffee, tea, sisal and sugar. Given careful reading and frequent references to earlier parts of the book and to the splendid series of coloured maps, these syntheses are immensely valuable. The following is a sample of them:

> . . . *African and Afro–Arabic peasant societies in areas of rainfed agriculture in the coastal lowland:* The habitat of the African and Afro–Arabic peasant societies in the coastal lowlands is separated from the Kenyan core area by the poor, arid areas of the Nyika. In historical times the population of this region had few contacts with the interior of the country, for not only the inhospitability of the Nyika itself but the warlike attacks of the Masai and Galla made caravan traffic difficult. Nevertheless, the coastal population maintained cultural and economic links with the peoples of the Arab and Indian culture areas. Numerous ruins and historic finds testify to the Arab dominance of the coast, and for 200 years, –

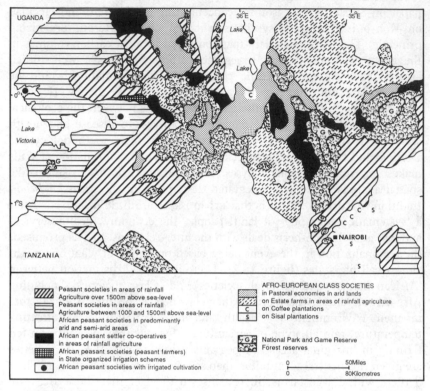

Figure 15.7   Part of the Diesfeld-Hecklau 'life-style regions' map of Kenya
Source: Diesfeld and Hecklau (1978)

that is from 1492 to 1692 – the Portuguese maintained a base at Mombasa for the sea-route around Africa to India, which they then once more lost to the Arabs. Even today there is only the one major link from the coast to the highlands, namely that from Mombasa to Nairobi. This major connection consists of an extraordinarily busy main road, the railway already mentioned, and the air route.

Morgan divides the Kenyan coast into a northern, sparsely settled section and a southern, relatively well-populated one, the economic centre of which is Mombasa, with good reason. But the agriculturally usable area, with in the main 6 to 8 humid months, is very narrow and only extends about 30 to 60 km from the coast into the interior. At this point the aridity limit for agriculture is to be found and linked with it the settlement margin for the peasant population. The ecological potential of this region is not yet fully utilized. For the development of the area a further build-up in population density would be desirable. In most places the population density remains below 100 persons to the square kilometre, only rising to values of up to 400 persons per square kilometre in the northern catchment area of Mombasa. These people are not families engaged solely in farming, however; many Africans from this district commute to Mombasa to work.

The form of agricultural land use differs from that of all the others in Kenya on account of the cultivation of fruit trees, in which the coconut palm is the most characteristic, although mangoes, citrus, and cashew trees are also widespread. The population's staple foodstuff is maize, and in the drier areas, cassava; cash crops include not only the tree crops mentioned above but also cotton.

Animal husbandry, and in particular the keeping of cattle, is made difficult by ticks and tsetse flies.

Shifting cultivation including burning the cleared bush still appears to be the most widely practised form of agriculture. Cultivation is also carried on beneath the tree crops. The strong Arab influence finds its expression in the land tenure: as early as the colonial period most agriculturally useful land was recognized as private property at a time when property titles in the European sense did not exist in the other African peasant societies. The size and structure of holdings also differ from those of the purely African peasant areas. In some places the peasant holdings are interspersed with large farming units, among which the sugar, sisal, and coconut plantations are of special economic importance. Many members of the farming population have found additional employment through tourism.

Besides malaria, which is particularly common in this hot and humid coastal strip, a special role is played by the *Wuchereria bancrofti* filariasis (though at first sight not much in evidence), and by *S. haematobium* schistosomiasis. So too infectious hepatitis appears remarkably frequently in the Annual Returns of Diseases of the hospitals. Hookworm infestation predominates over that of roundworm and tapeworm. The settlement schemes and irrigation schemes established at Taveta, Voi, and Galole (Hola) in the coastal hinterland have promoted the occurrence of these diseases. By comparison with the northern part of the coastal area, leprosy predominates in the southern half – a fact attributed by some authors to the immigration or settlement of population groups particularly susceptible to leprosy infection.

The provision of medical services is particularly effective in the coastal strip. Here, too, the concentration of the population along a narrow strip with good transport links along the coast have combined to increase it. In the face of this, the sparse population of the coastal hinterland suffers from similar disadvantages to those people living along the Tana River; exceptions to this are the townships of Galole, Voi, Taita, Taveta, and Wesu.

Irrigation schemes in the Yala Swamps area: A small irrigation scheme has already been completed near Bunyala, namely the Bunyala Irrigation Scheme. The Yola river which now runs into Lake Kanyaboli and the adjoining Yala Swamps is to be diverted by a canal. It is hoped that by lowering the water-level of the lake, about 200 ha of the swamps can be drained and then cultivated and irrigated using water from the canal. If the plan succeeds, part of the Yola Canal water will be led through the old river bed back to the lake, from whence it will hopefully distribute across the entire drained area of the former Yola Swamps through a system of canals. It will then be used for the irrigation of the newly-won fields. About 16 000 ha of land could be cultivated in this manner, and the development works are already in progress.

Particular health risks are common in such co-operative irrigation projects at altitudes below 1500 m. Apart from what has been previously mentioned, there is a danger of artificially creating breeding places for the mosquito vectors of malaria and the snails which act as intermediate hosts of schistosomiasis. The malaria situation is largely under control, partly because these areas are in any case holo-endemic and stable, and their new settlers already possess more or less distinct, acquired immunity or premunition. On the other hand suitable larvicidal and chemoprophylactic measures applied by the Ministry of Health's Division of Vector-Borne Diseases in the controlled settlement areas restrict the vectors of malaria and have reduced gradually the role of parasites among the population. The danger is essentially one of re-introduction from outside by new settlers, of the development of resistance of the mosquito vectors and malaria plasmodia towards the chemical substances applied, or of economic and organisational difficulties in keeping up the control measures which are demanding of personnel and finance.

A problem much more difficult to control is schistosomiasis. In every irrigation scheme, whether already in existence or still at the preparatory stage, there is the potential danger of intensive schistosomiasis transmission. In the area of the Mwea Tebere Irrigation Scheme, following massive snail infestation and infection of the population, the application of modern molluscicides at first succeeded in breaking the transmission cycle. The population received systematic treatment, with the result that the problem is now largely under control.

In the remaining projects no efforts have as yet been made in this respect. The snails are known to be intermediate hosts and the newly settled population is as infected by natural contact as is the autochthonous population. So far systematic control measures have not been introduced, although very important investigations have been carried out on the spot instead, with the result that the scientific basis for control at an appropriate time is at least available.

It is only in the Perkerra Irrigation Scheme that schistosomiasis does not occur, although the shores of nearby Lake Baringo are infested. Ecological conditions in the inner area of the irrigation scheme are not favourable to snails.

. . . *Afro-European class societies engaged in pastoral economy in arid areas:* Although large pastoral farms may occur in areas of rain-fed agriculture where mixed farming is possible or is actually carried out, by far the greatest number and acreage of ranches is found in those areas where agriculture is not feasible for climatic reasons. One of these is the Laikipia Plateau, another the area of pastoral farming north and south of Lake Naivasha in the East African Rift Valley. The amount of precipitation in these areas reaches an annual mean of less than 700 to 800 mm over a period in the main less than three humid months. The basis of foodstuffs for the cattle is the natural vegetation, supplemented in only a few, intensively managed, farms by the cultivation of green fodder based on irrigation. According to the ecological map drawn up by Pratt, Greenway and Gwynne by far the greatest part of the ranches is located in ecological zones 4 and 5. In ecological zone 4 vegetation consists of 'dry forms of woodland and savanna (often on *Acacia-Themeda* association), or equivalent bushland'. In ecological zone 4 less than 4 ha of grazing are required for the rearing of one unit of cattle. But the carrying capacity of the pasture is greatly reduced by the overgrowth of bush. Pasture also reacts sensitively to over-grazing. Ecological zone 5 is characterized by Pratt et al. as follows: 'The woody vegetation being dominated by *Commiphora*, *Acacia* and allied genera, often of shrubby habit. Perennial grasses such as *Cenchrus cillaris* and *Chloris roxburghiana* can dominate, but succumb readily if the ranch is managed harshly'. Here more than 4 ha are needed to support one unit of cattle. A rational utilisation of the grazing potential requires rotational grazing over large areas. Under these ecological conditions and management form on the large pastoral farms the population density must be low indeed. In the Laikipia Plateau it is less than 10 persons per square kilometre, and in the contiguous areas to north and south it even falls below four persons per square kilometre. So too, in the East African Rift Valley the population density is very low. Around Lake Naivasha it is below twenty and between Lake Naivasha and Lake Nakuru below ten persons to the square kilometre.

The farm units are extraordinarily large; they are still almost exclusively owned by Europeans, although their operation depends on African labour. The Africans live in small farm settlements, which, due to the size of the farm units are far away from one another. The living standard of the stockmen on the farms is low, their sanitary conditions are as a rule poor, and, as almost everywhere among the Kenyan Africans, their staple food is maize. The health services are poor, the vast distances within the areas making access to the scanty medical facilities very difficult.

The large pastoral farms have by no means fully exploited the natural potential. Only about half the grazing is divided up into enclosed pastures and the remaining half is not even made use of everywhere. There are great reserves to be found here, probably on account of the lack of capital or the absence of markets sufficient for the proper development of these farms. On the other hand, some areas with large pastoral farms have seen the pastures overgrown by bush encroachment. This phenomenon of bush invasion Troup explained as resulting from the prohibition of the annual burning, the annihilation of game, the small number of goats, and in some cases over-grazing.

Rotational grazing, bush clearance, seeded grass, fodder cropping, and possibly, if irrigation proved favourable, even hay and silage making – all offer possibilities for improving the animals' feeding basis and the realization of any significant improvement in the carrying capacity of Kenya's pastoral areas. The supply of animal protein to the growing population urgently requires fast and energetic development of pastoral farming in Kenya.

In a climatically favourable area above the altitude at which malaria is endemic, health conditions are good. The disease pattern is consequently determined more by the ubiquitous infectious diseases like tuberculosis, poliomyelitis, and hepatitis than by specifically tropical ones. Among the farming community, however, a life style increasingly orientated towards the monetary economy increases the danger of malnutrition among children in circumstances under which neither sufficient production for domestic consumption nor much inclination to buy any additional and necessary foodstuffs are observable.

Micro-scale Studies from a Developed Country

Turning to the developed countries, it seems right to start again with Dr William Pickles of Wensleydale: he still offers an example to general practitioners and to any geographer who can gain access to a GP's records, while of course preserving confidentiality in handling them. Some flavour of his work may be gained from the quotation from his 1948 paper in the *New England Journal of Medicine*, opposite the title page of this book, or his older and longer *Epidemiology in Country Practice*, or the passage in chapter 6 on contact tracing and the diffusion of hepatitis.

A study in urban medical geography, on Exeter, is in Griffiths (1971a), and she followed this up with a detailed study of one of the wards of the city, Wonford, with relatively unfavourable mortality experience (1971b). The ward-wise statistical analysis is of course subject to the so-called 'ecological fallacy' (see chapter 1), but there is no reason to doubt the substance of Dr Griffith's findings. In within-city differences, on wide consensus, there are environmental factors at work, just as say in Girt's study of bronchitis mentioned in chapter 5, but they are very largely related to socioeconomic differences. To quote Griffiths:

> Thus for each major category where the number of deaths is sufficient for the SMR [Standardized Mortality Ratio] to have meaning, the level of mortality in Wonford Ward is in close agreement with the known social class pattern of that disease. It is unfortunate that the social class structure of each age–sex group is not known and that mortality cannot be standardized for social class as well as age. If this could be done, it seems probable that much of the excess mortality in Wonford Ward would be accounted for.

And again:

> The inhabitants of Wonford Ward were moved from slums to new houses supplied with every necessity; but they inherited much from their past. Perhaps their health was impaired in their youth; perhaps they have maintained their former habits and way of life just as they have recreated overcrowded conditions in their new environment. All evidence seems to endorse other findings concerning rehoused populations and it seems as if 'the evil of slums could not be repaired in a period short of the life of one generation, if not several.'

While a Marxist might have phrased this differently, the consensus is strong – and also consistent with Third World urban studies even with different, though overlapping, environmental variables. See also Howe's (1972b) comparative study of London and Glasgow, and a valuable series of papers on the East Midlands (*East Midlands Geographer* 1976).

England and Wales as a Meso-scale Study of Regional Disparity

On a national but still a meso-scale, by world standards, the present author has twice attempted to pull together a picture of England and Wales covering some indices of health need, mainly from mortality mapping by Howe (1970) and health service provision, mainly from a pioneering book on regional variations in Britain (Coates and Rawstron 1971); my 1978 book almost coincided with completion of a valuable PhD thesis on infectious diseases, including diffusion studies and also a regionalization of England and Wales (Johnson 1978). My concern was primarily with teaching rather than original research and to assist the Open University's distant undergraduates reading a course on decision-making in Britain to try out some testing for themselves of a hypothesis that in general health and ill-health conditions suggest that the north and west of England and Wales are disadvantaged, compared with the south and east of England, as in figure 15.8 of male deaths from all causes, or figure 4.9 earlier in this book. Others of Howe's maps appear to confirm this, such as those for bronchitis, tuberculosis (but not lung cancer), stomach and uterus cancer (but not breast cancer), and, though less strongly, maps for heart disease and strokes; the maps for diabetes, pneumonia and gastric and duodenal ulcers do not show the bias to the north and west, nor lung and breast cancer as noted earlier, and it should be stressed that the heavy concentration of population in Greater London often shows its own pattern with high rates in less prosperous areas (Learmonth 1972b, 1978). The maps of health provision, still of historical interest, showed much more fluctuating patterns, still some legacies from active or wealthy local authorities in earlier times, and in some, such as dental services, a relation to the location of dental schools. The picture has been changing, with efforts to even out availability of general practitioners for many years, and more recently the attempt to improve the basis of allocations following the Resources Allocation Working Party (RAWP).

More recent mapping of mortality does not seem to alter the general picture, such as that in Howe (1979), or the atlases by Gardner et al. (1983, 1984). It is often said that these patterns reflect socioeconomic factors, as in the study of Exeter by Griffiths noted earlier in this chapter. It is difficult to believe that the north and west of England and Wales

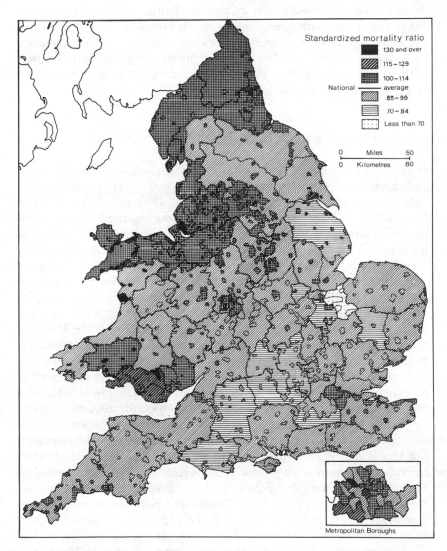

Figure 15.8 Mortality, all causes, males, England and Wales, 1959–1963
Source: Howe (1970)

have higher proportions of lower socioeconomic groups such as to cause
such repetitive patterns of bias towards high rates in the north and west.
And the exceptions with high rates equally strong in the south and east,
are equally worth probing. As with the Exeter data, there is a great need
for mapping standardized by socioeconomic group as well as by age and
sex even granting that problems of small sample size will arise. As in

Howe's more recent work, it is wise to concentrate on premature deaths rather than total death rates. On the health provision data, the 'inverse care law' mentioned in chapter 16 does not seem to operate regionally, but research may be required on unmet need, along the lines of Pyle's work on Chicago (also cited in chapter 16) or on delays in treatment, or generally consumer-oriented research.

France: a Regional Study using Three Scales of Analysis

From France it is possible to illustrate the ingenious use of mainly quite traditional techniques of cartographic analysis and correlation at the three scales discussed, micro-, meso- and macro- (Picheral 1976). Though Picheral's main focus is on the Midi region fronting the Mediterranean, he consistently puts this meso-region in the macro-regional context of the whole of France, while also coming down to micro-scale (admittedly for a large city) in detailed mapping of Marseilles, particularly for infant mortality as a key indicator of all-round health and well-being. The maps and graph in figures 15.9a,b,c, 15.10a and b, 15.11 and 15.12 may give some flavour of his approach, often mapping what he sees as two variables together. Thus at the beginning of the book, in asking if the Midi is a sick region on the evidence of its high consumption of medical services, he maps and graphs their costs against age and against urbanization: the Midi turns out to combine high overall usage with under-consumption by agricultural workers and under-provision in small towns. Mortality from all causes was excessive in some areas, especially after the extreme asperities of the 1939–45 war: isolated and relatively backward areas especially experienced a sort of retreat from post-war underdevelopment, and this is well illustrated by figure 15.9, showing the retreat of infant mortality rates approaching those of some Third World countries today. To follow infant mortality a little further, figure 15.12 stresses another element reminiscent of the Third World, the poor life-chances of poor immigrant groups in the *bidonvilles* (literally 'petrol-can towns') in parts of the periphery of Marseilles. Here Picheral pleads that as well as Maximilien Sorre's pathogenic complexes – noted in chapter 1 – there is a complementary concept, the socio-pathogenic complex.

Picheral goes on to describe what he calls bastions and refuges of infectious and parasitic diseases: these are of course more important in developing than in developed countries, and this brings out two important aspects of the Midi – the retreat of 'post-war underdevelopment' from backward, isolated tracts, and the transitional position of Mediterranean Europe between temperate Europe and the sub-tropical Middle East and North Africa. Examples include malaria, long important especially in

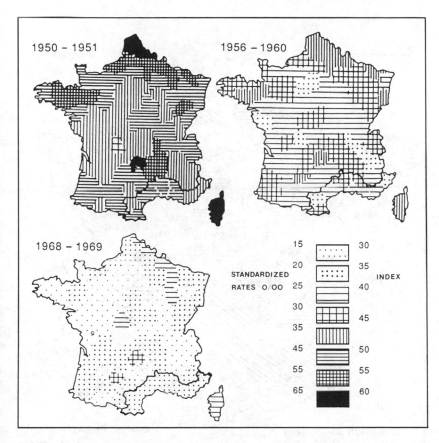

Figure 15.9   Infant mortality, France, 1950–1951, 1956–1960, 1968–1969
Source: Picheral (1976)

Corsica and still calling for post-eradication vigilance; visceral and dermal leishmaniases, with two vector sandflies, *Phlebotomus* spp.; two rickettsias, Marseilles fever (*R. conori*, its reservoir in dogs, rabbits and rodents with tick or flea vectors, and Q fever, *Coxiella* burneti with its reservoir in cattle, sheep, goats and some birds, and transmission by contact with the animal or its excreta or from its milk and so, like brucellosis from *B. melitensis*, found in areas of archaic or unhygienic farming); leptospirosis, linked with rice-fields in this region, presumably the virus from infected rodents' urine entering the tepid water in flooded fields, then entering small wounds in the workers' skin; typhoid and paratyphoid, as diseases of deprived people in unhygienic environments, as also polio, especially in *bidonvilles* where levels of vaccination may be low.

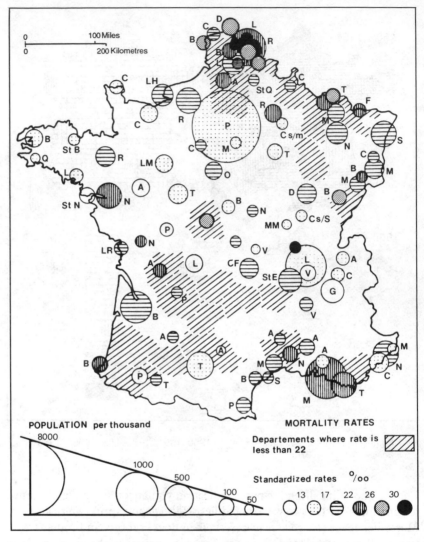

Figure 15.10 (a) Infant mortality, urban France 1968–1969
Source: Picheral (1976)

Picheral then moves on to 'the rise of the degenerative diseases', showing that the Midi does share this trend, though less affected than, say, the industrial north-east of France. His first example is, paradoxically, an infection, tuberculosis, shown in dramatic retreat from the grim post-war picture, though with residual foci in some urban and industrial areas on the mainland and some rural ones in Corsica, the differing life-chances

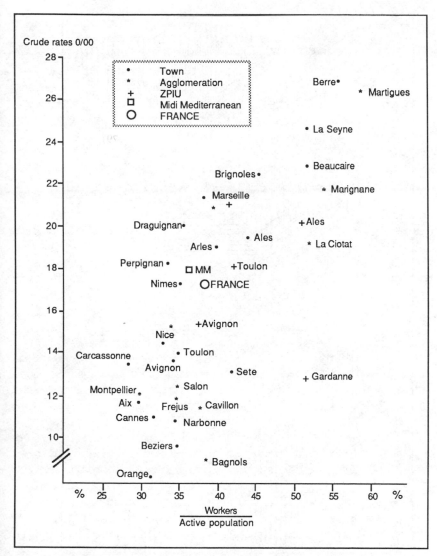

Figure 15.10 (b)   Graph of urban infant mortality, France, 1968–1969, plotted against proportions of industrial workers in the population
Source: Picheral (1976)

of particular social groups being both mapped and tabulated. Alcoholism is important in itself and for the later discussion of liver cirrhosis: the Midi people, generally and characteristically hardworking and quite abstemious in drinking mainly with meals, yet include pockets of people with high proportions of alcoholism pure and simple – in some rural

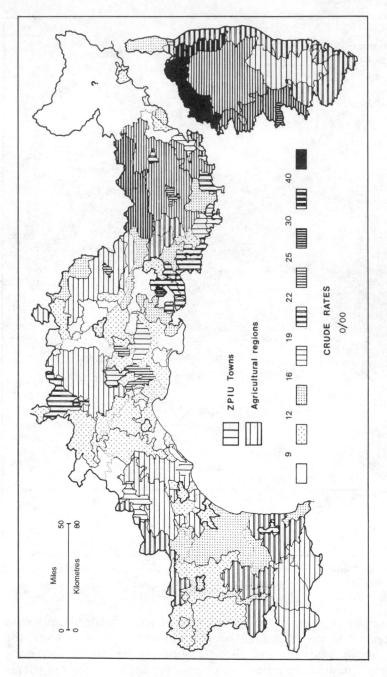

Figure 15.11 Infant mortality, le Midi (France) 1965–1969
Source: Picheral (1976)

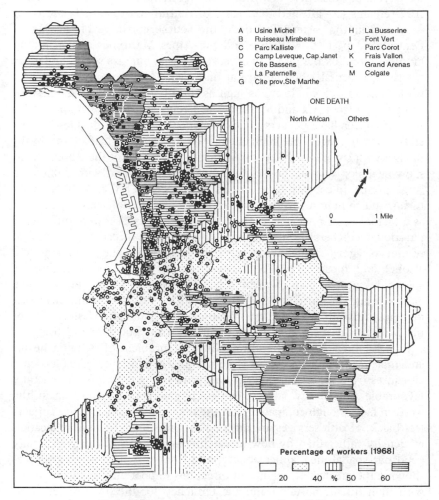

A   Usine Michel   H   La Busserine
B   Ruisseau Mirabeau   I   Font Vert
C   Parc Kalliste   J   Parc Corot
D   Camp Leveque, Cap Janet   K   Frais Vallon
E   Cite Bassens   L   Grand Arenas
F   La Paternelle   M   Colgate
G   Cite prov.Ste Marthe

ONE DEATH

North African   Others

N

0   1 Mile

Percentage of workers [1968]

20   40   %   50   60

Figure 15.12 Infant mortality, Marseilles, 1965–1969
Source: Picheral (1976)

areas of viticulture in Languedoc, Vaucluse and the Alpes Maritimes, while alcoholism linked with cirrhosis focuses rather on poor areas of industrial cities with more indiscriminate drinking including spirits – the costs and social selectivities, mainly of factory workers, are analysed. *Maladies d'usure* (degenerative diseases) include diabetes, where the Midi is, atypically, higher than in most parts of France, and the black spots within the region seem to be linked with high consumption of fats (but margarine and vegetable oil rather than butter?), sugar and alcohol. Then for circulatory disorders the Midi, sharing the national and international rise, remains less affected than parts of central and eastern France, but with foci in the eastern Pyrenees, the southern fringes of the Massif Central and parts of Vaucluse and the Alpes Maritimes and including mining and industrial rather than service towns, but also some rural areas where agricultural labourers are at high risk. A last example is cancer: while cancers as a whole are as high as in much of northern and eastern France only from Aix and Marseilles to Fréjus and St Tropez, particular sites of cancer have pockets of high incidence in the Midi. Oesophagus and stomach cancers are high mainly in the western half of the Midi, though with some exceptions for stomach cancer east of the Rhone delta, showing links with alcoholism (and liver cirrhosis) and with vulnerable rural groups; in contrast lung cancers are associated rather with manufacturing and mining towns, without of course excluding cigarette-smoking as a factor. After reviewing genetic factors, here as elsehwere difficult to pin down, Picheral sums up that the cancers, affected by place of residence, age, occupation, life style including diet and addictions like alcohol and tobacco, can be treated seriously as a social disease. A splendid synthetic map of within-region departures from average in age of death and in mortality from tuberculosis, alcoholism and cirrhosis, diabetes, tumours and circulatory failure brings out the western half of the Midi as the main area of premature death in the prime of life.

Picheral then tackles the always difficult problem of defining health and *faute de mieux* combines a large number of mortality variables from all causes from infant mortality to cancer of the oesophagus. A generally favourable but locally adverse situation emerges – mainly again the western half, though compared with the national level the picture appears less black. Health services are mapped in some detail though by location or density rather than by flow or catchment area. Provision is generally good but spatial inequalities appear, and Corsica is used as an example, showing the greater importance of infections in poor and backward areas, with high infant mortality and the tendency for the 'inverse care law' (not by that name!) to operate in backward areas or again in poor areas with many industrial workers in Marseilles, including *bidonvilles*.

Finally Picheral puts his study into a perspective in geography, along with sister disciplines, notably medical sociology, pleads again for his concept of the socio-pathogenic complex as modifying Sorre's, and evokes two final perspectives, that of Mediterranean geography and of fresh health legislation in France in 1970, just prior to publication. It is a conspectus almost contemporaneous with that of Pyle on Chicago, more traditional but equally imaginative in methodology, and quite as remarkable overall. By way of up-dating, a principal source must lie in the same author's edited volumes (Picheral 1981; *Géosanté* 1984), and from an interdisciplinary viewpoint, such sources as the special issue of *Social Science and Medicine* (1985), or Steudler (1986) in another Special Issue on Europe. A valuable historical dimension is in Comiti (1981); see also Hatton et al. (1984).

Some Other Macro-scale Studies

Moving to a macro-scale, efforts to prepare atlases for western Europe, or for the European Community, have so far not succeeded. There are intriguing glimpses. Northern Ireland may, like Scotland, share in many of the characteristics of the north and west of England and Wales, but in the Republic of Ireland the gradients indicated by Pringle (1985) show a bias towards unfavourable conditions in the south and east. In the Low Countries mortality rates are found to increase from north to south and east and into northern France (Mackenbach 1986; van Poppel 1981; WHO 1981). Some mapping by countries' major statistical divisions is extremely suggestive, but tantalizing: even on traditional mapping techniques and *a fortiori* by computer graphics, it should be possible to achieve much more detailed and down-to-earth mapping before encountering the small-sample problem. Figure 15.13 shows something of the potential – and the questions raised! Naumov and Lazanov (1970) give a general survey of Bulgaria.

Conclusion

This chapter of regional case studies has attempted to pull together the picture of health and disease, and health services also where the sources permit, on three scales that I have termed micro, meso and macro. One set of examples draws on studies from the Third World, from India and Africa in particular, and another set deals with the developed countries of western Europe and especially the UK and France. A number of approaches to regionalization are illustrated, from sub-regional division as in the study of Chandigarh Dun to a life-style division, of course carrying some spatial connotation, as in the study of Kenya, from synthesis based on existing atlases – and a little hypothesis testing – as in the UK study to the traditional but compelling explanatory description very much in the best tradition of French geography. The pages of *Social Science and Medicine* alone, including special issues or sections on Latin America, are sufficient to make it clear that the approaches demonstrated could be matched from all the Americas – North, South and the Central and Caribbean, if space permitted in this short book. The ecological

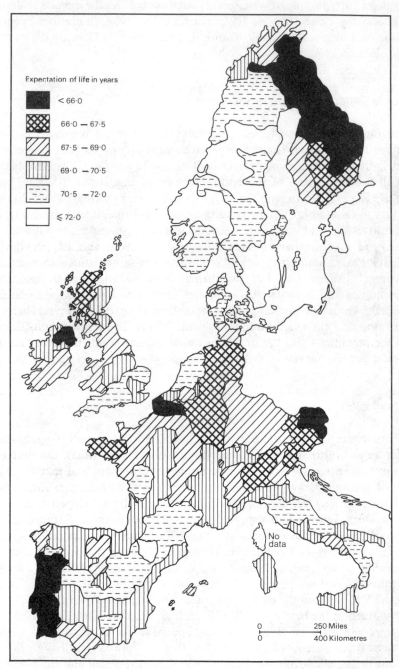

Figure 15.13 Expectation of life, Western Europe
Source: van Poppel (1981)

material from Latin America is particularly rich and fascinating. And Australia and New Zealand are rich in sources also.

There is for some people a worthwhile gain in understanding the medical geography of a country or even the world if regional analysis and synthesis are attempted, so that one can see the whole picture of health and ill-health in its environmental context and judge the response of the health services, broadly defined, to the felt need. Some of the studies are by biomedical researchers rather than by or with geographers but a geographical eye certainly helps, and if professional geographers do not lose sight of the benefits of training and practice in synthesis, they should be able to contribute to regionalizing Health for All.

16 Ecological Medical Geography and the Geography of Public Health

Are there Trends towards a New Holism in Health Geography?

This book has been concerned with links between geography and disease ecology. However, it seems wrong to conclude without some indications of other geographical studies relating to health, and some assessment of how far we may expect to see integration between streams of research that so far have been separate, even disparate, despite a common concern with health. One such stream, dealing with the geography of health care, already has whole volumes devoted to it; a second, concerning geography and traditional medicine, could well be the subject of a substantial volume, and though it has not yet been written, so far as I know, a number of special issues of *Social Science and Medicine* have been devoted to this or cognate studies; a third stream concerns geography and health education (or health promotion though I dislike the term on the grounds that education may produce more lasting or internalized effects): this interdisciplinary field I think may have great importance in future, though, so far, geographical contributions might fill a substantial pamphlet rather than a book. In this concluding chapter each of these three must be contained within a paragraph or two, but I hope with enough starting points for students who are drawn to them, or to more integrated studies than have yet been achieved. See Mayer (1982), Picheral (1982), and also K. Jones, G. Moon and Meade et al. (both in press at the time of writing), who attempt an integrated text.

The Geography of Health Care

For some 15 years after the National Health Service in the UK was set up in 1947–8, general appreciation of the free-at-point-of-access provision perhaps blinkered British geographers to the need for geographical analysis of health care. Perhaps one or two workers saw that optimal or sub-optimal location techniques might be applicable to choosing sites for hospitals or ambulance stations (Massam 1975), and Coates and Rawstron (1971) had made us aware of regional disparities in welfare and social provision. However, it was the phase of acute awareness of social (and ethnic) disparities in the USA in the late 1960s and early 1970s that brought forward this branch of geography, with the quadrennial International Geographical Congress in Canada in 1972 as a particular platform for its dissemination. The corresponding Congress in 1976 in Moscow, incidentally, gave the international community a strong impression that in the USSR medical geography, though a strong and, as already noted, an applied field, was primarily nosogeography not at all concerned with questions like optimal location which were left to administrators. The last decade may well have seen a change in this. In the Association of American Geographers' powerful and influential College Geography series, Pierre de Vise's (1973) text on misused and misplaced hospitals and doctors still captures the atmosphere, heady, radical and iconoclastic; or see Shannon and Dever's short book (1974) for a more conventional account. However, from the very dynamic flow of work on Chicago, including, for instance, Morrill and Earickson (1969) on an experimental location model, I have chosen as an example for discussion Pyle's (1971) paper on heart disease, stroke and cancer in the city, already cited for its use of trend surfaces in forecasting (figures 16.1(a) to (c), with captions to outline the steps in Pyle's analysis and synthesis). Though a pioneering paper in several ways, it comes as close to integration of the geography of need, of disease, and of health care locational analysis, as anything I know. However, note that Pyle used crude mortality rates, not standardized mortality ratios or age-specific mortality rates: these suited his purpose of mapping future need, and he did not try to study causes of spatial differences in the three disease patterns. Thus, though advancing farther than almost anyone towards integration of the nosogeography and the health care streams of research, he did not go quite all the way. Cancers as a whole, interestingly enough, he found more useful for his project than trend surface mapping and forecast surfaces of cancers of individual sites in the body, stomach, lung etc. – probably mainly because of the problem of small sample size that constantly recurs as one

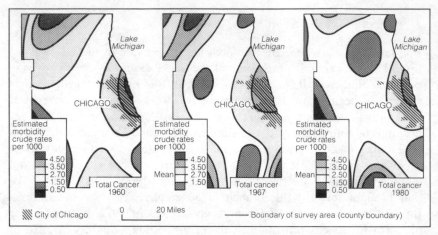

Figure 16.1 (a) Trend surfaces of total cancers, Chicago, with isopleths or 'contours' for 1960, 1967 and (forecast in 1971) for 1980
Source: Pyle (1971)

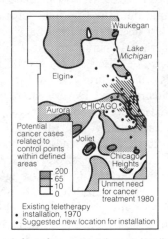

Figure 16.1 (b) Unmet need, from forecast total cancers allowing for forecast facility provision based on existing trends, 1980
Source: Pyle (1971)

approaches the micro-scale for any comparatively rare occurrence. An interesting stated assumption is that by his forecast date of 1980 the colour of one's skin would not matter for location of health facilities in Chicago, and Pyle himself in a retrospective comment says that his 1971 paper was regarded as feasible in principle but not in the current financial climate. And a point of great significance, I believe, is the unstated

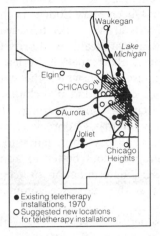

Figure 16.1 (c)   Existing and new facility locations for 1980
Source: Pyle (1971)

assumption in this and I think in much health care geography, that there will be no major 'breakthrough' in prevention of the diseases studied, here heart disease, stroke and cancer. While this assumption may well be shared by many biomedical workers, it must be considered along with the estimate that a large proportion – some say up to 80 per cent – of cancers, for instance, may be linked with environmental causes and so in principle preventible, and with *some* proportion of strokes and heart disease also avoidable. It is above all because this assumption can and probably should be questioned that I believe that the two streams of medical geography should come much closer together than they have been in recent years, and hence, too, my inclusion of paragraphs on geography and health education.

Since this period of intellectual ferment in American health care geography, the financial and political climate there has changed (Mayer 1985) and, despite differences between countries in health care systems, broadly comparable pressures exist in many of them. There has been a spate of publications from geographers and other social scientists, professional administrators and politicians more or less well informed, more or less biased, for instance in many issues of *Social Science and Medicine*. Here I select only two books on health care geography for brief discussion.

Authors from Canada and from the UK collaborate in Joseph and Phillips (1984), a wide-ranging and yet down-to-earth treatment of accessibility to and utilization of health facilities with many detailed examples; and complementary to it is Eyles and Woods (1983) from a strong research team at Queen Mary College in the University of London. Though Eyles and Woods draw on specific research mainly covering the North East Thames Regional Health Authority (Eyles et al. 1982), their broader title is justified: their book is at least partly a search for a philosophical base for research in which the structure and values in the societal matrix must be crucial, and it includes a powerful plea for the complete fusing of disciplines and the removal of boundaries between them. (This is a viewpoint that I appreciate, yielding to no-one in my enthusiasm for interdisciplinary approaches to our complex field, yet believing that a geographer does better to approach with a particular trained competence *and* a determination to keep in touch with developments in geography over the years: see comment in the conclusions to chapter 1 and to this chapter.)

Other important series of papers include those from Haynes and Bentham (1979) on the impacts of hospital centralization in East Anglia, and from Mohan and others (1984a,b) on the spatial effects of private hospital development in Britain. Some of the many papers comparing health systems in different countries are by geographers, such as that by Mohan and Curtis (1984) and this may prove an increasingly fruitful research topic. Note also the valuable series of papers by Knox, alone or with co-authors, including Knox (1979) and Knox and Pacione (1980); Whitelegg (1982) is also germane.

The 'Inverse Care Law' and the Modern Usage of 'Political Economy'

The works reviewed include many references to the 'inverse care law' enunciated by a radical general practitioner from Glyncorwg in South Wales (Hart 1971): that the greater the need for health care the less is the provision. This thinking grades into a health and health-care aspect of the modern usage of the term 'political economy', rather different from that of Adam Smith and the classical and laissez-faire economists, except for a common declared interest in the greatest good of the greatest number. In the health context, health and disease, and health care too, are seen in the whole-society context, in a particular sort of holism – though to a Marxist the only one? There is a large literature, some explicitly or implicitly Marxist, some liberal though still structuralist in the sense that changes in the structure of society are seen as the only remedy for health problems analysed. Geographical contributions that reflect something of the spectrum include Brownlea's (1981) paper 'From public health to political epidemiology', Jones (1985) on what he called 'critical epidemiology' and Eyles (1982) with a particularly sharp exposition of health care seen as fetishized into a commodity in capitalist (and capitalist-influenced?) societies. This strand of thinking is taken further in Eyles and Woods (1985) on an 'inverse interest law': that given the medical power structure, the causes of ill-health that cause the greatest demand on health services, like chronic mental conditions and disabilities of the aged, arouse least interest and attract the lowest level of funding. For some medical geographers, these arguments lie outside the limits of our discipline: it is perhaps fair to say that with some exceptions, including one or two papers cited above, the spatial working-out of the ideas is not yet fully accomplished. This may be one reason why some of their leading protagonists believe that boundaries between the social sciences ought to be fused and forgotten?

Health Care Geography and Traditional Medicine in the Third World

This heading is not to be taken as implying that developed countries do not have any traditional medicine (on Europe, for instance, see Vaskilampi et al. (1982)). That must exist everywhere, with its own traditional herbs etc., channels of transmission of knowledge, its own successes and failures; it may even be increasing in some communities as part of the trend towards various forms of 'alternative medicine' and 'holistic medicine'. And even conventional scientific medicine has its myths? (Posner 1977, 1984). However, the literature to date is stronger in suggesting that the Third World has more powerful and immanent traditional medicine, some with a strong scholarly tradition as in Indian and Chinese medicine, some the folk medicine common everywhere but usually stronger than in western countries, some concerned with spirit-possession and spiritual healing, some with the witch-doctors, spells, potions and incantations (see Worsley 1982). There is a good measure of agreement that, given the immense health and resource problems of the Third World, there is an urgent need to effect some integration of western 'scientific' medicine and traditional medicine (see, for instance, Bannerman (1983)). To reinforce this point I have chosen from the now considerable literature just a few papers for brief mention, one from India (Ramesh and Hyma 1981a), and one based mainly on African first-hand experience but concerned with the less developed countries as a whole (Good 1980, 1987b) and see also Good et al. (1979), Stock (1981), Pearce (1982)).

India is remarkable in that though there are tensions between western and traditional medicine, there is – as in China also – government support and recognition (though these are regarded as inadequate in degree in

India by the authors cited); and there are many more practitioners than would be found in most societies who are trained and qualified in both paradigms. See also Qureshi and Kharbanda (1980), Fendall (1981), ICMR (1982). We owe to Dr Hyma and Professor Ramesh a unique insight into the operation and spatial arrangement of three forms of traditional medicine found in the million-city of Madras (figure 16.2): these are the India-wide Sanskrit-based Ayurveda, a somewhat comparable

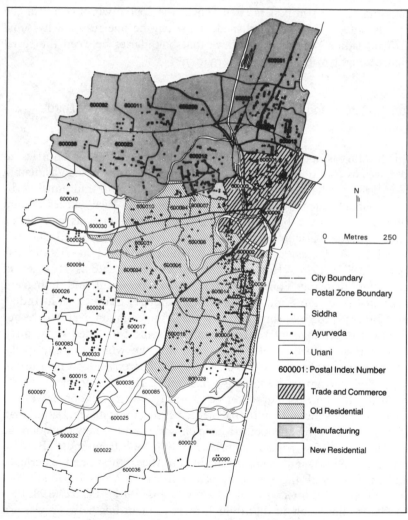

Figure 16.2   Traditional medicine in Madras
Source: Hyma and Ramesh (1980)

South Indian system, Siddha, and the Moslem medicine (with Greek roots!) Unani. In this survey they had, respectively, 36, 36 and 10 per cent of the practitioners, and it is very significant that 10 per cent practised integrated medicine. Women practitioners were very few indeed, but increasing. There was a very wide range of prosperity and sophistication of consultation area, from open shop to well-equipped surgery and pharmacy, and a wide range in catchment areas too, the subject of further studies by the two authors. The map showed Hyma and Ramesh that in the within-city pattern, traditional medicine was by no means incompatible with industry. (I am reminded of a report by the social anthropologist of Bangalore slums, Gertrude Woodruff, in her PhD thesis for Radcliffe College, Harvard, of the treatment, indeed cure on some criteria, of a case of spirit-possession of a woman slum-dweller, by two *pujaris*, the junior of whom was a mechanic in the aircraft factory.) The authors go on to plead for more government support (with less lip-service?) and much greater integration of the traditional and the western approach.

Professor Good uses the widest possible canvas and quotes a spectrum of references to match: he regards the integration of traditional healer into health programmes as vital. This is not, of course, to accept everything in traditional medicine uncritically: like western medicine it too has its iatrogenic casualties, like the blindness already cited from McGlashan (1969) and Queguiner (1981). Figures 16.3 and 16.4 demonstrate visually the framework of integration he envisages.

Medical Geography and Health Education

Links with health education are as yet few. Budd and Budd (1981) present in a set of geographical papers a survey that lies between political geography, medical geography, mass communication studies and perhaps the modern usage of 'political economy' noted above; in the event it proved not strongly spatial, but should be considered by geography students interested in this aspect. In the context of the change towards prevention and health education signalled by a government paper (DHSS 1976), it analyses impacts of a campaign using the mass media to encourage healthier life styles. Tables present numerical data on age, sex and social class; on levels of credibility attached by respondents to various sources of health information, by age, sex and social group; on contacts with general practitioners – frequency, travel time, mode of transport, ease of travel and degree of satisfaction with the GP; and on degree of concern for various illnesses (cancer, coronary heart disease, rheumatism and arthritis, mental illness and bronchitis), by age group and social

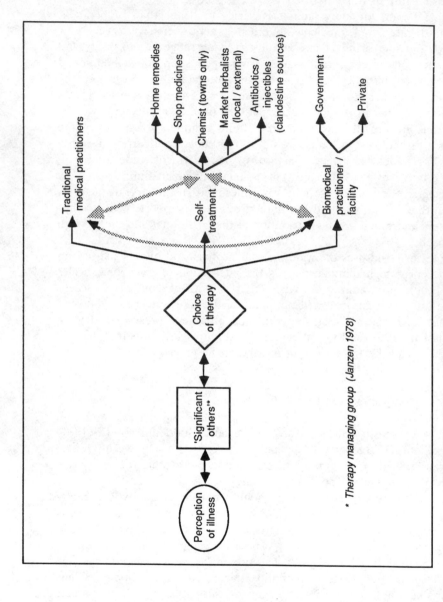

Figure 16.3　Choice between two types of medicine, traditional and western
Source: Good (1987b)

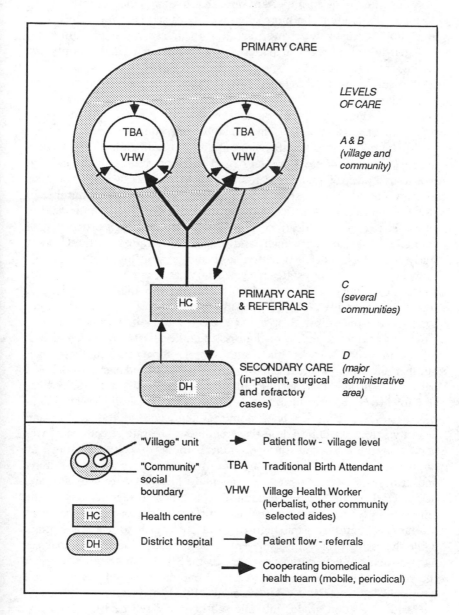

PRIMARY CARE

LEVELS
OF CARE

A & B
(village and
community)

PRIMARY CARE
& REFERRALS

C
(several
communities)

SECONDARY CARE
(in-patient, surgical
and refractory
cases)

D
(major
administrative
area)

"Village" unit — Patient flow - village level

"Community"
social
boundary

TBA   Traditional Birth Attendant

VHW   Village Health Worker
(herbalist, other community
selected aides)

HC   Health centre

DH   District hospital — Patient flow - referrals

Cooperating biomedical
health team (mobile, periodical)

Figure 16.4   Possible pattern of integration between traditional and western medicine
Source: Good (1987)

class. The finding is an important one, that dissemination of information through GPs tends to be more effective than use of the mass media. It is possible, even likely, that an areally broader survey might bring out stronger spatial or regional patterns, but even for a single county the findings are significant.

The Budds' work, developed further, clearly has practical potential. Realized application in health education is seen at work in a paper from Portsmouth Polytechnic (Moon and Jones 1985; Jones and Moon, in press; and see figure 16.4). Census analysis and computer mapping were used to 'target' limited health visitor and other health education resources to *people in areas of concentration* of risk of hypothermia in the elderly. In a second piece of action research an initial stage was by cluster analysis to bring out areas in Gosport where clustering occurred of a number of socioeconomic characteristics known from earlier research in Sheffield to be associated with cot deaths – population mobility, high proportion of young (16–19) married women, and high fertility ratios. In the Gosport study some areas stood out in terms of numbers of births (figure 16.5): Rowner, with a large estate of armed-services, mainly naval, families; and some clusters in the east of the borough with high proportions of single-parent families. The dot maps in figure 16.5 of total births not cot deaths make the point. Gosport was selected for initial work using the 'Sheffield composite index' of high-risk families. Data are gathered first by the midwife, later by the health visitor, concerning mother's age, number of previous pregnancies, duration of second stage of labour, baby's weight at birth, hospital admission if any, difficulty in feeding, and any attacks of breathlessness or cyanosis from lack of oxygen. High-risk babies are identified on a points system, and additional care and health visiting concentrated on these families. The rate of cot deaths was halved in the first year of operation, without of course raising any implication that all cot deaths are due to the factors used in the study and two years later the rate had fallen by four-fifths. Researchers and health workers alike were particularly concerned to identify any of the tendency to 'victim-blaming' that can surface all too easily; in the event the families identified as at high risk did not appear to feel any stigma, while the caring professions were enthusiastic that the additional analyses had assisted the general level of care in the whole community, not just the high-risk families. See also OPCS/London School of Hygiene and Tropical Medicine (1982), Tildon et al. (1983).

Health education grades into the self-help and self-health movement, and there are many relevant papers in *Social Science and Medicine*, the *World Health Forum* and the journal of the UK College of Health, *Self Health*. An Australian project with a strong geographical component, in a huge modern suburb in South Brisbane, is described in Brownlea et

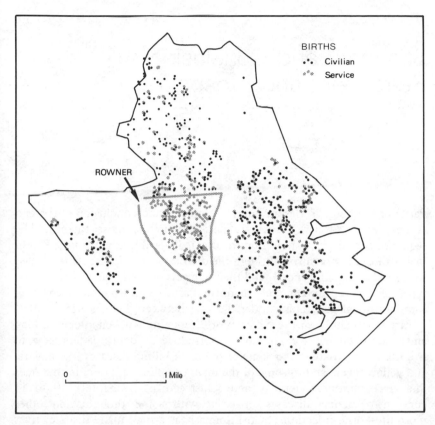

BIRTHS
•‚• Civilian
‚•‚ Service

ROWNER

0   1 Mile

Figure 16.5 Targeting resources against cot deaths: a dot map of total service and civilian births in Portsmouth, a naval port. Other analyses helped to draw attention to areas of single-parent families
Source: Moon and Jones (1985)

al. (1976–7). However, see Najman et al. (1983) on some of the impediments to progress. On mass screening in preventive medicine, Sir Richard Doll (1983) regards pre-natal screening as generally useful, post-natal as more doubtful; he is lukewarm on breast cancer screening, and on screening following blood in stools (against cancer of the colon); but he is strongly in favour of screening for cervical cancer and of blood pressure in the elderly. Interestingly enough the trend in eastern Europe seems to be towards annual health examination for all, Bulgaria for instance following USSR in this (Apostolov et al. 1980).

Summary and Conclusion: Retrospect and Prospect

Part I of the book carries an interim summary and conclusion at the end of chapter 8, so here it is only necessary to condense further. The sequence goes from chapter 1 on the divided world that is yet One World to a pathogenic organism, through the discussion of what are often called western diseases, in general, and then in terms of cartography and several types of geographical model, to finish Part I with chapter 8 covering some historical geography under the title Between Two Worlds.

Part II is mainly on the Third World, opening with chapter 9, a long and mainly descriptive attempt to introduce student readers new to tropical disease patterns to some of the main killing diseases like malaria and yellow fever, and to some of the main crippling and debilitating ones like river blindness, leprosy and schistosomiasis. Chapters 10 to 14 concern particular diseases: malaria, with some thoughts on other mosquito-borne infections; schistosomiasis as a man-made disease; river blindness and the control campaign against it; and some cancers important in the tropics and with strong spatial patterns – liver cancer, cancer of the oesophagus, and Burkitt's lymphoma. Chapter 14 on the geography of hunger includes reminders of the recency of famine, and seasonal hunger too, in what are now the developed worlds, with brief accounts of some malnutritions, mineral deficiencies, toxic contaminants of some foods, and the merest indication of some of the problems of general or specific overnutrition. This concludes Part II, clearly less sophisticated in techniques reviewed than is Part I, but using some of the same approaches. On the other hand the writer has often found that the Third World has some lessons for us in western countries.

Part III comprises chapter 15, with some regional syntheses on different scales, micro, meso and macro, and, appropriately as the book approaches its conclusion, it includes examples from both developed and developing countries. The concluding chapter includes very brief reviews and examples of work in geography on health care, on traditional medicine, and on health education, as a perspective in which to place the ecological medical geography that is the prime object of the volume.

In retrospect then, I have tried to carry the idea of One World through the common experience of the three worlds – the developed capitalist or mixed-economy countries, the developed communist countries (including some state-capitalist ones, according to some Marxist scholars!), and the developing countries (some with mixed economies, some with socialist governments). Some of the common experience, chapter 8 suggests, chapter 14 too, depends on a sense of history: the dynamics of the demographic transition and the closely related epidemiological transition alike remind us that history carries lessons for the present and future, even though it is unlikely to repeat itself precisely.

Some workers believe that ecological medical geography can only be a purely academic pursuit, for its own sake, or to deepen understanding of population, welfare or social geography: that the individual geographer, with rare exceptions, lacks the broad biomedical training necessary for studies of spatial differences in disease patterns to be at all useful in practical terms. I hope that, to most readers, parts at least of this book may put a contrary case, that geographical techniques can fruitfully be used in epidemiology, pure and applied, and more frequently than they have in the past – except indeed for atlases and other maps. However, the majority of such diffident or pessimistic geographers would probably concede that geographers in research teams have shown themselves capable of contributing substantially to useful and applicable research: looking over the preceding chapters, it seems clear to me that the still few trained geographers involved in such team work contribute best when they are taken seriously as spatial analysts, and not simply considered as cartographers. (Cartography, after all, is a discipline in its own right!) Given this, useful, medically significant contributions, perhaps applicable in health education or preventive campaigns, are the more likely to emerge. In links between geography and disease ecology biogeography will often be crucial, but equally often it may be behavioural human geography (Gillett (1985) is a timely reminder!).

In my earlier book in 1978 I described two streams in medical geography as separate, in the main, but complementary – on the one hand the geographical perspective on disease ecology that is the main theme of the present volume and has many links with biomedical and related sciences; and on the other hand the health care stream briefly referred to – hardly outlined – in this chapter, linking with different sister disciplines like medical sociology, anthropology, economics and even political science, indeed with 'political economy' in its modern usage. It is, I think, the political economy school of thought that is particularly associated with the call for the fusing of the social sciences in research on health care, as some at least of the workers cited earlier would agree. This part of my 1978 book has been much quoted, mainly on the mistaken assumption that I approve of the dichotomy into the two streams that I perceived: I do not. This is perhaps clear from my references to Pyle's 1971 monograph earlier in this chapter. However, his work has not been followed up to any great extent: he himself has recorded that his findings have been regarded as feasible logistically but not in terms of current economic and political trends. Perhaps if Health for All by the year 2000 is to become a reality the two streams will have to merge and sweep aside obstacles in their path. If a book concentrating mainly on the disease ecology stream becomes out-of-date in five or ten years from now, giving way to a more holistic viewpoint, no one will rejoice more than the author.

As it happens the writing of the present book has been carried out *pari passu* with a small and mainly post-retirement part in the Open University course on Health and Disease (1985, Books I–VIII, and Reader dated 1984). Here too the plea for this sort of holism – differing from current interest in 'holistic medicine – is very strong, as is the case made against reductionist or single-cause attribution of disease while neglecting the whole-person and in particular the whole-society context. (Of course if the anti-reductionists brush aside conventional biomedical explanations too much, and attribute all health burdens to society, or to capitalism, then their analysis is no longer holistic.) This in places carries its own arguments for holism, for instance in the selective account of Professor J.M. Hunter's pilgrimage from daring hypothesist on a broad environmental front, about river blindness, through participation in a vast and imaginative international control project, to urgent advocacy of holistic views of disease associations and their societal matrix. The present writer's own concern with malaria was turned by a field trip in South India into a wider concern with other mosquito-borne diseases, biogeography and the little-studied behavioural geography of people's contact with mosquitoes being both involved: indeed the experience renewed my interest in the spatial patterns in the regional burden of disease as a whole, as outlined in chapter 15. There is, too, the dialectic between researchers putting their faith in vaccines for future control and those looking rather to biological and ecological approaches – to economic development too – in fact to more holistic methods (Lord 1983).

My own credo as medical geographer is a humble one. I approach an awesomely interdisciplinary field of study knowing that it involves many competences that I do not possess and now never will; so I approach as a human and regional geographer. I am not overly conscious of discipline boundaries or imperialisms, I hope, but I still approach *as* geographer. Pondering this from time to time over a good many years, I think that my stance arises because I know that I lack the gifts to approach as a polymath: all that I have to give to this highly interdisciplinary field is based on my (limited) competence within geography. But beyond my own individual case, I also believe that a geographer working in medical geography will normally contribute more if he or she maintains a foothold in the parent discipline, and makes the effort to keep in touch with its changing and developing techniques and philosophical approaches – paradigms if you will. I believe that this advice obtains whether the geographer is struggling alone with a piece of research, over-burdened by the several disciplines that must be mastered, more or less, or engaged in team-work with researchers from other disciplines and perhaps feeling over-borne by people who seem to possess stronger and more confident disciplines than geography has had at times over the last decade or two. So, with humility, I say 'Hold on to your discipline; we have something to contribute.' If this book demonstrates this I shall be richly rewarded.

References

Abbott, P. 1982: The art of medicine. *World Health Forum*, *3*, 194–5.

Abercrombie, M., Hickman, C.J. and Johnson, M.L. 1951: *A Dictionary of Biology*. Harmondsworth: Penguin.

Abstr. Hyg. especially 1978, *53* onwards. A general source.

Adams, J.G.U. 1985: *Risk and Freedom: the record of road safety regulation*. Cardiff: Transport Publishing Projects.

Adesina, H.O. 1981: A statistical analysis of the distribution characteristics of cholera within Ibadan city, Nigeria (1971). *Soc. Sci. Med. 15D*, 121–32.

_____ 1984a: The diffusion of cholera outside Ibadan city, Nigeria, 1971. *Soc. Sci. Med. 18*, 421–8.

_____ 1984b: Identification of the cholera diffusion process in Ibadan city, 1971. *Soc. Sci. Med. 18*, 429–40.

_____ 1984c: Explaining the incidence of cholera in Ibadan city, Nigeria, 1971. *Indian Geog. J. 59*, 22–8.

Agarwal, R.K., Jain, A.M., Dube, M.K. and Bhandari, B. 1980: Anaemia in protein-energy malnutrition in preschool children. *Indian J. Med. Res. 72*, 236–40.

Ahmed, H.A., Touw, J., Stoner, G.L. and Belehu, A. 1983: Immunoglobin A (Ig A) in nasal washings and saliva of leprosy patients. *International J. Leprosy 51*, 22–8.

Aiken, S.R. and Leigh, C.H. 1978: Dengue haemorrhagic fever in South-east Asia *Trans. Inst. British Geogrs 3*, 476–97.

_____ Frost, D.B. and Leigh, C.H. 1980: Dengue haemorrhagic fever and rainfall in peninsular Malaysia: some suggested relationships. *Soc. Sci. Med. 14D*, 307–16.

Akesode, F.A. and Ajibode, H.A. 1983: Prevalence of obesity among Nigerian school children. *Soc. Sci. Med. 17*, 107–11.

Akhtar, R. 1978: Goitre zonation in the Kumaon Himalayas. *Soc. Sci. Med. 12D*, 152–63.

_____ 1980: *Environment, Agriculture and Nutrition in Kumaon region*. New Delhi: Marwah Publications.

_____ 1982: Colonization and its impact on the incidence of malaria in the Tarai region of Uttar Pradesh, India. *Geographia Medica 12*, 59–77.

_____ 1983: India, a study in geocancerology with special reference to mouth cancer. IGU Working Group (1983) pp. 79–86.

_____ 1985a: Scope of geography of health and geomedical research in India. Akhtar and Learmonth (1985) pp. 3–21.

_____ 1985b: Geography of nutrition in the Kumaon Himalayas. Akhtar and Learmonth (1985) pp. 289–311.

_____ (ed.) 1987: *Health and disease in tropical Africa: geographical and medical viewpoints*. London: Harwood Academic Publishers.

_____ and Izhar, N. 1985: Inequalities in the distribution of health care in India. Akhtar and Learmonth (1985) pp. 437–60.

_____ and Learmonth, A. 1977: The resurgence of malaria in India 1965–76. *GeoJournal* 1(5), 69–80.

_____ 1979: Malaria annual parasite index maps of India by malaria control units 1965–76. *Research Paper No. 3 Social Science Faculty*, Milton Keynes: The Open University.

_____ 1982: Malaria returns to India. *Geog. Mag. 54*, 135–9.

_____ (eds) 1985: *Geographical Aspects of Health and Disease in India*. New Delhi: Concept Publishing.

Akinkugbe, F.M. 1980: Anaemia in a rural population in Nigeria (Ilora). *Annals Trop. Med. and Parasit. 74*, 625–33.

Alamgir, M. 1980: *Famine in South Asia: political economy of mass starvation*. Cambridge, Mass: Oelgeschlager, Gunn and Hain.

Alexander, J.T. 1980: *Bubonic Plague in Early Modern Russia: public health and urban disaster*. Baltimore: Johns Hopkins University Press.

Al-Fouadi, A. and Parkin, D.M. 1984: Cancer in Iraq: seven years' data from the Baghdad Tumour Registry. *International J. Cancer 34*, 207–13.

Allen-Price, E.D. 1960: Uneven distribution of cancer in West Devon, with particular reference to the divers water supplies. *The Lancet* i, 1235–8.

Alter, G. 1983: Plague and the Amsterdam annuitant: a new look at annuities as a source for historical demography. *Population Studies 37*, 23–41.

Alvarez, G. 1982: The neurology of poverty. *Soc. Sci. Med. 16*, 945–50.

Anantaraman, M. 1984: Is bilharzia likely to establish itself in India? *Indian Geog. J. 59*, 13–17.

Anderson, D. 1982: The monitoring of environmental mutagens/carcinogens: a perspective on tests predicting chemical mutagens/carcinogens in man. *Ecology of Disease 1*, 59–73.

Anderson, R.F. 1984: Temporal trends of cancer mortality in eastern New England compared to the nation 1950–75. *Soc. Sci. Med. 19*, 749–58.

Anderson, R.M. (ed.) 1982: *Population Dynamics of Infectious Diseases: theory and applications*. London: Chapman and Hall.

Angulo, J.J., Takiguit, C.K., Pederneiras, C.A.A., Carvalho-de-Souza, A.M., Oliveira-de-Souza, M.C. and Mcgale, P. 1979: Identification and process in the spread of a contagious disease. *Soc. Sci. Med. 13D*, 183–9.

Annals of Internal Med. 1985: International Conference on Acquired Immunodeficiency Syndrome 14–17 Apr. 1985, Atlanta, Georgia, 653–790.

Apeldoorn, G.J. 1981: *Perspectives on Drought and Famine in Nigeria*. London: George Allen and Unwin.

Apostolov, E., Golemanov, N., Netchaev, S. and Stančev, K. 1980: The Gabrovo health services development project – mass prophylactic screening in primary health care in Bulgaria. *World Health Forum 1*, 87–98.

Archives de l'Institut Pasteur de Tunis 1982: Communications sur la rage 59, 3–17.

Armijo, R. et al. 1981a: Epidemiology of gastric cancer in Chile. *International J. Epidemiology*. I Case-control study (R. Armijo, M. Orellana, E. Medina, A.H. Coulson, J.W. Sayre, R. Detels) 10, 53–6; II Nitrate exposure and stomach cancer frequency (R. Armijo, A. Gonzalez, M. Orellana, A.H. Coulson, J.W. Sayre, R. Detels) 10, 57–62.

———, Detels, R., Coulson, A.H., Medina, E., Orellana, M. and Gonzalez, A. 1981b: Epidemiology of gastric cancer in Chile. *Revista Médica de Chile 109*, 551–6.

Armor, D.J. 1978: *Alcoholism and Treatment*. New York: Wiley.

Armstrong, B. 1980: The epidemiology of cancer in the People's Republic of China. *International J. Epidemiology 9*, 305–15.

——— and Doll, R. 1975: Environmental factors and cancer incidence and mortality in different countries with special reference to dietary practices. *International J. Cancer 15*, 617–31.

Armstrong, R.W. 1973: Tracing exposure to specific environments in medical geography. *Geogr. Analysis 5*, 122–32.

——— 1976: The geography of specific environments of patients and non-patients in cancer studies, with a Malaysian example. *Econ. Geog. 52*, 161–70.

——— 1980: Geographical aspects of cancer incidence in Southeast Asia. *Soc. Sci. Med. 14D*, 299–306.

——— 1984: Exposure to air pollution zones in a tropical city. *Geographia Medica 14*, 49–64.

——— and Armstrong, M.J. 1983a: Environmental risk factors and nasopharyngeal carcinoma in Selangor, Malaysia: a cross-ethnic perspective. *Ecology of Dis. 2*, 185–98.

———, Yu, M.C. and Henderson, B.E. 1983b: Inhalants and salted fish as risk factors for nasopharyngeal carcinoma in Malaysian Chinese. *Cancer Res. 43*, 2967–70.

———, Chan Siew Eng, A. 1983c: Salted fish and nasopharyngeal carcinoma in Malaysia. *Soc. Sci. Med. 17*, 1559–67.

———, Kutty, M.K. and Armstrong, M.J. 1978: Self-specific environments associated with nasopharyngeal cancer in Selangor, Malaysia. *Soc. Sci. Med. 10*, 149–56.

Arroz, M.E. 1979: The spatial diffusion of infectious hepatitis. *Finisterra 13(27)*, 36–69.

Ashton, B., Hill, K., Piazza, A. and Zeitz, R. 1984: Famine in China 1958–61. *Population and Development Review 10*, 613–45.

Aspock, H. 1979: The biogeography of the arboviruses of Europe. *Geog. Zeitschr. 51*, 11–28.

Aston, A.R. and Brazier, P.H. 1979: Endemic goitre, the factors controlling iodine deficiency in soils. *Sci. of the Total Env. 11*, 99–104.

Audy, J.R. 1949: A summary topographical account of scrub typhus 1908–46.

Bull. Inst. Med. Res. Malaya No. 1 (new series), 1–82.

_____ 1968: *Red Mites and Typhus*. Heath Clark lectures 1965. London: University of London, The Athlone Press.

_____ 1971: Measurement and diagnosis of health. In P.E. Shephard and D. McKinley (eds) Environ/Mental: essays on the planet as a home. Boston: Houghton Mifflin.

Awad el Karim, M.A., Collins, K.J., Sukkar, M.Y., Omer, A.H.S., Amin, M.A. and Doré, C. 1981: An assessment of anti-schistosomal treatment on physical work capacity. *J. Trop. Med. Hyg. 84*, 67–72.

_____, El Hassan, B.M. and Hussein, K.K. 1985: Social and public health implications of water supply in arid zones of the Sudan. *Soc. Sci. Med. 20*, 393–8.

Baczkowski, D.M. 1980: Viral hepatitis in metropolitan Sydney. *Australian Geogr. 11*, 285–95.

Badger, G. 1981: Environmental factors in human cancer. *Search 12*, 22–9.

Bailey, N.T.J. 1967: *The Mathematical Approach to Biology and Medicine*. New York: Wiley.

_____ 1982: *The Biomathematics of Malaria*. The Biomathematics of Diseases, I. High Wycombe: Charles Griffin.

Bain, O. 1981: The genus *Onchocerca*: hypothesis on its evolution and a key to the species. *Annales de Parasitologie Humaine et Comparée 56*, 503–26.

Bain, R.J. 1979: Heart disease and geologic setting in Ohio. *Geology 7*, 7–10.

Baird, D. 1973: Environmental factors in relation to obstetrics. In G.M. Howe and J.A. Loraine (eds) 1973, pp. 169–84.

Baker, R. 1977: The Sahel: an information crisis. *Disasters 1*, 13–22.

Baker, S.R. 1980: Pitfalls in evaluation of cancer data for geographic analysis. In Melinda S. Meade (ed.) 1980, pp. 155–69.

Balint, M. 1957: *The Doctor, His Patient and the Illness*. Tunbridge Wells: Pitman Medical.

Banerjee, B. and Hazra, J. 1974: Geo-ecology of cholera in West Bengal. Calcutta: Jayati Hazra.

_____ 1982: Geo-ecology of leprosy with special reference to West Bengal. *Geographia Medica 11*, 116–40.

Banks, A.L. 1959: The study of the geography of disease. *Geog. J. 125*, 199–216.

Bannerman, R.H. and eight participants 1983: Traditional medicine in modern health care. *Hamdard 26*, 54–92.

Barata da Silveira, M.A. 1981: Fight against schistosomiasis. *Revista Brasileira de Medicina 38*, 691–9.

Barbosa, F.S. and Costa, D.P.P. 1981: A long-term schistosomiasis project with molluscicides in a rural area of Brazil. *Annals Trop. Med. Parasit. 75*, 41–52.

Barker, D.J.P. 1982: *Practical Epidemiology* 3rd edn. Edinburgh: Churchill Livingstone.

Barrett, F.A. 1980: Medical geography as a foster child. In M.S. Meade (ed.) (1980) pp. 1–15.

Bayliss, J.H. 1980: The extinction of bubonic plague in Britain. *Endeavour 4*(2), 58–66.

Bayoumi, A. 1981: The epidemiology of fatal motor accidents in Kuwait. *Accident Analysis and Prevention 13*, 339–48.

Beaglehole, R., Hay, D.R., Foster, F.H., and Sharpe, D.M. 1981: Trends in coronary heart disease mortality and associated risk factors in New Zealand. *New Zealand Med. J. 93*(10 June), 371–5.

Behbchani, A.M. 1983: The smallpox story: life and death of an old disease. *Microbiol. Reviews 47*, 455–509.

Bein, F.L. 1977: Peasant response to drought in the Sudanese Sahel *Great Plains. Rocky Mountain Geog. J. 6*, 137–46.

Bella, H., Marshall, T.F., Omer, A.H.S. and Vaughan, J.P. 1980: Migrant workers and schistosomiasis in the Gezira, Sudan. *Trans. Roy. Soc. Trop. Med. Hyg. 74*, 36–9.

Bellezza, G. 1983: L'Italia sulla frontiera sanitaria mondiale. In IGU Working Group on Geography of Health, Rome. 1983, pp. 199–227.

Bentham, G. 1985: Motor vehicle accidents: a rural epidemic? IBG/AAG symposium in medical geography, University of Nottingham 15–19 July.

Bentley, C.A. 1916: *Malaria in Bengal*. Calcutta: Government Printing Office.

Beresford, S.A.A. 1985: Is nitrate in the drinking water associated with the risk of cancer in the urban United Kingdom? *International J. Epidem. 14*, 57–63.

Bernus, E. 1977: Herdsmen and the drought in the African Sahel. *African Environment, Special Report 6*, 140–7.

Berry, L., Campbell, D.J. and Emker, I. 1977: Trends in man–land interaction in the West African Sahel. *African Environment, Special Report 6*, 83–91.

Bertini, B., Ber A., Posener, L.N. and Zelikson-Singer, S. 1971: Ethnic and constitutional differences and their relation to breast diseases in Israel. *British J. Cancer 25*, 428–40.

Bhatia, B.M. 1975: Famine and agricultural labour of India: a historical perspective. *Indian J. Industrial Relations 10*, 575–94.

Bickmore, D. and Stocking, B. 1982: Computer mapping and tropical disease. *J. Trop. Med. Hyg. 85*, 19–26.

Biellik, R.J. and Henderson, P.L. 1981: Mortality, nutritional status and diet during the famine in Karamoja, Uganda 1980. *Lancet* ii (12 Dec.) 1330–3.

Biggar, R.G., Gardiner, C., Lennette, E.T., Collins, W.E., Nkrumah, F.K. and Henle, W. 1981: Malaria, sex and place of residence as factors in antibody response to Epstein-Barr virus in Ghana, West Africa. *Lancet* ii (18 July) 115–8.

Bignall, J.R. 1982: Failure to control tuberculosis: a personal view. *International Union against Tuberculosis 57*, 122–5.

Black, D. 1986: *The Plague Years: a chronicle of AIDS, the epidemic of our times*. London: Picador/Pan Books.

Black, N., Boswell, D., Gray, A., Murphy, S. and Popay, J. (eds) 1984: *Health and Disease: a Reader*. Milton Keynes: The Open University Press.

Blaikie, P. 1978: The theory of the spatial diffusion of innovations: a spacious cul-de-sac. *Progress in Human Geography 2*, 268–95.

Blythe, C.R. 1986: Cancer of the oesophagus, with special reference to Scotland. M. Phil. thesis, The Open University, Milton Keynes MK7 6AA.

Bouchard, D.C. 1976: Spatial autocorrelation and health care data: a preliminary study. *Cahiers de Géog. de Québec 20*,(51), 521–38.

Bousfield, D. 1979: Snail-paced parasite that is marching through South America. *Nature 279* (5714), 573–4.

Bozzo, S.R., Novak, K.M., Galdos, F., Hakoopian, R. and Hamilton, L.D. 1979: Mortality, migration, income and air pollution. *Soc. Sci. Med. 13D*, 95–110.

Bradley, A.K. 1972: The effect of disease on rural economy, social structure and settlement: a case study of onchocerciasis in the Hawal valley, Nigeria. WHO Mimeo. WHO/ONCHO/72.93.

_____ 1981: Local perceptions of onchocerciasis in the Hawal valley, Nigeria. *GeoJournal 5*, 357–62.

_____, Gilles, H.M. and Shehu, U. 1977: Malumfashi Endemic Disease Project I: Some ecological and demographic considerations. *Annals Trop. Med. Parasit. 71*, 443–9.

Bradshaw, E. and Schonland, M. 1974: Smoking, drinking and oesophageal cancer in African males of Johannesburg, South Africa. *British J. Cancer 30*, 157–63.

_____, Harington, J.S. and McGlashan, N.D. 1983: Geographical distribution of lung and stomach cancers in South Africa. *South African Med. J. 64*, 655–73.

_____ 1985: Cancers in South Africa, 1949–79. *South African Med. J. 68*, 455–65.

_____, McGlashan, N.D., Fitzgerald, D. and Harington, J.S. 1982: Analyses of cancer incidence in black gold miners from southern Africa. *British J. Cancer 46*, 737–48.

Brancato, M.A. 1983: Il diabete come malattia sociale in Italia. In *IGU Working Group on Geography of Health*, 1983, pp. 415–24.

Brandling-Bennett, A.D., Doberstyn, E.B. and Pinichpongse, S. 1981: Current epidemiology of malaria in Southeast Asia. *Southeast Asian J. Trop. Med. Public Health 12*, 289–97.

Bray, R.S. 1981: Malignant tertian malaria and pregnancy. *Postgraduate Doctor – Africa 3*, 250–5.

_____ 1982: The zoonotic potential of reservoirs of leishmaniasis in the Old World. *Ecol. of Dis. 1*, 257–67.

Brennan, L. 1984: The development of the Indian Famine Code. In Currey and Hugo (eds) 1984, pp. 91–111.

Brenner, M.H. and Mooney, A. 1983: Unemployment and health in the context of economic change. *Soc. Sci. Med. 17*, 1125–38.

Brilliant, G.E. and Brilliant, L.B. 1985: Using social epidemiology to understand who stays blind and who gets operated on for cataract in a rural setting. *Soc. Sci. Med. 21*, 553–8.

Brinkmann, U.K. 1982: *Medicine in Developing Countries*. Vol. 14 *Onchocerciasis in West Africa*. Frankfurt-am-Main: Peter Lang.

British J. Hosp. Med. 1982: Screening. *27*, 577–607.

Brock, J.F. 1954: Survey of the world situation on kwashiorkor. *Annals New*

York Acad. Sci. 57 Art. 6, 696–713.

Brodsky, H. 1984: The bystander in highway injury accidents. *Soc. Sci. Med. 19*, 1213–6.

Brooks, R.H. and Colley, D.G. 1976: The role of migrants in the spread of Schistosomiasis *mansoni* or, what nine million Brazilians have and you don't. In R.J. Tata (ed.) Latin America: search for geographic explanations. *Proceedings of 5th Conference of Latin Americanist Geographers, Boca Raton, Fa.* Chapel Hill NC: University of North Carolina, pp. 89–96.

Brothwell, D. 1981: Microrevolutionary change in the human pathogenic treponemes: an alternative hypothesis. *International J. Systemic Bacteriol. 31*, 82–7.

Brown, A.W.A. and Deom, J.O. 1973: Health aspects of man-made lakes. In W.C. Ackermann, G.F. White, E.B. Worthington (eds) *Man-made lakes, their problems and environmental effects*. Geophysical Monographs Series, vol. 17. Washington, DC: American Geophysical Union, pp. 755–64.

Brownlea, A.A. 1967: An urban ecology of infectious disease: City of Greater Wollongong–Shellharbour. *Australian Geogr. 10*, 169–87.

_____ 1972a: Modelling the geographic epidemiology of infectious hepatitis. In N.D. McGlashan (ed.) 1972, pp. 279–302.

_____1972b: Environmental impact and epidemiologic monitoring. Paper to meeting of the Medical Geography Commission of the International Geographical Union, Guelph, Canada, August 1972.

_____ 1978: Personal communication.

_____ 1981: From public health to political epidemiology. *Soc. Sci. Med. 15D*, 57–67.

_____, Condon, M., Feuerring, K., Landbeck, M., Taylor, C. and Walker, W. 1976–77: *Health servicing urban children project* vols I and II. Nathan, Brisbane: Griffith University, School of Australian Environmental Studies.

Brubaker, G., Geser, A. and Pike, M.C. 1973: Burkitt's lymphoma in the North Mara district of Tanzania 1964–70: failure to find evidence of time–space clustering in a high risk isolated rural area. *British J. Cancer 28*, 469–72.

Bruce-Chwatt, L.J. 1965: Paleogenesis and paleo-epidemiology of primate malaria. *Bull. WHO 32*, 363–87.

_____ 1970: Global view of malaria control and eradication by attack on the vector. *Misc. Pubn Entom. Soc. America 7*, 7–23.

_____ 1976: Ague as malaria: an essay on the history of the two medical terms. *J. Trop. Med. Hyg. 79*, 168–76.

_____ 1980: *Essential Malariology*. London: Heinemann Medical.

_____ 1983: Malaria and pregnancy. Editorial, *British Med. J. 286* (7 May), 1457–8.

_____ 1984: Malaria: from eradication to control. *New Scientist* 19 Apr., 17–20.

_____, Zulueta, J. de 1980: *The rise and fall of malaria in Europe*. Oxford: WHO/ Oxford University Press.

Brummer-Korvenkontio, M., Oker-Blom, N., Petterson, R., Saikhu, P., Swedmyr, A. and Wahlberg, P. 1984: Kumlinge disease: tick-borne meningo-encephalitis in the Åland islands and southwestern Finland. *Nordisk Med. 99*, 282–4.

Bryson, R.A. and Murray, T.J. 1977: *Climates of Hunger: mankind and the world's climates*. Madison Wis.: University of Wisconsin Press.

Budd, A. and Budd, J.L.S. 1981: Politics, health and the mass media: a geographical perspective from Leicestershire. In Leicester Geographical Essays *Leicester University Department of Geography Occasional Paper no. 1*, pp. 19–36.

Bulatao-Jayme, J., Almero, E.M., Castro, C.A., Jardeleza, T.R. and Salamat, L.A. 1982: A case-control dietary study of primary liver cancer risk from aflatoxin exposure. *International J. Epidem. 11*, 112–9.

Bull. WHO 1981: The ecology of influenza viruses: a WHO Memorandum, *59*, 869–73.

Bundy, D.A.P. 1984: Caribbean schistosomiasis. *Parasit. 89*, 377–406.

Burgess, E.W. 1925: The growth of the City. In R.E. Park and E.W. Burgess (eds), *The City*. Chicago: University of Chicago Press, pp. 47–62.

Burkitt, D. 1962: A children's cancer dependent on climatic factors. *Nature 194*, 232–4.

———— 1973: Diseases of modern development. In G.M. Howe and J.A. Loraine (eds) 1973, pp. 140–4.

————, Morley, D. and Walker, A. 1980: Dietary fibre in under- and overnutrition in childhood. *Arch. Dis. Childhood 55*, 803–7.

Byrne, B. 1984: Viral polyarthritis. Correspondence, *Med. J. Australia 140*, 445–6.

Cahiers ORSTOM Série Entomologie et Parasitologie 1980: Laveran symposium on the biology, epidemiology and immunology of malaria, Strasbourg 2–3 May 1980 *18*, 81–186.

Caldwell, J.C. 1975: The Sahelian drought and its demographic implications. Overseas Liaison Committee Paper, American Council on Education *8*, 1–88.

Caldwell, J.R., Theisen, V., Kaunisto, C.A., Reddy, P.J., Smythe, P.S. and Smith, D.W. 1983: Psychosocial factors influence control of moderate and severe hypertension. *Soc. Sci. Med. 17*, 773–82.

Caltabiano, A. 1983: Osservazione geografiche sul morbo di Hansen in passato e oggi. In *IGU Working Group on the Geography of Health*, pp. 297–310.

Cambon-Thomsen, A., Prevost, P., Sevin, A. and Ohayon, E. 1984: Génétique et géographie: les marqueurs génétiques dans les Provinces Françaises. In *Géosanté* 1984, pp. 43–68.

Carney, W.P., Banzon, T., de Veyra, V., Daño, E. and Cross, J.H. 1980: Intestinal parasites on man in northern Bohol, Philippines, with emphasis on schistosomiasis. *Southeast Asian J. Trop. Med. Public Health 11*, 473–9.

Casadei, E., Pereira, C.R. and Bruheim, S. 1982: Contamination with aflatoxins of basal foods in Mozambique. *Revista Méd. de Moçambique 1*, 23–31.

Catford, J.C. and Ford, S. 1984: On the state of public ill health: premature mortality in the United Kingdom and Europe. *British Med. J. 289* (15 Dec.), 1668–70.

CEGET (Centre d'Etudes de Géographie Tropicale) 1983: *de L'Epidémiologie à la Géographie Humaine*. Bordeaux, le CEGET (CNRS) Domaine Universitaire de Bordeaux 33405 Talence CEDEX.

Chakraborty, S., Dutta, M., Srivastava, L., Barui, K.C. and Mandal, S.P. 1982: Current outbreaks of kala-azar in Malda and Murshidabad districts of West

Bengal: an epidemiological evaluation. *J. Commun. Dis. 14*, 263–73.

Chamberlain, R.W. 1982: Arbovirology – then and now. *American J. Trop. Med. Hyg. 31*, 430–7.

Chambwe, A. 1982: Behavioural patterns of alcohol use among selected groups of young people in Britain and Zimbabwe. *Central African J. Med. 28*, 131–6.

Chandler, A.C. 1926–8: The prevalence and epidemiology of hookworm and other helminthic infections in India. *Indian J. Med. Res. 14* and *15*, 185–94 and later.

Chapin, G. and Wasserstrom, R. 1981: Agricultural production and malaria resurgence in Central America and India. *Nature 293* (5829), 181–5.

_____ 1983: Pesticide use and malaria resurgence in Central America and India. *Soc. Sci. Med. 17*, 273–90.

Chappell, J.M.A. and Webber, M.J. 1970: Electrical analogues of spatial diffusion processes. *Regional Studies 4*, 25–39.

Charmot, G. 1983: Aspects géographiques de la chloroquino-résistance de *Plasmodium falciparum*. In CEGET 1983, pp. 83–95.

Cheesmond, A. 1980: Migrant workers and schistosomiasis in the Gezira, Sudan. *Trans. Roy. Soc. Trop. Med. Hyg.* 691–2 (correspondence).

Cheesmond, A.K. and Fenwick, A. 1981: Human excretion behaviour in a schistosomiasis endemic area of the Gezira, Sudan. *J. Trop. Med. Hyg. 84*, 101–7.

Chilvers, C. and Adelstein, A. 1978: Cancer mortality: the regional pattern. *Popn Trends 12*, 4–9.

China, Malaria Commission, Committee of Medical Sciences 1983: Epidemiological status of malaria in the People's Republic of China in 1981 and suggestions for control. *J. Parasit. and Parasitic Dis. 1*, 1–4.

Choubey, K. 1985: Diseases of Sagar City in the light of environment and nutritional deficiency factors: a case study of medical geography. In Akhtar and Learmonth, 1985, pp. 275–87.

Choudhury, N., Saxena, N.B.L., Dwivedi, S.R. and Khamre, J.S. 1983: Study of the outbreak of Japanese encephalitis in Goa. *J. Commun. Dis. 15*, 111–20.

Chretien, J., Holland, W., Macklem, P., Murray, J. and Woolcock, A. 1984: Acute respiratory infections in children: a global public health problem. *New England J. Med.* 310/15 982–4.

Christie, A.B. 1977: Smallpox. In G.M. Howe (ed.) 1977, pp. 255–70.

_____ 1981: Infection in Britain yesterday. *J. Roy. Coll. Physicians London 15*, 95–7.

_____ 1982: Plague: review of ecology. *Ecol. of Dis. 2*, 111–5.

Chung, R. 1970: Space–time diffusion of the Transition Model: the twentieth century patterns. In C.J. Demko, H.M. Rose and G.A. Schnell (eds), *Population Geography: a reader*. New York: McGraw Hill, pp. 220–39.

Citron, K.M., Raynes, R.H. and Borrie, J.R.H. 1981: *Tuberculosis Today*. London: HMSO.

Cleek, R.K. 1979: Cancers and the environment: the effect of scale. *Soc. Sci. Med. 13D*, 241–7.

Cliff, A.D. and Haggett, P. 1985: *The spread of measles in Fiji and the Pacific: spatial components in the transmission of epidemic waves through island communities*

Department of Human Geography Publication HG/18 Research School of Pacific Studies, The Australian National University, Canberra.

_____, Ord, J.K. and Versey, G.R. 1981: *Spatial diffusion: an historical geography of epidemics in an island community.* Cambridge University Press, Cambridge Geographical Studies No. 14.

_____ 1984: Island epidemics. *Scientific American 250*(5), 110–17.

_____ and Ord, J.K. 1985: Forecasting the spread of an epidemic. In O.D. Anderson et al. (eds) *Time series analysis: theory and practice.* Proceedings conference Toronto 1983. Amsterdam: North Holland/Elsevier.

Cliff, J. and Zinkin, P. 1983: Vaccination and epidemiology of measles in Maputo, Mozambique. *Revista Méd. de Moçambique 1*, 121–5.

Clough, P.W.L. 1983: Nitrates and gastric carcinogens. *Minerals and the Environment 5*, 91–5.

Clugston, G.A. 1981: The effect of malnutrition on brain growth and intellectual development. *Trop. Doctor 11*, 32–8.

Clyde, D.F. 1980: *Two centuries of health care in Dominica.* New Delhi: Mrs Sushima Gopal, Kailash Apartments, New Delhi 110 048 India.

_____ 1985: *Health in Grenada: a social and historical account.* London: Vade-Mecum Press.

Coates, B.E. and Rawstron, E.M. 1971: *Regional Variations in Britain: studies in economic and social geography.* London: Batsford.

Coates, D. and Redding-Coates, T.A. 1981: Ecological problems associated with irrigation canals in the Sudan with particular reference to the spread of bilharziasis, malaria and aquatic weeds and the ameliorative role of fishes. *International J. Environmental Studies 16*, 207–22.

Cockburn, A. 1963: *The Evolution and Eradication of Infectious Disease.* London: Oxford University Press.

Cohen, N., Measham, A.R. and Akbar, J. 1983: Smoking and respiratory disease symptoms in rural Bangladesh. *Public Health* (London) 97, 338–46.

_____, Jalil, M.A., Rahman, H., Matin, M.A., Sprague, J., Islam, J., Davison, J., Leemhuis de Regt, E. and Mitra, M. 1985: Landholding, wealth and risk of blinding malnutrition in rural Bangladeshi households. *Soc. Sci. Med. 21*, 1269–72.

Cohen, S. (ed.) 1982: Malaria. *British Med. Bull. 38*, 115–218.; also Edinburgh: Churchill Livingstone.

Colledge, M. 1982: Economic cycles and health: towards a sociological understanding of the impact of the recession on health and illness. *Soc. Sci. Med. 16*, 1919–27.

Collins, J.J. 1982: The contribution of medical measures to the decline of mortality from respiratory tuberculosis: an age–period–cohort model. *Demography 19*, 409–27.

Collis, C.H., Cook, P.J., Foreman, J.K. and Palframan, J.F. 1971: A search for nitrosamines in East African spirit samples from areas of varying oesophageal cancer frequency. *Gut 12*, 1015–18.

Combes, C. 1982: Trematodes: antagonism between species and sterilizing effects on snails in biological control. *Parasitology 84* 4, 151–75.

Comiti, V.-P. 1981: Evolution de la pathologie française au XXe siècle. In H.

Picheral (ed.) 1981, pp. 11–28.

Commoner, B. 1977: Cost-risk-benefit analysis of nitrogen fertilization: a case history. *Ambio 6*, 157–61.

Communicable Disease Surveillance Centre UK 1985: Sexually transmitted disease surveillance in Britain: 1983. *British Med. J. 291* (24 Aug.), 528–30.

Cook, G.A. and Draper, G.J. 1984: Trends in cervical cancer and carcinoma *in situ* in Great Britain. *British J. Cancer 50*, 367–75.

Cook, I.F. 1985: Hepatitis B and AIDS in Africa. *Med. J. Australia 142*(12), 661 (correspondence).

Cook, P. and Burkitt, D. 1970: *An epidemiological study of seven malignant tumours.* London: Medical Research Council mimeo.

_____, Collis, C.H., Foreman, J.K. and Palframan, J.F. 1971: *Cancer of the oesophagus and alcoholic drinks in East Africa.* Cambridge University Expedition to East Africa of 1969, mimeo.

Cook-Mozaffari, P., Azordegan, F., Day, N.E., Ressicaud, A., Sabai, C. and Aramesh, B. 1979: Oesophageal cancer studies in the Caspian littoral of Iran: results of a case-control study. *British J. Cancer 39*, 293–309.

_____ and van Rensburg, S. 1984: Cancer of the liver. In R. Doll (ed.) 1984, pp. 342–5.

Cook, W.L., Wachsmuth, K., Feeley, J. and Huq, I. 1983: The question of classical cholera. *Lancet* i (16 Apr.) 879–80.

Cooper, R. 1981: Rising death rates in the Soviet Union. The impact of coronary heart disease. *New England Med. J. 304/21*, 1259–65.

_____ 1982: Smoking in the Soviet Union. *British Med. J. 285* (21 Aug.), 549–51.

_____, Schatzkin, A. and Sempos, C. 1984: Rising death rates among Polish men. *International J. Health Services 14*, 289–302.

Cornet, L., N'Guessan, H.-A., Mobiot, L.-M., Kadio, R., Douane, P.-G. and Dick, R. 1983: Approche épidémiologique du cancer de l'oesophage en Côte d'Ivoire. *Bordeaux Médicale 16*, 219–22.

Cossar, J.H., Dewar, R.D., Reid, D. and Grist, N.R. 1983: Travel and health: illness associated with winter package holidays. *J. Roy. Coll. GPs 33*, 642–5.

Costa, M.F.F.F. de L., Katz, N. and Dias, J.C.P. 1980: Re-infection of patients in *Schistosoma mansoni* endemic areas after specific treatment. IV: Observations in Belo Horizonte, Brazil. *Revista do Inst. de Med. Trop. de São Paulo 22*, 97–107.

Cotter, J.V. and Patrick, L.L. 1981: Disease and ethnicity in an urban environment. *Annals Assoc. American Geogrs 71*, 40–9.

Cousens, S.H. 1960a: The regional pattern of emigration during the great Irish famine 1846–51. *Trans. Inst. British Geogrs 28*, 119–34.

_____ 1960b: Regional death rates in Ireland during the great famine. *Popn Studies 19*, 55–73.

Craft, A.W., Openshaw, S. and Birch, J.M. 1985: Childhood cancer in the Northern Region 1968–82: incidence in small geographical areas. *J. Epidem. Commun. Health 39*, 53–7.

Craig, M. 1985: The diffusion of cholera in rural Bangladesh: beyond a descriptive epidemiology? In IBG/AAG Symposium on Medical Geography, 1985.

_____ 1986: Bari-level analysis of the distribution of cholera in Matlab thana, Bangladesh and the mode of transmission debate. IBG Conference University of Reading, January 1986.

Craighead, J.E. 1981: Viral diabetes in man and experimental animals. *American J. Med. 70*, 127–34.

Cravioto, J. and De Licardie, E.R. 1976: Malnutrition in early childhood. *Food and Nutrition 11*(4), 2–11.

Creighton, C. 1894: *A History of Epidemics in Britain*. Cambridge University Press. Reprinted with additional material by D.E.C. Eversley, E.A. Underwood and L. Ovenall. London: Cass, 1965.

Crews, D.E. and MacKeen, P.C. 1982: Mortality related to cardiovascular disease and diabetes mellitus in a modernizing population. *Soc. Sci. Med. 16*, 175–81.

Crimmins, E.M. 1981: The changing pattern of American mortality decline. 1940–77. *Popn and Development Rev. 7*, 229–54.

Crockett, G.S. and Simpson, K. 1953: Malaria in neighbouring London. *British Med. J.* 21 Nov., 1141.

Cross, E.R., Sheffield, C., Perrine, R. and Pazzaglia, G. 1984: Predicting areas endemic for schistosomiasis using weather variables and a Landsat data base. *Military Med. 149*, 542–4.

Crow, B. 1985: Famine and plenty. Unit 24 in Course D205 *Changing Britain, changing world: geographical perspectives*. Milton Keynes: Open University Press.

Cummins, R.O. 1983: Recent changes in salt use and stroke mortality in England and Wales. *J. Epidem. and Commun. Health 37*, 25–8.

Cumper, G.E. 1984: *Determinants of Health Levels in Developing Countries*. Letchworth: Research Studies Press.

Currey, B. 1980: Famine in the Pacific: losing the chance for change. *GeoJournal 4*, 447–66.

_____ 1981: Fourteen fallacies about famine. *Ceres* Mar.–Apr., 20–5.

_____ 1984: Coping with complexity in food crisis management. In Currey and Hugo (eds) 1984, pp. 183–202.

_____ 1986: Webs of survival: towards greater specificity in famine warning systems. IBG Conference University of Reading January 1986. In press with *Disasters*.

_____ and Hugo, G. (eds) 1984: *Famine as a Geographical Phenomenon*. Dordrecht: D. Reidel Publishing/The GeoJournal Library.

_____ 1984: Famine as a geographical phenomenon. In Currey and Hugo (eds) 1984, pp. 1–6.

Curtis, C.F. and White, G.B. 1984: *Plasmodium falciparum* transmission in England: entomological and epidemiological data relative to cases in 1983. *J. Trop. Med. Hyg. 87*, 101–14.

Cutler, P. 1986: The spread of famine in northern Ethiopia 1981–85. IBG Conference University of Reading January 1986.

Dadzie, K.Y., Rolland, A. and Thylefors, B. 1984: The evolution of ocular onchocerciasis in the Volta river basin area over a period of five years of vector control. *Tropen med. u. Parasit. 35*, 41–6.

Damien Foundation 1981: *Atlas of Leprosy*. Brussels: Damien Foundation.

Dando, W.A. 1980: *The Geography of Famine*. London: Arnold/USA Halstead/ Wiley.

Daniels, V.G. 1985: *AIDS: the Acquired Immune Deficiency Syndrome*. Lancaster: MTP Press.

Darby, H.C. 1940a: *The Medieval Fenlands*. b: *The draining of the fens. Cambridge University Press.*

——— 1983: *The changing Fenland*. Cambridge University Press.

Daschaudhuri, P.C. 1978: Mosquito research in India. *Sci. and Culture 44*, 209–15.

——— 1980a: Encephalitis in India. Calcutta: *Indian Statistical Institute Technical Report 2/80*.

——— 1980b: On the biology of the malaria vectors of Calcutta. Calcutta: *Indian Statistical Institute Technical Report Entom. 1/80*.

Davey, S.C. and Giles, G.G. 1979: Spatial factors in mental health in Tasmania. *Soc. Sci. Med. 13D*, 87–94.

Davey, T.H. and Lightbody, W.P.H. 1956: *The Control of Disease in the Tropics*. London: H.K. Lewis.

Davies, P. and Walsh, D. 1983: *Alcohol Problem and Alcohol Control in Europe*. London: Croom Helm.

Davis, A. 1984: Minimal requirements for planning control projects. *Arzneimittel Forschung 34* (II,9b), 1239–40.

Day, L.H. 1984: Death from non-war violence: an international comparison. *Soc. Sci. Med. 19*, 917–27.

Day, N.E. 1984: The geographic pathology of cancers of the oesophagus. *British Med. Bull. 40*, 329–34.

De, J. and Gollerkiri, R.S. 1984: Morbidity of infectious hepatitis in Vadadora. *Annals. Nat. Assoc. Geogrs India 4/2*, 56–65.

Dean, K.G. 1979: Measuring stress. *Area 11*, 313–4.

Dear, M. 1981: Assigning service-dependent elderly to appropriate treatment settings. *Soc. Sci. Med. 15D*, 405–16.

Defoe, D., 1724: A Tour through England and Wales, vol. I reprint. London: Dent-Everyman 1928.

Carvalho, S. de, 1977: Endoecology and cancer. *Méd. Biol. Env. 5*, 35–43.

Deinhardt, F. and Gust, I.D. 1982: Viral hepatitis. *Bull. WHO 60*, 661–91.

Delange, F. and Ahluwalia, R. (eds) 1983: *Cassava toxicity and thyroid: research and public health issues*. Proceedings of a workshop, Ottawa, Canada 31 May–2 Jun. 1982. Ottawa: International Development Research Centre.

DeMaeyer, E.M., Lowenstein, F.W. and Thilly, C.H. 1979: *The Control of Endemic Goitre*. Geneva: WHO.

Derrick, E.H. 1961: The incidence and distribution of scrub typhus in northern Queensland. *Australian Annals Med. 10*, 256–67.

de Santis, G. and Grasselli, E.L. 1983: L'infestazione malarica tra squilibri ambientali e insediamenti umani. In IGU Working Group on Geography of Health 1983, pp. 241–56.

Devadas, R.P. and Saroja, S. 1980: Prevalence of vitamin A deficiency among rural children. *Indian J. Nutr. and Dietetics 17*, 401–7.

de Vise, P. 1973: *Misused and misplaced hospitals and doctors: a locational analysis of the urban health care crisis.* Washington DC: Association of American Geographers Commission on College Geography Resource Paper no. 22.

De Zulueta, J., Mujtaba, S.M. and Shah, I.H. 1980: Malaria control and long-term periodicity of the disease in Pakistan. *Trans. Roy. Soc. Trop. Med. Hyg.* 74, 624–32.

DHSS (Department of Health and Social Security) 1976: *Prevention and health: everybody's business.* London: HMSO.

―――― 1980a: *Inequalities in health: report of a research working group.* London: HMSO.

―――― 1980b: *Rickets and osteomalacia: report of the working party on fortification of food with vitamin D.* Committee on medical aspects of food policy. London: HMSO.

Diesfeld, H.J. 1965a: Vorkommen, Häufigkeit und Mehrfachbefall von Darmparasiten in Ethiopien. *Zeitschr. f. Tropenmed. u. Parasit.* 16, 411–22.

―――― 1965b: Amöbiasis im tropischen Hochland. *Zeitschr. f. Tropenmed u. Parasit.* 16, 402–10.

―――― 1978: Personal communication.

―――― 1980: Importation of tropical diseases and prophylaxis in international tourism. *Gesundheitswesen* 42, 497–502.

―――― 1982: Holiday tours to the tropics – health counselling for mass tourism. *Arbeitsmed. Socialmed. Präventivmed.* 17, 197–200.

―――― and Hecklau, H. 1976: Model for a geomedical monograph. In Jusatz (ed.) 1976, pp. 71–88.

―――――――― 1978: *Kenya.* Geomedical monograph series. Regional studies in geographical medicine 5. Berlin: Springer.

Dobson, M. 1980: 'Marsh fever' – the geography of malaria in England. *J. Hist. Geog.* 6, 357–89.

―――― 1982: When malaria was an English disease. *Geog. Mag.* 54, 94–9.

Dockery, D.W., Ware, J.H., Ferris, B.G., Jr, Speizer, F.E., Cook, N.R. and Herman, S.M. 1982: Change in pulmonary function in children associated with air pollution episodes. *J. Air Pollution* 32, 937–42.

Doll, R. 1983: Prospects for prevention (review). *British Med. J.* 286 (5 Feb.), 445–53.

―――― (ed.) 1984: The geography of disease. *British Med. Bull.* 40, 307–408.

―――― and Hill, A.B. 1952: A study of the aetiology of carcinoma of the lung. *British Med. J.* 2, 1271.

―――― and Peto, R. 1981: The causes of cancer: quantitative estimates of avoidable risks of cancer in the United States. *J. Nat. Cancer Inst.* 66, 1191–308. (see also critical comment by J. Clemmesen, A. Neilsen 'Morbidity versus mortality' 69, 549, and the authors' rejoinder 549–50).

Donaldson, L.J. and Clayton, D.G. 1984: Occurrence of cancer in Asians and non-Asians. *J. Epidem. and Commun. Health* 38, 203–7.

Doumenge, J.-P. 1984: Unité et diversité des systèmes pathogènes des schistosomiases en Afrique. In *Géosanté* symposium 1984, pp. 519–29.

―――― Cheming, C., Villenave, D. and Guerin, B. 1983: Intérêt et limites d'une cartographie des schistosomiases humaines dans le monde. In CEGET 1983, pp. 169–76.

Dorland's Illustrated Medical Dictionary 1974: Philadelphia: Saunders.

Dowlatshahi, K. and Miller, R.J. 1985: Role of opium in esophageal cancer: a hypothesis. *Cancer Res. 45*, 1906–7 (correspondence).

Dowler, J.C. 1982: Case study no. 6: toxic-shock syndrome and 'tampon disease'. *Environmental monograph*, Institute for Environmental Studies University of Toronto, 3, 173–80.

Dube, N. and Youde, L. 1981: Etude de la distribution spatiale des principales causes de mortalité dans la ville de Québec (1976–78). *Cahiers de Géographie du Québec 25*(66), 413–32.

Duke, B.O.L. 1981: Geographical aspects of onchocerciasis. In *Institut de Médecine Tropicale Prince Léopold* 1981, pp. 179–86.

Dunlop, E.M.C. 1983: Venereal disease: chlamydial genital infection and its complications. *British J. Hosp. Med. 29*, 6–11.

Dustin, J.-P. and Lavoipierre, G.J. 1981: Food aid as capital investment. *World Health Forum 2*, 106–13.

Dutt, A.K., Akhtar, R. and Dutta, H.M. 1980: Malaria in India with particular reference to two west-central States. *Soc. Sci. Med. 14D*, 317–30.

_____ and Dutta, H.M. 1984: Diseases in South and Southeast Asia with special reference to India. *Indian Geog. J. 59*, 141–7.

_____ 1985: Environmental determinism and the resurgence of malaria in Sri Lanka. IBG/AAG Symposium on Medical Geography, University of Nottingham, July.

Dutta, H.M. and Dutt, A.K. 1978: Malarial ecology: a global perspective. *Soc. Sci. Med. 12*, 69–84.

Eckert, E.A. 1982: Spatial and temporal distribution of plague in a region of Switzerland. *Bull. Hist. Med. 56*, 175–94.

Edmondson, C.M. 1977: The politics of hunger: the Soviet response to famine. *Soviet Studies 29*, 506–18.

Edmundson, W. 1980a: Adaptation to undernutrition: how much food does man need? *Soc. Sci. Med. 14D*, 119–26.

_____ 1980b: Applied nutritional geography: priorities and praxis. *Soc. Sci. Med. 14D*, 133–7.

Elton, P. 1982: The measurement of distance when testing hypotheses of contagion. *Soc. Sci. Med. 16*, 1065–6.

Epidemiological Bull. 1981a: Status of plague in the Americas *2*(3), 5–8.

_____ 1981b: Dengue in the Americas. *2*(4), 1–4.

_____ 1984: Years of potential life lost – Brazil 1980. *5*(5), 3–7.

EURO Reports and Studies 1982: Legionnaires' disease. Report on a WHO working group, Baden, Austria, 19–21 Oct. 81. No. 72, 1–29.

Evans, D., Bowie, M.D., Hansen, J.D.L., Moodie, A.D. and van der Spuy, H.I.J. 1980: Intellectual development and nutrition. *J. Paed. 97*, 358–63.

Evenson, R.E., Popkin, B.M. and King-Quizon, E. 1979: Nutrition, work and demographic behaviour in rural Philippine households: a synopsis of several Laguna household studies. *Yale University, Economic Growth Center, Discussion Paper* 308, 1–76.

Eyles, J. 1982: Health and medicine in urban society: the social construction and fetishism of health. Dept. of Geography, Queen Mary College, University of London *Occasional Paper* 20, 13–34.

————, Smith, D.M. and Woods, K. 1982: Spatial resource allocation and state practice: the case of health service planning in London. *Reg. Studies 16*, 239–52.

———— and Woods, K.J. 1983: *The Social Geography of Medicine and Health.* London: Croom Helm.

———— 1985: An inverse interest law? In IBG/AAG Symposium on Medical Geography, University of Nottingham, July.

Fallon, R.J. 1982: *Legionella* infections in Scotland. *J. Hyg. UK 89*, 439–48.

———— 1983: Legionellosis and allied infections. *J. Infect. 6*, 13–16.

———— 1985: Meningococcal infections in Scotland 1984. *Commun. Dis. in Scotland 19*, vii–xii.

————, Brown, W.M. and Lore, W. 1984: Meningococcal infections in Scotland 1972–82. *J. Hyg. UK 93*, 167–80.

Farid, M.A. 1980: The malaria programme – from euphoria to anarchy. *World Health Forum 1*, 8–22.

Farooqi, M.Y., Nasir, J. and Fatima, T. 1981: The potentiality of vitamins and minerals in the agricultural output of Orissa. *Geogr. Observer 17*, 21–5.

Farrag, O.L. 1983: The status of child nutrition in the Gulf Arab States. *J. Trop. Paed. 29*, 325–9.

Faulk, W.P., Mata, L.T., and Edsall, G. 1975: Effects of malnutrition on the immune response in humans: a review. *Trop. Dis. Bull. 72*, 89–103.

Favier, A. and Thouvenot, C. 1980: Eléments de cartographie alimentaire. *Annales de Géog. 493*, 273–89.

Feachem, R.G. 1984: Interventions for the control of diarrhoeal diseases among young children: promotion of personal and domestic hygiene. *Bull. WHO 62*, 467–76.

————, Garelick, H. and Slade, J. 1981: Enteroviruses in the environment. *Trop. Dis. Bull. 78*, 186–230.

———— et al. 1981–82: Environmental Aspects of Cholera Epidemiology: I R.G. Feachem, 1981. A review of selected reports of endemic and epidemic situations during 1961–80. *Trop. Dis. Bull. 78*, 676–98.

II————, Miller, C. and Draser, B. 1981: Occurrence and survival of *Vibrio cholerae* in the environment. *Trop. Dis. Bull. 78*, 866–80.

III———— 1982: Transmission and control. *Trop. Dis. Bull. 79*, 2–47.

Fendall, N.R.E. 1981: Ayurvedic medicine and primary health care. *Trop. Doctor 11*, 81–5.

Fenwick, A., Cheesmond, A.K. and Amin, M.A. 1981: The role of field irrigation canals in the transmission of *Schistosoma mansoni* in the Gezira scheme, Sudan. *Bull. WHO 59*, 777–86.

————————, Kardaman, M., Amin, M.A. and Manjing, B.K. 1982: Schistosomiasis among labouring communities in the Gezira irrigated area, Sudan. *J. Trop. Med. and Hyg. 85*, 3–11.

Ferguson, A.G. 1977: Probability mapping of the 1975 cholera epidemic in Kisumu district, Kenya. *J. Trop. Geog. 44*, 23–32.

———— 1981: Local mobility and the spatial dynamics of measles in a rural area of Kenya. *GeoJournal 5*, 315–22.

Ffrench, G.E. and Hill, A.G. 1971: *Kuwait: urban and medical ecology: a geomedical study.* Geomedical monograph series vol. 4, New York, Heidelberg: Springer.

Fine, P.E.M. 1982: Leprosy: the epidemiology of a slow bacterium. *Epidem. Review 4*, 161–88.

――――― 1986: Comment on Hunter et al. (1984a) *Trop. Dis. Bull. 83* (402), 145–6.

Firth, R. 1959: *Social Change in Tikopia.* London: George Allen and Unwin.

Foba-Pagou, R., Kegoum, E., Same-Ekobo, A., Eben-Moussi, E., Faucher, P., Carrie, J. and Ripert, C. 1980: An epidemiological study of intestinal helminthiases (ascariasis, *Necator* infection, taeniasis, schistosomiasis) in the town of Maroua (North Cameroon). Results of treatment with mebendazole. *Bull. de la Soc. Path. Exotique et de ses Filiales 73*, 171–8.

Forman, D., Al-Dabbagh, S. and Doll, R. 1985: Nitrates, nitrites and gastric cancer in Great Britain. *Nature 313* (25 Feb.) 620–5.

Forsyth, D.M. 1982: Comment on Cheesmond et al. (1981). *Trop. Dis. Bull. 79* (400), 170.

――――― 1983: Comment on Kloos et al. (1982). *Trop. Dis. Bull. 80* (1040), 288–9.

Foster, H.D. 1979: The geography of stress. *Area 11*, 107–8.

Fox, A.J., Jones, D.R. and Goldblatt, P.O. 1984: Approaches to studying the effect of socioeconomic circumstances on geographic differences in mortality in England and Wales. *British Med. Bull. 40*, 309–14.

Fox, J.P., Hal, C.E., Cooney, M.K. and Foy, H.M. 1982a: Influenza virus infections in Seattle families 1975–79. I. Study design, methods and the occurrence of infections by time and age. *American J. Epidem. 116*, 212–17.

――――― , Cooney, M.K., Hall, C.E. and Foy, H.M. 1982b: Idem. II Pattern of infection in invaded households and relation of age and prior antibody to occurrence of infection and related illness. *American J. Epidem. 116*, 228–42.

Freeman, H.E., Klein, R.E., Townsend, J.W. and Lechtig, A. 1980: Nutrition and cognitive development among rural Guatemalan children. *American J. Public Health 70*, 1277–85.

Fries, J.F. 1985: The compression of morbidity. *World Health Forum 6*, 47–51.

Fritz, C. 1980: *Combating nutritional blindness in children. A case study of technical assistance in Indonesia.* Oxford: Pergamon.

Fukushima, M., Ogagaki, T., Twiggs, L.B., Clark, B.A., Zachow, K.R. and Ostrow, R.S. 1985: Histological types of carcinoma of the uterine cervix and the detectability of human papillomavirus DNA. *Cancer Res. 45*, 3252–5.

Fulford, K.W.N., Catterall, R.D., Hoinville, E., Lim, K.S. and Wilson, G.D. 1983: Social and psychological factors in the distribution of STD in clinic attenders. I Demographic and social factors. II Personality disorders, psychiatric illness and abnormal sexual attitudes. III Sexual activity. *British J. Venereal Dis. 59*, 376–85 and 386–93.

Furmenko, I.P., Grosheva, T.N. and Luzhkov, B.N. 1982: Complex social and hygienic characteristics of cardiovascular pathology in the rural population. *Sovetskoe Zdravookhranenie 10*, 25–30.

Gaitan, G. 1983: Endemic goiter in western Colombia. *Ecol. of Dis. 2*, 295–308.

Garcia, R.V. and Escudero, J.C. 1982: *Drought and Man: the 1972 case history. Vol. 2 The constant catastrophe; malnutrition, famines and drought.* Oxford: Pergamon.

Gardner, M.J. 1984: Mapping cancer mortality in England and Wales. *British Med. Bull* (Churchill Livingstone) *40*, 320–8.

———, Winter, P.D., Taylor, C.P. and Acheson, E.D. 1983: *Atlas of Cancer Mortality in England and Wales*. Chichester: Wiley.

———, Winter, P.D. and Barker, D.J.P. 1984: *Atlas of Mortality from Selected Diseases in England and Wales*. Chichester, Wiley.

Gatenby, P.C. 1982: Patterns of cardiovascular disease mortality in the Glasgow region. *Ecol. of Dis. 1*, 75–85.

Gatus, B.J. and Rose, M.R. 1983: Japanese B encephalitis: epidemiological, clinical and pathological aspects. *J. Infection 6*, 213–8.

Gavrilov, L.A., Gavrilova, N.S. and Semyonova, V.G. 1985: Epidemiological approach to the biology of human life span. *Geographia Medica 15*, 40–64.

Geddes, A. 1942: The population of India: variability in change as a regional demographic index. *Geog. Rev. 32*, 562–73.

——— 1982: *Man and Land in South Asia*. New Delhi: Concept Publishing.

GeoJournal 1981: Studies in medical geography in Africa, 5. No. 4 special issue 298–400.

Géosanté 1984: Symposium de géographie de la santé. 25th Congress, International Geographical Union, Montpellier, Université Paul Valéry.

Gerber, L.M. 1983: Gains in life expectancies if heart disease and stroke were eliminated among Caucasians, Filipinos and Japanese in Hawaii. *Soc. Sci. Med. 17*, 349–53.

Gerrard, N. 1981: The tuberculosis environment. *Geog. Mag. 53*, 641–4.

Geser, A., Brubaker, G. and Olwitt, G.W. 1980: The frequency of Epstein-Barr virus infection and Burkitt's lymphoma at high and low altitudes in East Africa. *Rev. d'Epidemiol. et de Santé Publique 28*, 307–21.

Ghadirian, P., Stein, G.F., Goradetzky, C., Roberfroid, M.B., Mahon, G.A.T., Bartsch, H. and Day, N.E. 1985: Oesophageal cancer studies in the Caspian sea littoral of Iran: some residual results, including opium use as a risk factor. *International J. Cancer 35*, 593–7.

Ghana Health Assessment Team 1981: *International J. Epidem. 10*, 73–80.

Ghannoum, M.A., Moore, K.E., Al-Dulaimi, M. and Nasr, M. 1981: The incidence of water-related diseases in the Brak area, Libya from 1977 to 1979, before and after the installation of water treatment plants. *Zentralblatt f. Bakter. Mikrobiol. u. Hyg. 173B*, 501–8.

Gibson, D.M. and Rowland, D.T. 1984: Community vs institutional care: the case of the Australian aged. *Soc. Sci. Med. 18*, 997–1004.

Giggs, J. 1973a: High rates of schizophrenia among immigrants in Nottingham. *Nursing Times* 20 Sep., 1210–2.

——— 1973b: The distribution of schizophrenics in Nottingham. *Trans. Inst. British Geogrs 59*, 57–76 (see also ibid. 1975 *64*, 149 for comment by Gudgin and 150–6 for rejoinder by Giggs).

——— 1983: Schizophrenia and ecological structure in Nottingham. In McGlashan and Blunden (eds) 1983, pp. 197–222.

——— 1984: The incidence of primary acute pancreatitis in Greater Nottingham. In *Géosanté* 1984, pp. 460–85.

———, Ebdon, D.S. and Bourke, J.B. 1980: The epidemiology of acute pancreatitis in the Nottingham Defined Population Area. *Trans. Inst. British Geogrs* 5, 229–42.

———, Mather, P.M. 1983: Perspectives on mental health in urban areas. *Nottingham Monographs in Applied Geography no. 3.* Department of Geography, University of Nottingham.

Gilbert, E.W. 1958: Pioneer maps of health and disease in England. *Geog. J.* 124, 172–83.

Giles, G.G. 1983: The utility of relative risk ratio in geographical epidemiology: Hodgkin's disease in Tasmania. In McGlashan and Blunden (eds) 1983, pp. 361–74.

Gilles, H.M. 1964: *Akufo: an environmental study of a Nigerian village community.* University of Ibadan Department of Preventive and Social Medicine/Liverpool School of Tropical Medicine.

Gillett, J.D. 1985: The behaviour of *Homo sapiens*, the forgotten factor in the transmission of tropical disease. *Trans. Roy. Soc. Trop. Med. Hyg.* 19, 12–20.

Gilli, G., Corrao, C. and Favilli, S. 1984: Concentrations of nitrates in drinking water and incidence of gastric carcinomas: first descriptive study of the Piemonte region, Italy. *Sci. of the Total Env.* 34, 35–48.

Gillies, M.E. and Paulin, H.V. 1983: Variability of mineral intakes from drinking water: a possible explanation for the controversy on the relationship of water quality to cardiovascular disease. *International J. Epidem.* 12, 45–50.

Gillis, C.R. 1977: Malignant neoplasms. In Howe (ed.) 1977, pp. 507–34.

Girt, J.L. 1972: Simple chronic bronchitis and urban ecological structure. In McGlashan (ed.) 1972, pp. 211–31.

——— 1974: The geography of non-vectored infectious diseases. In J.M. Hunter (ed.) *The geography of health and disease.* Department of Geography Studies in Geography no. 5. Chapel Hill NC: University of North Carolina.

——— 1978: A programming model of the spatial and temporal diffusion of contagious disease. *Soc. Sci. Med.* 12D, 173–81.

Glantz, M.H. 1977a: Nine fallacies of natural disaster: the case of the Sahel. *Climatic Change* 1, 69–84.

——— 1977b: *The Politics of Natural Disaster: the case of the Sahel drought.* New York: Praeger.

Glezen, W.P., Couch, R.B. and Six, H.R. 1982: The influenza herald wave. *American J. Epidem.* 116, 589–98.

Glick, B. 1979a: The spatial autocorrelation of cancer mortality. *Soc. Sci. Med.* 13D, 123–30.

——— 1979b: Distance relationships in theoretical models of carcinogenesis. *Soc. Sci. Med.* 13D, 253–6.

——— 1979c: Tests for space–time clustering used in cancer research. *Geogr. Analysis* 11, 202–8.

——— 1980: The geographic analysis of cancer occurrence: past progress and future directions. In Meade (ed.) 1980, pp. 170–93.

——— 1982: The spatial organization of cancer mortality. *Annals American Assoc. Geogrs* 72, 471–81.

Goel, K.M., Sweet, E.M., Campbell, S., Attenburrow, A. and Logan, R.W.

1981: Reduced prevalence of rickets in Asian children in Glasgow. *Lancet* ii (22 Aug.) 405–7.

Goll, P.H. 1982: Seasonal changes in the distribution of *Biomphalaria sudanica sudanica* (Martens) in Lake Zwai, Ethiopia. *Annals Trop. Med. and Parasit.* 76, 159–64.

Golledge, R.G., Parnicky, J.J. and Raynor, J.N. 1979: An experimental design for assessing the spatial competence of mildly retarded populations. *Soc. Sci. Med. 13D*, 291–5.

Good, C.M. 1980: Ethnomedical systems in Africa and the LDCs: key issues for the geographer. In Meade (ed.) 1980, pp. 93–116.

_____ 1987a: Community health in tropical Africa: is medical pluralism a hindrance or a resource? in Akhtar (ed.) 1987, pp. 13–50.

_____ 1987b: Ethnomedical systems in Africa: patterns of traditional medicine in rural and urban Kenya. New York: Guilford Publications (in the Press).

_____, Hunter, J.M. and Katz, S.H. 1979: The interface of dual systems of health: toward health policy initiatives in Africa. *Soc. Sci. Med. 13D*, 141–54.

Gopalan, R. 1968: Dietary patterns of children developing kwashiorkor as against marasmus in poor Indian families. In R.A. McCance and E.M. Widdowson (eds) *Calorie deficiencies and protein deficiencies*. Proceedings of a colloquium held in Cambridge, April 1967. London: J. and A. Churchill.

Gordon, T. and Kannel, W.B. 1983: Drinking habits and cardiovascular disease: the Framingham study. *American Heart J. 105*, 667–73.

Gori, G.B. and Richter, B.J. 1978: Macroeconomics of disease prevention in the United States. *Science 200* (4346), 1124–30.

Gotanègre, J.-F. 1984: La bilharziose, l'eau et la démographie sur les hautes terres volcaniques du Rwanda septentrional (Afrique). In *Géosanté* 1984, pp. 530–43.

Gould, P. and Rogier, A. 1984: Famine as a spatial crisis. In Currey and Hugo (eds) 1984, pp. 135–54.

Gramiccia, G. 1981: Health education in malaria control – why has it failed? *World Health Forum 2*, 385–93.

Grange, J.M. 1980: *Mycobacterial Diseases*. London: Arnold.

Grantham-McGregor, S., Stewart, M.E. and Schofield, W.N. 1980: Effect of long-term psychosocial stimulation on mental development of severely malnourished children. *Lancet* ii (11 Oct.), 785–9.

Greenberg, M.R. 1984: Changing cancer mortality patterns in the rural United States. *Rural Sociol. 49*, 143–53.

_____ 1985: Disease competition as a factor in ecological studies of mortality. IBG/AAG Symposium on Medical Geography, University of Nottingham, July.

Greenough, R. 1975: Famine mortality, destitution and victimisation: Bengal 1943–46. 14th annual Bengal studies conference. University of Iowa.

Greenwood, B.M., Blakebrough, I.S., Bradley, A.K., Wale, S. and Whittle, H.C. 1984: Meningococcal disease and season in sub-Saharan Africa. *Lancet* i (16 June), 1339–42.

_____, Bradley, A.K. and Wall, R.A. 1985: Meningococcal disease and season in sub-Saharan Africa. *Lancet* ii (12 Oct.), 829–30 (correspondence).

Gregory, J.W. and Piche, V. 1983: Inequality and mortality: demographic hypotheses regarding advanced and peripheral capitalism. *International J. Health Services 13*, 89–106.

Greig, W.R., Thomson, J.A. and McGirr, E.M. 1973: The environment and thyroid disorders. In Howe and Loraine (eds) 1973, pp. 154–68.

Griffiths, M. 1971a: A geographical study of mortality in an urban area. *Urban Studies 8*, 111–20.

———— 1971b: A case study in medical geography, Wonford Ward, Exeter. In K.J. Gregory and W. Ravenhill (1971) Exeter essays in honour of Arthur Davies. University of Exeter.

Grigg, D. 1981: The historiography of hunger: changing views on the world food problem. *Trans. Inst. British Geogrs 6*, 279–92.

———— 1985: *The World Food Problem 1950–80*. Oxford: Basil Blackwell.

Grove, A.T. 1977: Desertification in the African environment. *African Environment Special Report 6*, 54–64.

———— 1978: Geographical introduction to the Sahel. *Geog. J. 144*, 407–15.

The Guardian 1985: AIDS Extra 1 and 2, 5–6 Nov.; Open Space 4 Feb. 1986.

Guiguemde, T.R., Sokal, C.D. and Roux, J. 1983: Dracunculiasis: a public health problem? *Méd. d'Afrique Noire 30*, 419–26.

Gupta, P.C., Bhonsle, R.B., Mehta, F.S. and Pindborg, J.J. 1984: Mortality experience in relation to tobacco chewing and smoking habits from a 10-year follow-up study in Ernakulam district, Kerala. *International J. Epidem. 13*, 184–7.

Gwynne, M. 1985: Use of imagery to assess degradation. Symposium: Geographical background to Africa's crisis, Royal Geographical Society 25 Nov. 85.

Haas, J.D. and Harrison, G.G. 1977: Nutritional anthropology and biological adaptation. In B.J. Siegel, A.R. Beals and S.A. Tyler (eds), *Annual Review of Anthropology*. Palo Alto, Calif.: Annual Reviews Inc., pp. 69–101.

Habibi, A. 1979: Aspect socio-économique de certains cancers en Iran. *Méd. Biol. Env. 7*, 28–31.

———— 1982: Particularités épidémiologiques de certains cancers au Proch-Orient. *Méd. Biol. Env. 10*, 56–9.

Hackett, L.W. 1937: *Malaria in Europe*. London: Oxford University Press.

Haddock, K.C. 1981: Control of schistosomiasis: the Puerto Rican experience. *Soc. Sci. Med. 15D*, 501–14.

Hägerstrand, T. 1952: The propagation of innovation waves. *Lund studies in geography B4*, 3–19.

———— 1967: Innovation diffusion as a spatial process.

Haggett, P. 1965: *Locational Analysis in Human Geography*. London: Arnold.

———— 1972: Contagious processes in a planar graph: an epidemiological application. In McGlashan (ed.) 1972, pp. 307–24.

———— 1976: Hybridizing alternative models of an epidemic diffusion process. *Econ. Geog. 52*, 136–46.

Hall, G.B., Hughes, R. and Dear, M.J. 1984: Predicting community reaction to mental health facilities. *J. American Planning Assoc. 50*, 37–47.

Halstead, S.B. 1981: The Alexander D. Langmuir lecture. The pathogenesis of dengue: molecular epidemiology in infectious disease. *American J. Epidem.* *114*, 632–48.

Hann, H.W.L., Kim, C.Y., London, W.T., Whitford, P. and Blumberg, B.S. 1982: Hepatitis B and primary hepatocellular carcinoma: family studies in Korea. *International J. Cancer, 30*, 47–51.

Hardy, J.L., Rosen, L., Kramer, L.D., Presser, S.B., Shroyer, D.A. and Turell, M.J. 1980: Effect of rearing temperature on transovarial transmission of St Louis encephalitis virus in mosquitoes. *American J. Trop. Med. Hyg. 29*, 963–8.

Hare, E.H., Moran, P.A.P. and Macfarlane, A. 1981: The changing seasonality of infant death in England and Wales 1912–78, and its relation to seasonal temperature. *J. Epidem. and Commun. Health 35*, 77–82.

Harinasuta, T., Dixon, K.E., Warrell, D.A. and Doberstyn, E.B. 1982: Recent advances in malaria with special reference to Southeast Asia. *Southeast Asian J. Trop. Med. and Public Health 13*, 1–34.

Harrison, G. 1978: *Mosquitoes, Malaria and Man – a history of the hostilities since 1880.* London: John Murray.

Harriss, B. 1985: Famine in Africa: are there any solutions? *J. Trop. Med. and Hyg. 88*, 185–8.

Hart, G.D. (ed.) 1983: *Disease in Ancient Man: an international symposium.* Ontario: Clarke Irwin.

Hart, J.T. 1971: The inverse care law. *Lancet* i, 405–12.

Hatton, F., Maujol, L. and Bouvier-Colle, M.H. 1984: Mortalité en France: évolution des disparités. In *Géosanté 1984*, pp. 105–20.

Haviland, A. 1892: *Geographical Distribution of Disease in Great Britain.* 2nd edn Part 1. London: Swan Sonnenschein.

Haworth, J. 1985: Comment on Ityavyar (1984). *Trop. Dis. Bull. 82* (2159), 622–3.

Hayakawa, N. and Kurihara, M. 1981: International comparison of trends in cancer mortality for selected sites. *Soc. Sci. Med. 15D*, 245–9.

Haynes, R. 1983: The geographical distribution of mortality by cause in Chile. *Soc. Sci. Med. 17*, 355–64.

_____ 1984: Regional associations between cancer mortality and urbanization in China. In *Géosanté 1984*, pp. 327–52.

Haynes, R.M. and Bentham, C.G. 1979: Accessibility and the use of hospitals in rural areas. *Area 11*, 186–91.

Hazra, J. 1984a: Spatial pattern of cancers in India with special reference to West Bengal. *Indian Geog. J. 59*, 55–63.

_____ 1984b: Heart disease in a rural community in West Bengal, India. In *Géosanté 1984*, pp. 295–307.

_____ and Banerjee, B. 1979: Medical geography of West Bengal. *Trans. Inst. Indian Geogrs 1*, 47–55.

He, S.Y., Gu, B.L. Tong, W.Y., Gao, Q., Zhao, B., Qin, S. and Fang, S. 1983: Survey on the effect of control of schistosomiasis in 99 production brigades of 10 counties in Jiangsu Province. *J. Parasit. and Parasit. Dis. 1*, 27–31.

Heath, E. 1981: North-South: a programme for survival. *Geog. J. 147*, 298–306.

Hecklau, H. 1978: Model for an economic and social–geographical classification of Kenya. *GeoJournal* 2, 311–19.

Helgason, T., Ewen, S.W.B., Ross, I.S. and Stowers, J.M. 1982: Diabetes produced in mice by smoked/cured mutton. *Lancet* ii (6 Nov.), 1017–22.

Henderson, A. 1984: Immunization against Japanese encephalitis in Nepal: experience of 1152 subjects. *J. Roy. Army Med. Corps 130*, 188–91.

Hendrickse, J.G. 1984: The influence of aflatoxins on child health in the tropics with special reference to kwashiorkor. *Trans. Roy. Soc. Trop. Med. and Hyg.* 78, 427–35.

_____, Coulter, J.B.S., Lamplugh, S.M., Macfarlane, S.B.J., Williams, T.E., Omer, M.I.A. and Suliman, G.I. 1982: Aflatoxins and kwashiorkor, a study in Sudanese children. *British Med. J. 285* (25 Sep.), 843–6.

Henry, N.F. 1981: Socio-spatial dimensions of health-seeking behavior in an urban elderly population. In J.W. Frazier and B.J. Epstein (eds) *Proc. of Applied Geog. Conferences* v. 4. Dept. of Geography, State University of New York, Binghamton.

Herbert, D.T. and Hijazi, B. 1984: Ill-health and health-care in Khartoum/Omdurman, *Soc. Sci. Med. 18*, 335–43.

Herzlich, C. and Pierret, J. 1985: The social construction of the patient: patients and illnesses in other ages. *Soc. Sci. Med. 20*, 145–51.

Hethcote, H.W., Yorke, J.A. and Nold, A. 1982: Gonorrhoea modelling: a comparison of control methods. *Math. Biosciences 58*, 93–109.

Hetzel, B.S. 1983: Iodine deficiency disorders (IDD) and their eradication. *Lancet* ii (12 Nov.), 1126–9.

Hill, A.G. (ed.) 1985: *Population, Health and Nutrition in the Sahel: issues in the welfare of selected West African communities*. London: Routledge and Kegan Paul.

Hillier, S.M. and Jewell, J.A. 1983: *Health Care and Traditional Medicine in China 1800–1982*. London: Routledge and Kegan Paul.

Hillyer, G.V. 1981: Can we vaccinate against schistosomes? An update five years later. *Bol. Assoc. Méd. de Puerto Rico 73*, 150–61.

Hinds, M.W., Stemmermann, G.N., Yang, H.-Y., Kolonel, L.N., Lee, J. and Wegner, E. 1981: Differences in lung cancer risk from smoking among Japanese, Chinese and Hawaiian women in Hawaii. *International J. Cancer* 27, 297–302.

Hinz, E. 1984: Vegetation, Nutzpflanzen und Endemien. In Jusatz and Wellmer (eds) 1984, pp. 32–44.

Hirsch, A. 1881: *Handbuch der historisch-geographischen Pathologie* translated as *Handbook of geographical and historical pathology* by C. Creighton. London: Sydenham Society, 1883–86.

Hoffman, D.B. Jr. and Warren, K.S. 1978: *Schistosomiasis IV: Condensations of the selected literature 1963–75*. Washington DC: Hemisphere Publishing.

Hogan, R.C. and 11 others 1977: Sahel nutrition surveys 1974 and 1975. *Disasters 1*, 117–24.

Hogbin, V. 1985: Railways, disease and health in South Africa. *Soc. Sci. Med. 20*, 933–8.

Holt, P.H. 1981: Comment on C.H. O'Neill et al. 1980. *Trop. Dis. Bull. 78* (1234), 511.

Holtermann, S. and Burchell, A. 1981: The costs of alcohol misuse. London: DHSS, *Government Economic Services Working Paper No. 37*.

Hoogstraal, H. 1981: Changing patterns of tick-borne disease in modern society. *Annual Rev. Entom. 26*, 75–99.

Hope, I.A., Hall, R., Simmons, D.Ll., Hyde, J.E. and Scaife, J.G. 1984: Evidence for immunological cross reaction between sporozoites and blood stages of a human malaria parasite. *Nature 308* (8 Mar.), 191–4.

Hope-Simpson, R.E. 1984: Age and secular distributions of virus-proven influenza patients 1961–76 in Cirencester: epidemiological significance discussed. *J. Hyg. UK 92*, 303–36.

Horstmann, D.M. 1982: Control of poliomyelitis: a continuing paradox. *J. Infect. Dis. 40*, 540–51.

_____, Quinn, T.C. and Robbins, F.C. (eds) 1984: International Symposium on Poliomyelitis Control, Washington 14–17 Mar. 1983. *Reviews of Infect. Dis.* 6 Supplement, pp., S301–600.

Howe, G.M. 1970: *National atlas of disease mortality in the United Kingdom*. London: Royal Geographical Society/Nelson (This subsumes the 1963 atlas)

_____ 1972a; 1976: *Man, Environment and Disease in Britain: a medical geography of Britain through the ages*. Newton Abbott: David and Charles; New York: Barnes and Noble; Harmondsworth: Penguin.

_____ 1972b: London and Glasgow: a comparative study of mortality patterns. *International Geography* (International Geographical Union) Toronto: University of Toronto Press, vol. 2, 1214–7.

_____ 1979: Mortality from selected malignant neoplasms in the British Isles: the spatial perspective. *Geog. J.* (Royal Geographical Society) *145*, 401–15; *Soc. Sci. Med. 15D* 1981, 199–211.

_____ 1983: Spatial appraisal of ischaemic heart disease and lung–bronchus cancer in Glasgow, Scotland. In IGU Working Group 1983, pp. 47–56.

_____ (ed.) 1977: *A World Geography of Human Diseases*. London: Academic Press.

_____ (ed.) 1986: *Global Geocancerology: a world geography of human cancers*. Edinburgh: Churchill-Livingstone.

_____, Burgess, L. and Gatenby, P. 1977: Cardiovascular disease. Howe (ed.) 1977, pp. 431–76.

_____ and Loraine, J.A. (eds) 1973: *Environmental Medicine*. London: Heinemann Medical.

Hoyt, H. 1939: The structure and growth of residential neighbourhoods in American cities. Washington DC: Federal Housing Administration.

Hudson, T. and Genesse, J. 1982: Hansen's disease in the United States. *Soc. Sci. Med. 16*, 997–1004.

Hugo, G.J. 1984: The demographic impact of famine: a review. In Currey and Hugo (eds) 1984, pp. 7–31.

Hunt, L.M. 1985: Relativism in the diagnosis of hypoglycemia. *Soc. Sci. Med. 20*, 1289–94.

Hunter, G.W. III, Yokogawa, M., Akusawa, M., Sano, M., Araki, K. and Kobayashi, M. 1982: Control of schistosomiasis japonica in the Nagatoishi area of Kurume, Japan. *American J. Trop. Med. and Hyg. 31*, 760–70.

———— 1984: Control of schistosomiasis japonica in Japan: a review. *Japanese J. Parasit. 33*, 341–51.

Hunter, J.M. 1966: River blindness in Nangodi, Northern Ghana: a hypothesis of cyclical advance and retreat. *Geog. Rev. 56*, 398–416.

———— 1973: On the merits of holism in understanding societal health needs. *Centennial Rev. 17*, 1–19.

———— 1980: Strategies for the control of river blindness. In Meade (ed.) 1980, pp. 38–76.

———— 1981a: Past explosion and future threat: exacerbation of red water disease (*Schistosomiasis haematobium*) in the Upper Region of Ghana. *GeoJournal 5*, 305–13.

———— 1981b: Progress and concerns in the World Health Organization onchocerciasis control program in West Africa. *Soc. Sci. Med. 15D*, 261–75.

———— and Young, J. 1971: Diffusion of influenza in England and Wales. *Annals Assoc. American Geogrs 61*, 627–53.

————, Rey, L. and Scott, D. 1982: Man-made lakes and man-made diseases: towards a policy resolution. *Soc. Sci. Med. 16*, 1127–45.

———— and Thomas, M.O. 1984a: Hypothesis of leprosy, tuberculosis and urbanization in Africa. *Soc. Sci. Med. 19*, 27–57.

———— and Arbona, S. 1984b: Disease rate as an artifact of the health care system: tuberculosis in Puerto Rico. *Soc. Sci. Med. 19*, 997–1008.

———— 1985a: Field testing along a disease gradient: some geographical dimensions of tuberculosis in Puerto Rico. *Soc. Sci. Med. 21*, 1023–42.

————, Shannon, G.W. and Sambrook, S.L. 1985b: Rings of madness: service areas of 19th century asylums in North America. IBG/AAG symposium on medical geography, University of Nottingham.

Huq, A., West, P.A., Small, E.B., Huq, M.I. and Colwell, R.R. 1984: Influence of water temperature salinity and pH on survival and growth of toxigenic *Vibrio cholerae* serovar 01 associated with live copepods in laboratory microcosms. *Applied and Environmental Microbiol. 48*, 420–4.

Hutchins, P., Hindocha, P., Phillips, A. and Walker-Smith, J. 1982: Traveller's diarrhoea with a vengeance in children of UK immigrants visiting their parents' homeland. *Arch. Dis. Childhood 57*, 208–11.

Hutt, M.S.R. 1979: The geography of cancer. *The Practitioner 222*, 181–90.

———— and Burkitt, D.P. 1986: *The geography of non-infectious disease*. Oxford University Press.

Hyma, B. and Ramesh, A. 1977: Cholera and malaria incidence in Tamilnadu, India. *Department of Geography Publication Series no. 9*, University of Waterloo, Canada.

———— 1980: The reappearance of malaria in Sathanur reservoir and environs: Tamil Nadu, India. *Soc. Sci. Med. 14D*, 337–44.

———— and Chakrapani, K.P. 1983: Urban malaria control situation and environmental issues, Madras City, India. *Ecol. of Dis. 2*, 321–35.

IARC (International Agency for Research on Cancer) 1982: Evaluation of the carcinogenic risk of chemicals to humans. Some aromatic amines, anthraquinones and nitroso compounds, and inorganic fluorides used in drinking water and dental preparations. *IARC Monographs 27*, 1–341. Lyon, France.

Iarotski, L.S. and Davis, A. 1981: The schistosomiasis problem in the world: results of a WHO questionnaire survey. *Bull. WHO 59*, 115–27.

IBG/AAG (Institute of British Geographers/Association of American Geographers) 1985:*Symposium on medical geography*. Department of Geography, University of Nottingham 15–19 July 1985.

Ibrahim, F. 1978: Anthropogenic causes of desertification in western Sudan. *GeoJournal 2*, 243–54.

ICMR (Indian Council of Medical Research) 1974: *Lathyrism – a preventable paralysis*. Hyderabad: National Institute of Nutrition, pp. 1–20.

_____ 1982: Traditional medicine. *Indian J. Med. Res. 76* (Supplement), 1–148.

_____ 1983: *Proceedings of the Indo–UK Workshop on leishmaniasis, Patna 6–10 Dec. 1982*. New Delhi: ICMR.

Ignatyev, Ye.I. 1966: Medical geography and practice. In *Mélanges de Géographie, physique, humaine, économique, appliquée, offerts à M. Omer Tulippe, Liége: T.II Géographie | conomique, Géographie Appliquée, Regionalisation et Théorie*. Gembloux, Belgium, Editions J. Ducolot. pp. 491–8.

IGU (International Geographical Union) Working Group on the Geography of Health 1983: *Primo Seminario Internazionale di Geografia Medica, Roma, 4–7 Nov. 82*. Perugia: Editrice RUX.

Inaba, Y., Maruchi, N., Matsuda, M., Yoshihara, N. and Yamamoto, S.I. 1984: A case-control study of liver cancer with special emphasis on the possible aetiological role of schistosomiasis. *International J. Epidem. 13*, 408–12.

Innes, F. 1979: Spatial patterns of cardiovascular diseases in Windsor, Ontario. University of Windsor Department of Geography, *Project Report 606*-1397–47.

Institut de Médecine Tropicale Prince Léopold 1981: International colloquium on onchocerciasis and other human filariases. *Ann. Soc. Belge. Méd. Trop. 61*, 145–54.

International Agency for the Prevention of Blindness (eds) 1980: *World Blindness and its Prevention*. v. I and II. Oxford University Press.

Inua, M., Duggan, M.B., West, C.E., Whittle, H.C., Kobge, O.I., Sandford-Smith, J.H. and Glover, J. 1983: Post-measles corneal ulceration in children in northern Nigeria: the role of vitamin A, malnutrition and measles. *Ann. Trop. Paediatrics 3*, 181–91.

Ityavyar, D.A. 1984: A traditional midwife practice, Sokoto state, Nigeria. *Soc. Sci. Med. 18*, 497–501.

Iyun, B.F. 1984: Tuberculosis: an urban health hazard in Nigerian cities – a case study of Ibadan City. In *Géosanté Symposium 1984*, pp. 255–71.

Jarcho, S. and van Burkalow, A. 1952: A geographical study of 'swimmers' itch' in the United States and Canada. *Geog. Rev. 42*, 212–26.

Jayant, K., Balakrishnan, V. and Sanghvi, L.D. 1971: A note on the distribution of cancer in some endogamous groups in western India. *British J. Cancer 25*, 611–9.

Jensen, O.M. 1982: Nitrate in drinking water and cancer in northern Jutland, Denmark with special reference to stomach cancer. *Ecotoxicology and Envir. Safety 6*, 258–67.

Jindal, S.K., Malik, S.K., Dhand, R., Gujral, J.S., Malik, A.K. and Datta, B.N. 1982: Bronchogenic carcinoma in northern India. *Thorax 37*, 343–7.

Jobin, W.R. 1978: Tropical disease, bilharzia and irrigation systems in Puerto

Rico. *J. Irrig. and Drainage Div. American Assoc. Civil Eng. 104*(IR3) *Proc. Paper* 14026, 307–22.

Johnson, B.K. and Chanas, A.C. 1981: The potential for the spread of arboviruses into new areas and for their subsequent persistence. A review. *Abstr. Hyg. and Commun. Dis.* 56, 165–80.

Johnson, I. 1978: A geography of infectious diseases in England and Wales. University of Bradford PhD thesis.

Joly, O.G., Lubin, J.H. and Caraballoso, M. 1983: Dark tobacco and lung cancer in Cuba. *J. National Cancer Inst.* 70, 1033–9.

Jones, E. and Grupp, F.W. 1983: Infant mortality trends in the Soviet Union. *Popn and Dev. Rev.* 9, 213–45; (and see comment by M. Feshbach 1984: *Popn and Dev. Rev.* 10, 87.).

Jones, K. 1985: Towards a critical epidemiology. IBG/AAG symposium on medical geography, University of Nottingham, July 1985.

_____ and Moon, G. *Health, Society and Medicine: an introduction to medical geography.* London: Routledge and Kegan Paul, in press.

Jones, P., Hamilton, P.J., Bird, G., Fearns, M., Oxley, A., Tedder, R., Cheinsong-Popov, R. and Codd, A. 1985: AIDS and haemophilia: morbidity and mortality in a well defined population. *British Med. J.* 291 (14 Sep.), 695–9.

Jordan, P. 1981 Targetted treatment of schistosomiasis. *Lancet* i (28 Mar.) 718 (correspondence).

_____ 1985: *Schistosomiasis: the St. Lucia Project.* Cambridge University Press,

_____ and Webbe, G. 1982a: *Schistosomiasis: Epidemiology, Treatment and Control.* London: Heinemann Medical.

_____, Unrau, G.O., Bartholomew, R.K., Cook, J.A. and Grist, E. 1982b: Value of individual household water supplies in the maintenance phase of a schistosomiasis control programme in Saint Lucia, after chemotherapy. *Bull. WHO 60*, 583–8.

Joseph, A.E. and Boeckh, J.L. 1981: Locational variation in mental health care utilization dependent upon diagnosis: a Canadian example. *Soc. Sci. Med. 15D*, 395–404.

_____ and Hall, D.B. 1985: The locational concentration of group homes in Toronto. *Professional Geogr.* 37, 143–55.

_____ and Phillips, D.R. 1984: *Accessibility and utilization: geographical perspectives on health care delivery.* London: Harper and Row.

Joshi, M.J. 1982: *Surgical Diseases in the Tropics.* Delhi: Macmillan India.

_____ and Deshpande, C.D. 1972: Geographical distribution of some diseases common in southern Asia. *Geog. Medica 3*, 5–29.

_____ 1985: The pattern of disease distribution and ecology in southern Asia with special reference to India. In Akhtar and Learmonth (eds) 1985, pp. 49–70.

Journal of the Geological Society 1980: Thematic set of papers on geology and health. *137*, 525–87.

Jusatz, H.J. 1982: 150 years of pandemics of Asiatic cholera 1831–1981. *Zentralblatt f. Bakter., Mikrobiol. u. Hyg. 252*, 257–67.

_____ 1984: Grundlagen und Grundbegriffe der Geomedizin. In H.J. Jusatz and H. Wellmer (eds), *Theorie und Praxis der Medizinschen Geographie und Geomedizin*. Wiesbaden: Franz Steiner, pp. 11–24.

_____ and Wellmer, H. 1982: Recreational danger from virus infection after tick bite. *Arbeitsmed. Sozialmed. Präventivmed. 17*, 200–2.

Kagami, M. 1983: Regional variance of cerebrovascular disease in Japan. *Ecol. of Dis. 2*, 277–83.

Kalimuddin, M.D., Narayan, K.G. and Choudhary, S.P. 1982a: Serological evidence of Japanese encephalitis virus activity in Bihar. *International J. Zoonoses 9*, 39–44.

_____ 1982b: Possible relation of seropositivity to Japanese encephalitis in pigs with the 1978 epidemic of human encephalitis in Bihar. *Trans. Roy. Soc. Trop. Med. and Hyg. 76*, 639–40.

Kanter, H. 1967: *Libya*. Geomedical monograph series, regional studies in geographical medicine 1. Berlin: Springer.

Kaper, J.B., Bradford, H.B., Roberts, N.C. and Falkow, S. 1982: Molecular epidemiology of *Vibrio cholerae* in the US Gulf Coast. *J. Clin. Microbiol. 16*, 129–34.

Kasili, E.G. 1983: Coping with cancer in sub-Saharan Africa. *World Health Forum 4*, 149–52.

Katz, S.L., Krugman, S. and Quinn, T.C. (eds) 1983: International symposium on measles immunization, Washington USA 16–19 Mar. 1982. *Reviews of Infect. Dis. 3*, 389–625.

Kay, B.H., Barker-Hudson, P., Stallman, N.D., Wilmers, M.A., Marks, E.N., Holt, P.J., Muscio, M. and Goldman, B.M. 1984: Dengue fever: reappearance in northern Queensland after 26 years. *Med. J. Australia 140*, 264–8.

Keen, H. 1982: Preventive measures in diabetes. *World Health Forum 3*, 181–4.

_____ and Ekoe, J.M. 1984: The geography of diabetes mellitus. *British Med. Bull. 40*, 359–65.

Keig, G. and McAlpine, J.R. 1980: The influence of age in analysis of mortality variation between population groups. *Soc. Sci. Med. 14D*, 165–8.

Keil, U. 1979: Water hardness, content of electrolytes and trace elements and cardiovascular diseases. *Geogr. Zeitschr. 51*, 59–76.

Keller, W. and Fillmore, C.M. 1983: Prevalence of protein-energy malnutrition. *World Health Stats Quart. 36*, 129–67.

Kemp, I.W. and Smith, D.C. 1982: Breast cancer in Scotland. *Health Bull. 40*, 183–8.

Kendrick, B.L. 1980: A spatial, environmental and socioeconomic appraisal of cancer in New Zealand. *Soc. Sci. Med. 14D*, 205–14.

Khan, A.M., Khan, A.Q., Dobrzynski, L., Joshi, G.P. and Myat, A. 1981: A Japanese encephalitis focus in Bangladesh. *J. Trop. Med. and Hyg. 84*, 41–4.

Khan, M.U., Shahidullah, M., Ahmed, W.U., Barua, D.R., Begum, T., Purification, D. and Rahman, N. 1984: Changes in the trend of shigellosis in Dhaka: family study on secondary infection, clinical manifestation and sensitivity pattern: 1980. *Trans. Roy. Soc. Trop. Med. and Hyg. 78*, 151–6.

Killick-Kendrick, R. and Ward, R.D. (reporters) 1981: Ecology of *Leishmania*

(Workshop). *Parasitology 82*/4, 143–52.

King, H., Zimmet, P., Raper, L.R. and Balkau, B. 1984: Risk factors for diabetes in three Pacific populations. *American J. Epidem. 119*, 396–409.

Klatzmann, J. 1979: World food typology. *Economie Rurale 129*, 3–10.

Klein, J.O., Waldvogel, F. and Weuta, H. (eds) 1984: Workshop on problems of bacterial meningitis, 4 Feb. 1984, Wiesbaden. *Infection* (1, Supplement) *12*, S1–S77.

Kloos, H. 1985: Water resources development and schistosomiasis in the Awash valley, Ethiopia. *Soc. Sci. Med. 20*, 609–25.

_____ and Thompson, K. 1979: Schistosomiasis in Africa: an ecological perspective. *J. Trop. Geog. 48*, 31–46.

_____, Sidrak, W., Michael, A.A.M., Mohareb, E.W. and Higashi, G.I. 1982: Disease concepts and treatment practices relating to schistosomiasis haematobium in Upper Egypt. *J. Trop. Med. and Hyg. 85*, 99–107.

_____, Higashi, G.I., Cattani, J.A., Schlinski, V.D., Mansour, N.S. and Murrell, K.D. 1983: *Soc. Sci. Med. 17*, 545–62.

Klovdahl, A.S. 1985: Social networks and the spread of infectious diseases: the AIDS example. *Soc. Sci. Med. 21*, 1203–16.

Knox, P.L. 1978: The intraurban ecology of primary health care: patterns of accessibility and their policy implications. *Env. and Planning 10*, 415–35.

_____ 1979: Medical deprivation, area deprivation and public policy. *Soc. Sci. Med. 13D*, 111–21

_____ 1981: Convergence and divergence in regional patterns of infant mortality in the United Kingdom from 1949–51 to 1970–72. *Soc. Sci. Med. 15D*, 323–8.

_____ and Pacione, M. 1980: Locational behaviour, place of preferences and the inverse care law in the distribution of primary health care. *Geoforum 11*, 43–55.

Koate, P., Diouf, S., Sylla, M.O., Diop, G. and Goeh, E. 1981: Meteorological variations and acute coronary insufficiency. *Dakar Médical 26* (special issue), 38–57.

Kondrashin, A.V. 1983: Malaria in southern Asia 1: Factors related to the epidemiological aspects of the present state of malaria in India. *Medits. Parazit. i Parazitarnye Bol. 61*, 29–34.

_____ and Orlov, V.S. 1985: Malaria in southern Asia 4. Migration of population in India and its role in the epidemiology of malaria. *Medits. Parazit. i Parazitarnye Bol. 63* 2, 46–51.

Kono, S., Ikeda, M. and Ogata, M. 1983: Salt and geographical mortality of gastric cancer and stroke in Japan. *J. Epidem. and Commun. Health 37*, 43–6.

Korenburg, E., Černý, V. and Daniel, M. 1984: Occurrences of ixodid ticks – the main vector of tick-borne encephalitis in urbanized territory. *Folia Parasitologia 31*, 365–70.

Krastev, R. 1979: Mortality by malignant neoplasms of breast and uterus. *Méd. Biol. Env. 7*, 46–52.

Kratochvil, O. 1983: Disease knows no frontiers. *Geographica Medica 13*, 47–52.

Kreier, J.P. (ed.) 1980: *Malaria.* Vol. 1 *Epidemiology, chemotherapy, morphology and metabolism.* Vol. 2 *Pathology, vector studies and culture.* Vol. 3 *Immunology and immunization.* New York: Academic Press.

Kulmanov, M.E. 1985: Contamination with aflatoxins of food raw material, food and feeds in the Kazakh SSR during 1981–82. *Voprosy Pitaniya 3*, 63–6.

Kumaraswamy, K. 1984: Patterns of cholera incidence in Madras City 1946–80. *Indian Geog. J. 59*, 29–45.

Küstner, H.G.V., Gibson, I.H.N., Carmichael, T.R. et al. 1981: The spread of cholera in South Africa. *South African Med. J. 60*, 87–90.

Kuwert, E., Mérieux, C., Koprowski, H. and Bögel, K. (eds) 1985: *Rabies in the Tropics*. Berlin: Springer.

Kvale, K.M. 1981: Schistosomiasis in Brazil: preliminary results from a case study of a new focus. *Soc. Sci. Med. 15D*, 489–500.

Kwofie, K.M. 1976: A spatio-temporal analysis of cholera diffusion in western Africa. *Econ. Geog. 52*, 127–35.

Laird, M. and Miles, J.W. (eds) v. I 1983; v. II 1985: *Integrated mosquito control methodologies*. London: Academic Press.

Lal, R.B. and Roy, S.C. 1937–38: Epidemic dropsy. *Indian J. Med. Res. 25*, 163–76 and later articles.

_____ and Seal, S.C. 1949: *General health survey, Singur Health Centre*. Calcutta: Government of India Press.

Lam, N. Siu-Ngan 1986: Geographical patterns of cancer mortality in China. *Soc. Sci. Med. 23*, 241–7.

Lancet 1982: Prevention of coronary heart disease in the United Kingdom. i. (10 Apr.) 846–7.

Landy, D. 1985: Pibloktoq (hysteria) and Inuit nutrition: possible implications of hypervitaminosis A. *Soc. Sci. Med. 21*, 173–85.

Langer, P. 1960: History of goitre. In WHO 1960, pp. 9–25.

Lawther, P.J. 1982: Pollution of the air by industry and its effect on habitation. *Ekistics 49*(296), 395–8.

Learmonth, A.T.A. 1957: Some contrasts in the regional geography of malaria in India and Pakistan. *Trans. Inst. British Geogrs 23*, 37–59.

_____ 1958: Medical geography in Indo-Pakistan: a study of twenty years' data. *Indian Geog. J. 33*, 1–59.

_____ 1959: Geography and health in the tropical forest zone. In R. Miller and J. Watson (eds) *Geographical essays in memory of Alan G. Ogilvie*. Edinburgh: Nelson, pp. 195–220.

_____ 1971: Demographic regions of the Indian sub-continent. In The Open University Course D100, *The population explosion: an interdisciplinary approach* (units 32–36). Milton Keynes: Open University Press, pp. 33–67.

_____ 1972a: Atlases in medical geography. In N.D. McGlashan (ed.) 1972, pp. 133–52.

_____ 1972b: Regional disparities in the health sector. In Open University Course D203, *Decision Making in Britain, Part V. Health*. Milton Keynes: Open University Press, pp. 19–77.

_____ 1977: Malaria. In G.M. Howe (ed.) 1977.

_____ 1978: *Patterns of Disease and Hunger*. Newton Abbot: David and Charles.

_____ 1980: Reflections on the regional geography of disease in late colonial South Asia. *Soc. Sci. Med. 14D*, 271–6.

_____ and Learmonth, A.M. 1955: Aspects of village life in Indo-Pakistan.

Geography 40, 145–60.

—— and Grau, R. 1969: Maps of some standardised mortality ratios for Australia for 1965–66 compared with 1959–63. Canberra: *The Australian National University School of General Studies, Department of Geography Occasional Paper 8.*

—— and Akhtar, R. 1984: The malaria resurgence in India 1965–76: towards a diffusion simulation model. *Annals National Assoc. Geogrs, India 4*, 23–69.

—————— Malaria and other mosquito-borne diseases in India. *The Geographer* (Aligarh Muslim University), in press.

Lechat, M.F., Bouche, R., de Goyet, C. deV. and Boucquey, C. 1976: Epidémiologie de l'avitaminose A au Niger. *Ann. Soc. Belge Méd. trop. 56*, 333–42.

Leclerc, A., Lert, F. and Goldberg, M. 1984: Les inégalités social devant la mort en Grande Bretagne et en France. *Soc. Sci. Med. 19*, 479–87.

Leeson, G.W. 1981: The elderly in Denmark: consequences of a mortality decline. *European Demographic Inf. Bull. 12*, 98–100.

Le François, P., Chevassus, S., Benefice, A.E., Dyck, J.L. and Mairi, B. 1980: Vitamin A status of populations in three West African countries. *International J. Vitamin and Nutr. Res. 50*, 352–63.

Legon, C.D. 1952: The aetiological significance of geographical variations in cancer mortality. *British Med. J. 27*, 700–2.

Levin, D.L. (ed.) 1980: *Cancer epidemiology in the USA and USSR.* Washington: NIH Publication 80-2044.

Levy, C. 1980: The mortality from accidents of children and adolescents in eight developed countries. *Population 35*, 291–319.

Limper, A. 1984: Climatic-geographic analysis of the occurrence of epidemic cerebrospinal meningitis in West Africa. *Geogr. Zeitschr. 70*, 62–74.

Logie, F. 1984: Mortality from cardiovascular diseases in Belgium: an exploratory analysis. In *Géosanté Symposium 1984*, pp. 309–10.

Long, D.A. 1982: Aflatoxins and kwashiorkor. *British Med. J. 285* (23 Oct.) 1208–9 (correspondence).

Longmate, N. 1966: *King Cholera: the biography of a disease.* London: Hamish Hamilton.

Loomis, W.F. 1970: Rickets. *Scientific American* December, 77–91.

Lord, R.D. 1983: Ecological strategies for the prevention and control of health problems. *Bull. Pan American Health Organ. 17*, 19–34.

Lu, S.-H., Camus, A.-M., Tomatis, L. and Bartsch, H. 1981: Mutagenicity of extracts of pickled vegetables in Linhsien County, a high incidence area of esophageal cancer in northern China. *J. National Cancer Inst. 66*, 33–6.

Lucas, A.O. and Gilles, H.M. 1984: *A Short Textbook of Preventive Medicine for the Tropics*, 2nd edn. London: Hodder and Stoughton.

Lu Zhong-xian, Qiang Guang-yo and Dai Xiu-dao 1983: Management of human excreta. *World Health Forum 4*, 279–80.

McAlpin, M.B. 1979: Dearth, famine and risk: the changing impact of crop failures in western India, 1870–1920. *J. Econ. Hist. 39*, 143–57.

McCracken, K.W.J. 1981: Analysing geographic variations in mortality. *Area 13*, 203–10.

McCullough, F. and Combes, C. 1982: Observations on the epidemiology and control of schistosomiasis around the Mediterranean basin. *Revista Ibérica de Parasit.* Vo. Extra, 407–22.

McCullough, F.S. 1981: Biological control of the snail intermediate hosts of *Schistosoma* spp.; a review of its present status and future prospects. *Acta Tropica 38*, 5–13.

McCutchan, T.F., Dame, J.B., Miller, L.H. and Barnwell, J. 1984: Evolutionary relatedness of *Plasmodium* species as determined by the structure of DNA. *Science USA, 225,* (24 Aug.) 808–11.

Macdonald, G., Cuellar, C.V. and Foll, C.V. 1968: The dynamics of malaria. *Bull. WHO 38*, 743–55.

Macfarlane, J.T., Finch, R.G., Ward, M.J. and Macrae, A.D. 1982: Hospital study of adult community-acquired pneumonia. *Lancet* ii (31 Jul.) 255–8.

McGlashan, N.D. 1968: Esophageal cancer and contaminated spirits: an exercise in medical geography. *International Path.* 9, 50–3.

_____ 1969: Measles, malnutrition and blindness in Luapula province, Zambia. *Trop. Geogr. Med. 21*, 157–62.

_____ 1972: Food contaminants and oesophageal cancer. In N.D. McGlashan (ed.) 1972, pp. 247–57.

_____ 1976: Mapping rare sites of cancer: oesophageal cancer in Australia. *Med. Biol. Env. 4*, 87–97.

_____ 1977a: Spatial variations in cause-specific mortality in Australia. In N.D. McGlashan (ed.) 1977, pp. 1–28.

_____ 1977b: Viral hepatitis in Tasmania. *Soc. Sci. Med. 11*, 731–44.

_____ 1980: The social correlates of alcohol-related mortality in Tasmania 1971–78. *Soc. Sci. Med. 14D*, 191–203.

_____ 1981: Cancer mortality in the Commonwealth Caribbean. *West Indian Med. J. 30*, 142–8.

_____ 1982a: A West Indies geographic pathology survey: causes of death in some English-speaking Caribbean countries. Hobart: *University of Tasmania Department of Geography Occasional Paper no. 12.*

_____ 1982b: Causes of death in ten English-speaking Caribbean countries and territories. *Pan American Health Organ. 16*, 212–23.

_____ 1982c: Primary liver cancer and food-based toxins: a Swaziland review. *Ecol. of Dis. 1*, 37–44.

_____ 1983: The black heart in southern Africa: a geographical view of the future. *South African Med. J. 63*, 355–9.

_____ (ed.) 1972: *Medical Geography: Techniques and Field Studies.* London: Methuen/University Paperbacks.

_____ (ed.) 1977: Studies in Australian Mortality. Hobart: *University of Tasmania, Environmental Studies Occasional Paper no. 4.*

_____ and Blunden, J.R. (eds) *Geographical Aspects of Health: Essays in honour of Andrew Learmonth.* London: Academic Press,

_____ and Chick, N.K. 1974: Assessing spatial variations in mortality: ischaemic heart disease in Tasmania. *Australian Geogr. Studies 12*, 190–206.

_____ and Harington, J.S. 1976: Some techniques for mapping mortality. *South African Geog. J. 58*, 18–24.

_____ and Bradshaw, E. 1982: Eleven sites of cancer in black gold miners from southern Africa: a geographic enquiry. *British J. Cancer 46*, 947–54.

_____ and Grice, A.C. 1983: Sudden infant deaths and seasonality in Tasmania 1970–76. *Soc. Sci. Med. 17*, 885–8.

_____ and Mathur, H.S. 1984: Cancer pathologic regions: a Rajasthan example. In *Géosanté Symposium 1984*, pp. 353–69; also *Geographica Medica 14*, 4–19.

McKeown, T. 1976: *The Modern Rise of Population*. London: Arnold.

_____ 1985: Looking at disease in the light of human development. *World Health Forum 6*, 70–5.

McLaren, D.S. 1980: *Nutritional Ophthalmology* (2nd edn of *Malnutrition and the Eye*). London: Academic Press.

_____ 1981: *A Colour Atlas of Nutritional Disorders*. London: Wolfe Medical.

MacMahon, S.W. and Leeder, S.R. 1984: Blood pressure levels and mortality from cerebrovascular disease in Australia and the United States. *American J. Epidem. 120*, 865–73.

McNeill, W.H. 1977, 1979: *Plagues and Peoples*. Oxford: Blackwell/Harmondsworth: Penguin.

McQuade, W. 1980: Good news from the house on Lincoln Street. *Fortune 101*, 86–92.

McQueen, D.V. and Celentano, D.D. 1982: Social factors in the aetiology of multiple outcomes: the case of blood pressure and alcohol consumption patterns. *Soc. Sci. Med. 16*, 397–418.

Mackenbach, J.P. 1986: Personal communication.

Maddison, D. 1980: A medical school for the future: the Newcastle experiment. *World Health Forum 1*, 133–8.

Madsen, S.T. 1973: Scarlet fever and erysipelas in Norway during the last hundred years. *Infection 1*, 76–81.

Maegraith, B. 1965: *Exotic Diseases in Practice*: the clinical and public health significance of the changing geographical patterns of disease with particular reference to the importation of exotic infections into Europe and North America. London: Heinemann Medical.

_____ 1971:*Imported Disease in Europe*, 2nd edn. Basle: CIBA-Geigy.

_____ 1973: *One World*. Heath Clark Lectures 1970. University of London Athlone Press.

Magnus, K. (ed.) 1982: Trends in cancer incidence: causes and practical implications. Proceedings of symposium Oslo, Norway 6–7 Aug. Washington: Hemisphere Publishing.

Mahalanabis, D., Merson, M.H. and Barua, D. 1981: Oral rehydration therapy: recent advances. *World Health Forum 2*, 245–9.

Mahboub, E., Kmet, J., Cook, P.J., Day, N.E., Ghadirian, P. and Salmasizadeh, S. 1973: Oesophageal cancer in the Caspian littoral of Iran: the Caspian cancer registry. *British J. Cancer 28*, 197–214.

Mahler, H. 1981: The meaning of 'health for all by the year 2000'. *World Health Forum 2*, 5–22.

Malberg, J.W., Savage, E.P. and Osteryoung, J. 1978: Nitrates in drinking water and the early onset of hypertension. *Environmental Pollution 15*, 155–60.

Malek, E.A. 1980: *Snail-transmitted Parasitic Diseases*. Boca Raton, Fa.: CRC Press.
Maleville, J. 1976: Syphilis and endemic treponemiasis: geographical distribution and ecology. *Cahiers d'Outre-Mer 29*(113), 5–17.
Manchester, K. 1984: Tuberculosis and leprosy in antiquity: an interpretation. *Med. Hist. 28*, 162–73.
Mandara, M.P. and Mhalu, F.S. 1980–81: Cholera control in an inaccessible district in Tanzania: importance of temporary rural centres. *Med. J. Zambia 15*, 10–13.
Mangoud, A., Hillier, V.F., Leck, I. and Thomas, R.W. 1985: Space–time interaction in Hodgkin's disease in Greater Manchester. *J. Epidem. and Commun. Health 39*, 58–62.
Mann, I. 1966: *Culture, Race, Climate and Eye Disease: an introduction to the study of geographical ophthalmology*. Springfield, Ill.: C.C. Thomas.
Mann, J.M., Shandler, L. and Cushing, A.H. 1982: Pediatric plague. *Pediatrics 69*, 762–7.
Mann, P.H. 1965: *An Approach to Urban Sociology*, London: Routledge and Kegan Paul.
Mansour, N.S., Higashi, G.I., Schinski, V.D. and Murrell, K.D. 1981: A longitudinal study of *Schistosoma haematobium* infection in Qena governorate, Upper Egypt. I Initial epidemiological findings. *American J. Trop. Med. and Hyg. 30*, 795–805.
Marinkelle, C.J. 1980: The control of leishmaniases. *Bull. WHO 58*, 807–18.
Markides, K.S. and McFarland, C. 1982: A note on recent trends in the infant mortality–socioeconomic relationship. *Social Forces 61*, 268–76.
Marks, P.A. (ed.) 1981: *Cancer Research in the People's Republic of China and the United States of America: epidemiology, causation and new approaches to therapy*. New York: Grune and Stratton; London: Academic Press.
Marmot, M.G. 1984: Geography of blood pressure and hypertension. *British Med. Bull. 40*, 380–6.
Martinez-Palomo, A. 1982: *The biology of Entamoeba histolytica*. Chichester: Research Studies Press/Wiley.
Massam, B.H. 1975: *Location and Space in Social Administration*. London: Arnold.
Mathur, D.R., Joshi, R.M. and Mathur, A. 1985: Gonorrhoea in children due to PPNG and non-PPNG strains in Zaria. *European J. Sexually Trans. Dis. 2*, 143–5.
Mathur, K.K., Bagchi, S.K., Sehgal, C.L. and Bhardwaj, M. 1981: Investigation of an outbreak of Japanese encephalitis in Raipur, Madhya Pradesh. *J. Communicable Dis. 13*, 257–65.
Maupas, P., Goudeau, A., Drucker, J., Coursaget, P., Barin, F., Chiron, J.-P., Raynaud, B., Denis, F., Diop, B., Diop, T., Ndiaye, P.D. and Diop Mar, I. 1981: Relationship between hepatitis B virus and primary cancer of the liver. *Méd. d'Afrique Noire 28*, 225–35.
May, J.M. 1950: Medical geography: its methods and objectives. *Geog. Rev. 40*, 9–41; reprinted *Soc. Sci. Med. 11*, 715–30.
_____ 1950–55: *World Atlas of Diseases*. New York: American Geographical

Society; also in *Geog. Rev.* 1950–55, *40–45*.

_____ 1958: *The Ecology of Human Disease*. New York: M.D. Publications. (Pages on the Red river delta reprinted with illustrations in *Geog. Mag* 1982 *54*, 23–9).

_____ 1961–8: Series of volumes, all New York: Hafner, on *The Ecology of Malnutrition in*. . .: 1961 *The Far and Near East*; 1963 *Five Countries of Eastern and Central Europe*; 1965 *Middle Africa*; 1966 *Central and South-eastern Europe*; 1967 *Northern Africa*; 1968 *French-speaking Countries of West Africa and Madagascar*.

_____ and McLellan, D.L. 1970–74: Series continued: 1970 *Eastern Africa and Four Countries of West Africa*; 1971 *Seven Countries of Southern Africa and Portuguese Guinea*; 1972 *Mexico and Central America*; 1973 *The Caribbean*; 1974 *Eastern South America*; 1974 *Western South America*.

Mayer, J.D. 1980: Migrant studies and medical geography. In M.S. Meade (ed.) 1980, pp. 136–54.

_____ 1982: Relations between two traditions of medical geography: health systems planning and geographical epidemiology. *Progress in Human Geog*. 6, 216–30.

_____ 1983: The role of spatial analysis and geographic data in the detection of disease causation. *Soc. Sci. Med. 17*, 1213–21.

_____ 1985: International perspective on the health care crisis in the USA. In *IBG/AAG* 1985.

Mbalawa, G. 1981: Epidemiology of cancer in the Congo. *Afrique Medicale 20*, 593–6.

Meade, M.S. 1976: A new disease in Southeast Asia: man's creation of dengue haemorrhagic fever. *Pacific Viewpoint 17*, 133–46.

_____ 1977: Medical Geography as human ecology: the dimension of population movement. *Geog. Rev.* 67, 379–93.

_____ 1979: Cardiovascular mortality in the Southeastern United States: the coastal plain enigma. *Soc. Sci. Med. 13D*, 257–65.

_____ 1980a: Potential years of life lost in countries of Southeast Asia. *Soc. Sci. Med. 14D*, 277–81.

_____ 1980b: An interactive framework for geochemistry and cardiovascular disease. In M.S. Meade (ed.) 1980, pp. 194–221.

_____ 1983: Cardiovascular disease in Savannah, Georgia. In N.D. McGlashan and J.R. Blunden (eds) 1983, pp. 175–96.

_____ (ed.) 1980: Conceptual and methodological issues in medical geography. *University of North Carolina at Chapel Hill, Department of Geography Studies in Geography no. 15*.

_____, Florin, J.W., and Gesler, W.M., in the press. *Medical Geography*. New York, Guilford Press.

Médecine d'Afrique Noire 1982: Viral hepatitis. *29*, 709–57.

Médecine Tropicale 1980: Arbovirus diseases: part 1. *40*, 451–568.

_____ 1983: Tropical cancerology. *43*, 213–98.

Medical Journal of Australia 1983: Aspects of the cigarette epidemic. *70*, 207–25.

Meheus, A., Butera, S., Eylenbosch, W., Gatera, G., Kivits, M. and Musafili,

I. (eds) 1982: *Health and Disease in Rwanda*. Wilrijk, Belgium: Universitaire Instelling Antwerpen.

Mehta, F.S., Gupta, M.B., Pindborg, J.J., Bhonsle, R.B., Jalnawalla, P.N. and Sinor, P.N. 1982: An intervention study of oral cancer and precancer in rural Indian populations: a preliminary report. *Bull. WHO 60*, 441–6.

Melnick, J.L., Ochoa, S. and Oró, J. (eds) 1985: Viruses, onchogenes and cancer. *Progress in Med. Virology 32*, 1–211.

Melville, A.R. 1979: Onchocerciasis and agricultural development in West Africa. *Outlook on Agriculture 10*, 116–22.

Memik, F. 1979: Relatively higher incidence of esophageal and gastric carcinoma in Eastern Anatolia and some possible etiological factors. *Méd. Biol. Env. 7*, 1–2.

Menotti, A., Petrelli, G., Maggini, M., Poroghesi, F. and Conti, S. 1981: Relation between coronary risk factors and mortality for cancer in the Italian areas of the Seven Countries Study. *Ann. dell' Istituto Superiore di Sanita 17*, 151–61.

Mesle, F. 1983: Cancer and food: the case of cancers of the intestine and rectum. *Population 38*, 733–62.

_____ 1984: Cancers digestif et alimentation. *Géosanté Symposium 1984*, pp. 382–404.

Migascna, P., Rcausuwan, W. and Changbumrung, S. 1980: Nitrates and nitrites in local Thai preserved protein foods. *J. Med. Assoc. Thailand 63*, 500–5.

Milio, N. 1985: Health policy and the emerging tobacco reality *Soc. Sci. Med. 21*, 603–13.

Miller, C.J., Drasar, B. and Feachem, R.G. 1982: Cholera and estuarine salinity in Calcutta and London. *Lancet* i (29 May), 1216–8.

_____, Feachem, R.G. and Drasar, B.S. 1985: Cholera epidemiology in developed and developing countries: new thoughts on transmission, seasonality and control. *Lancet* i (2 Feb.), 261–3.

Miller, F. DeW., Hussein, M., Mancy, K.H., Hilbert, M.S., Monto, A.S. and Barakat, R.M.R. 1981: An epidemiological study of *Schistosoma haematobium* and *S. mansoni* in 35 rural Egyptian villages. *Trop. and Geogr. Med. 33*, 355–65.

Miller, J.C. 1982: The significance of drought, disease and famine in the agriculturally marginal zones of West Central Africa. *J. African Hist. 23*, 17–61.

Milne, D. 1984: The detection of mutagenic compounds in the aqueous environment. In M. Pacione and G. Gordon (eds) *Quality of life and human welfare*. Proceedings of 3rd Royal Scottish Geographical Society Symposium. Norwich; Geo Books, pp. 111–16.

Ministry of Agriculture Fisheries and Food 1970: *Manual of Nutrition*. London: HMSO.

Ministry of Transport (UK) 1967: *Road safety – a fresh approach*. London: HMSO Cmd.3339.

Mitchell, F.K. 1983: The plague in Cape Town in 1901 and its subsequent establishment as an endemic disease in South Africa. *South African Med. J.*

29 June Special Issue, 17–19.

Mitra, A. 1978: *India's Population: aspects of quality and control* Vols I and II. New Delhi: Abhinav Publications.

Miyawaki, N. and Sheng-Chih Chen 1981: A statistical consideration of the mapping of mortality. *Soc. Sci. Med. 15D*, 93–101.

MMWR (Morbidity and Mortality Weekly Report) 1980: Cholera – Florida. *29*, 601–2.

_____ 1981: Measles. *Texas 30*, 209–11.

_____ 1985: Self-reported behavioral change among gay and bisexual men – San Francisco. *34*, 613–5.

Moens, G.F.G. 1984: Some aspects of the geographical mortality pattern of the Brussels population in 1970. *Soc. Sci. Med. 18*, 59–62.

Mohammed, I. and Zaruba, K. 1981: Control of epidemic menigococcal meningitis by mass vaccination. *Lancet* ii (11 July), 80–3.

_____, Onyemelukwe, G.C., Obineche, E., Gupta, N. and Oyeyinka, G.O. 1984: Control of epidemic meningococcal meningitis by mass vaccination. II Persistence of antibody four years after vaccination. *J. Infect. 9*, 197–202.

Mohan, J. 1984a: Geographical aspects of private hospital developments in Britain. *Area 16*, 191–9.

_____ 1984b: Spatial aspects and planning implications of private hospital development in South East England 1976–84. *University of London, Birkbeck College Department of Geography Occasional Paper.*

_____ and Curtis, S. 1984: A comparative study of policies and techniques for health service resource distribution in Britain and France. In *Géosanté Symposium* 1984, pp. 544–53.

_____ and Woods, K. 1985: Restructuring the Welfare State? The social geography of health care under the British Conservative Government. *International J. Health Serv. 15*, 197–215.

Mollison, D. 1984: Simplifying simple epidemic models. *Nature* 310(5974), 224–5.

Molyneux, D.H. and Ashford, R.W. 1983: The Biology of *Trypanosoma* and *Leishmania*, Parasites of Man and Domestic Animals. London: Taylor and Francis.

Monnier, Y. 1980: Méningite cérébro-spinale, harmattan et déforestation. *Cahiers d'Outre-mer 33*, 103–22.

Moon, G. and Jones, K. 1985: Targetting resources for health education. IBG Conference Leeds, January. Symposium on medical geography.

Morrill, R.L. and Earickson, R.J. 1969: Locational efficiency of Chicago area hospitals: an experimental model. *Health Services Res. 4*, 128–41.

Morris, R.J. 1971: Cholera: the social disease. *New Society* 8 July, 52–6.

Morrow, R.H. Jr 1984: The application of a quantitative approach to the assessment of the relative importance of vector and soil transmitted diseases in Ghana. *Soc. Sci. Med. 19*, 1039–49.

_____, Smith, P.G. and Nimo, K.P. 1982: Assessing the impact of disease. *World Health Forum 3*, 331–5.

Morton, R.S. 1985: A clinical look at the morbus gallicus. *European J. Sexually Transmitted Dis. 2*, 133–40.

Moss, D.J., Burrows, S.R., Castelino, D.J., Kane, R.G., Pope, J.H., Rickinson, A.B., Alpers, M.P. and Heyward, P.F. 1983: A comparison of Epstein-Barr virus-specific T-cell immunity in malaria-endemic and non-endemic regions of New Guinea. *International J. Cancer 31*, 727–32.

Mott, K.E. and Cline, B.L. 1980: Advances in epidemiology survey methodology and techniques in schistosomiasis. *Bull. WHO 58*, 639–47.

Mougne, C., MacLellan, R. and Atsana, S. 1982: Smoking, chewing and drinking in Ban Pong, northern Thailand. *Soc. Sci. Med. 16*, 99–106.

Mourant, A.E., Kopeç, A. and Domaniewska-Sobczak, K. 1976: *The Distribution of the Human Blood Groups and Other Polymorphisms*. Oxford: Oxford University Press.

Muirhead-Thomson, R.C. 1968: *Ecology of Insect Vector Populations*. London: Academic Press.

_____ 1982: *Behaviour Patterns of Blood-sucking Flies*. Oxford: Pergamon.

Mukammal, E.I., McKay, G.A. and Neumann, H.H. 1983: A note on cardiovascular diseases and physical aspects of the environment. *International J. Biometeorology 28*, 17–28.

Mukerji, A.B. 1980: The disease ecology of a small cul-de-sac: Chandigarh Dun. *Soc. Sci. Med. 14D*, 331–6.

Mundo, F., Ines-Cuyegkeng, E. and Aviado, D.M. (eds) 1983: Primary maternal and neonatal health: a global concern. New York: Plenum Press.

Murdoch, J.McC. and Gray, J.A. 1973: Patterns of disease in developed countries in relation to environmental factors. In G.M. Howe and J.A. Loraine (eds) 1973, pp. 128–39.

Murray, M. 1967: The geography of death in the United States and the United Kingdom. *Annals Assoc. American Geogr. 57*, 301–14.

Museur, M. and Pirson, R. 1976: The consequences of drought on a Saharan region. *Rev. Belge de Géog. 100*, 293–311.

Najman, J.M. and 6 others 1983: Politics, policy and performance: the primary prevention of disease in two community health centres in Queensland. *Australian and New Zealand J. Sociol. 19*, 476–90.

Napalkov, N.P., Tserkovny, G.F., Merabishvili, V.N., Parkin, D.M., Smans, M. and Muir, C.S. 1983: *Cancer incidence in the USSR*. IARC Scientific Publications no. 48, 1–84. Lyon, France.

Narasimham, M.V.V.L., Krishna Rao, C. and Rao, C.K. 1983: Some clinical aspects of bancroftian filariasis in East Godavari District, Andhra Pradesh. *Indian J. Med. Res. 78*, 631–5.

Nasir, P. 1981: Freshwater larval trematodes. XXXVIII Some observations on biological control of *Schistosoma mansoni*. *Rivista di Parassit. 41*, 451–60.

Naumov, Y. and Lozanov, E. 1970: Medico-geographical characteristics of the territory of Bulgaria. *Proc. Postgrad. Med. Hist. ISUL* Sofia 17, 167–71.

Neequaye, J. 1984: Neonatal tetanus in Accra. *Lancet* ii (28 July) 224–5 (correspondence).

Neuberger, A. and Jukes, T.H (eds) 1982: *Human Nutrition. Current issues and controversies*. Lancaster: MTP Press.

Neumann, J. and Lindgren, S. 1979: Great historical events that were significantly affected by the weather: 4. The great famines in Finland and Estonia 1695–97. *Bull. American Meteorol. Soc. 60*, 775–87.

Newland, K. 1981: Infant mortality and the health of societies. *Worldwatch Paper 47*, 1–56.

_____ 1982: Condensed from 1981 paper. *World Health Forum 3*, 321–4.

Newman, J.L. 1980: Dietary behavior and protein–energy malnutrition in Africa south of the Sahara. In M.S. Meade (ed.) 1980, pp. 77–92.

Newton, B.A. (ed.) 1985: Trypanosomiasis. *British Med. Bull. 41*, 103–99.

Ngindu, A., Johnson, B.K., Kenya, P.R., Ngira, J.A., Ocheng, D.M., Nandura, H., Omondi, T., Jansen, A.J., Ngare, W., Kairti, J.N., Gatel, D. and Simgok, T.A. 1982: Outbreak of acute hepatitis caused by aflatoxin poisoning in Kenya. *Lancet* i (12 June), 1346–8.

Nguma, J.F., McCullough, F.S. and Masha, E. 1982: Elimination of *Biomphalaria pfeifferi*, *Bulinus tropicus* and *Lymnaea natalensis* by the ampulid snail *Marisa cornuaris* in a man-made lake in northern Tanzania. *Acta Tropica 39*, 85–90. (See comment by R.F. Sturrock 1982.)

Nicolas, G. 1977: Observations on certain socioeconomic factors of the famine for a sub-Saharan society. *African Environment Special Report 6*, 159–69.

Nielsen, L.T. 1979: Mosquitoes, the mighty killers. *National Geog. Mag. 156*, 427–40.

Nihei, N., Asami, S. and Tanaka, H. 1981; Geographical factors influencing the population numbers and distribution of *Oncomelania nosophora* and the subsequent effect on the control of schistosomiasis japonica in Japan. *Soc. Sci. Med. 15D*, 149–57.

Norman, L.G. 1962: *Road traffic accidents: epidemiology, control and prevention*. Geneva: WHO.

Normandeau, L. and Legare, J. 1979: Infant mortality in the Inuit of Quebec. *Canadian Rev. Sociol. and Anthropol. 16*, 260–74.

Notkola, V., Punsar, S., Karvonen, M.J. and Haapakoski, J. 1985: Socio-economic conditions in childhood and mortality and morbidity caused by coronary heart disease in adulthood in rural Finland. *Soc. Sci. Med. 21*, 517–23.

Nozais, J.-P., Doucet, J. and Dunand, J. 1980: A survey of schistosomiasis in Ivory Coast. *Méd. Tropicale 40*, 41–4.

_____, Dunand, J., Doucet, J. and Condat, M. 1981: Evaluation of the main intestinal parasites in 860 Ivory Coast children from thirteen different villages. *Méd. Tropicale 41*, 181–5.

Nuttall, G.H.F., Cobbett, T., Strangeways-Pigg 1901: The geographical distribution of anopheles in relation to the former distribution of ague in England. *J. Hyg. 1*, 25, 88–42.

Oganov, R.G., Glasunov, I.S., Chazova, L.V., Zhukovsky, G.S. and Baubiniene, A.V. 1985: Preventing cardiovascular disease in the USSR. *World Health Forum 6*, 243–5.

Ohin, A.J. 1979: Features of geographical distribution of cancer in Africa. *Méd. Biol. Env. 7*, 4–9.

Ohno, K. and Aoki, K. 1981: Cancer deaths by city and county in Japan

(1969–71): a test of significance for geographical clusters of disease. *Soc. Sci. Med. 15D*, 251–8.

O'Keefe, P. and Wisner, B. 1976: The World food crisis. *Issues* (Bradford) No. 1.

Olveda, R.M., Tiu, E., Fevidal, P. Jr., DeVeyra, F. Jr., Icatlo, F.C. Jr. and Domingo, E.O. 1983: Relationship of prevalence and intensity of infection to morbidity in schistosomiasis japonica: a study of three communities in Leyte, Philippines. *American J. Trop. Med. and Hyg. 32*, 1312–21.

Omran, A.R. 1971: The epidemiological transition: a theory of the epidemiology of population change. *Milbank Memorial Fund Quart. 49*, 6–47.

_____ 1977: Epidemiologic transition in the United States. *Popul. Bull. 32*, 4.

Omura, T., Hisamatsu, S., Takizawa, Y., Minowa, M., Yanagawa, H., Shigematsu, I. 1987: Geographical distribution of cerebrovascular disease mortality and food intakes in Japan. *Soc. Sci. Med. 24*, 401–9.

O'Neill, C.H. Hodges, G.M., Riddle, P.N., Jordan, P.W., Newman, R.H., Flood, R.J., and Toulson, E.C. 1980: A fine fibrous silica contaminant of flour in the high oesophageal cancer area of north-east Iran. *International J. Cancer 26*, 617–28. (See comment by P.H. Holt 1981.)

_____, Pan, Q.Q., Clarke, G., Hodges, G., Jordan, P, Newman, R., Liu, F.S., Ge, M., Chang, Y.M. and Toulson, E. 1982: Silica fragments from millet bran in mucosa surrounding oesophageal tumours in patients in northern China. *Lancet* i (29 May), 1202–6.

O'Neill, I.K., von Borstel, R.C., Miller, C.T., Long, J. and Bartsch, H. (eds) 1985: N-nitroso compounds: occurrence, biological effects and relevance to human cancer. Proc. VIIIth international symposium on N-nitroso compounds, Banff, Canada 5–9 Sep. 1983. Oxford University Press *IARC Scientific Publications no. 57*.

Oomen, J.M.V. 1981: Monitoring health in African dams. The Kamburu Dam (Kenya) as a test case. Erasmus University Rotterdam, Thesis.

OPCS (Office of Population Censuses and Surveys) 1983: *Communicable disease statistics*. London: HMSO, series MB2 no. 8, 9, 10.

_____, London School of Hygiene and Tropical Medicine 1982: Studies in sudden infant deaths. London: HMSO, *Studies on Medical and Population Subjects no. 45*.

Open University (UK) 1985: Course U205 *Health and Disease*, in eight books: I Studying health and disease; II Medical knowledge: doubt and certainty; III The health of nations; IV The biology of health and disease; V Birth to old age: health in transition; VI Experiencing and explaining disease; VII Caring for health: history and diversity; VIII Caring for health; dilemmas and prospects. Milton Keynes, Open University Press (see also N. Black et al. (eds) 1984).

Order of Christian Unity 1985: *Children and Contraception – failure of a policy*. London: OCU.

Orford, J. and Edwards, G. 1977: *Alcoholism*. Oxford University Press, *Maudsley Monographs Institute of Psychiatry no. 26*.

Orlov, V.S., Kondrashin, A.V. and Lovey, G.I. 1984: Malaria in southern India.

II Structure of malaria morbidity in India. *Med. Parazit. i Parazitarnye Bol. 62/3*, 40–5.

Osei, L. 1981: Yaws in rural Accra. *J. Hyg. Epidem. Microbiol. and Immunology 25*, 293–300.

Osmond, C., Gardner, M.J. and Acheson, E.D. 1982: Analysis of trends in cancer mortality in England and Wales during 1951–80 separating changes associated with period of birth and period of death. *British Med. J. 284* (3 Apr.), 1005–8.

Osuntokun, B.O. 1981: Cassava diet, chronic cyanide intoxication and neuropathy in the Nigerian Africans. *World Rev. Nutr. and Dietetics 36*, 141–73.

Pace, J.L. 1983: Treponematoses in Arabia. *Saudi Med. J. 4*, 211–20.

Pal, R. 1982: Disease vector control in the People's Republic of China. *Mosquito News 42*, 149–58.

Palagiano, C. 1984: Incidence of cancer in Italy. *Indian Geog. J. 59*, 64–6.

Panero, M. 1976: Différences territoriales d'incidence des tumeurs: essai d'analyse des données d'un registre du cancer. *Méd. Bio. Env. 4*, 7–9.

PANOS 1986: Dossier 1, 1986: *AIDS and the Third World*. London, PANOS in association with the Norwegian Red Cross.

Parkin, D.M. (ed.), 1986: *Cancer occurrence in developing countries*. IARC Scientific Publications no. 75, Lyon, WHO/IARC and Oxford, New York, Oxford University Press.

_____, Stjernswärd, J. and Muir, C.S. 1984: Estimates of the worldwide frequency of twelve major cancers. *Bull WHO 62*, 163–82.

Passmore, R. 1951: Famine in India: an historical survey. *Lancet 18 Aug.*, 303.

_____ 1982: Comment on Devadas (1980). *Trop. Dis. Bull. 79* no. 877, 323.

_____ 1983: Comment on Sommer (1982b). *Trop. Dis. Bull. 80*, no. 28, p. 27.

_____ 1984: Comment on Delange et al. (1983). *Trop. Dis. Bull. 1984, 81* no. 2290, 595–6.

Pattanayak, S. and Roy, R.G 1980: Malaria in India and the modified plan of operations for its control. *J. Communicable Dis. 12*, 1–13.

Patten, R.C. 1981: Aflatoxins and disease, *American J. Trop. Med. and Hyg. 30*, 422–5.

Patterson, K.D. 1985: Pandemic and epidemic influenza 1830–48. *Soc. Sci. and Med. 21*, 571–80.

_____ and Pyle, G.F. 1983: The diffusion of influenza in sub-Saharan Africa during the 1918–19 pandemic. *Soc. Sci. Med. 17*, 1299–1307.

Pavlovskiy, E.N., Petrishcheva, P.A., Zasukhin, D.N. and Olsofiev, N.G. (eds) 1955: *Natural nidi of human diseases and regional epidemiology*. Leningrad: Medgiz.

Pearce, T.O. 1982: Integrating Western orthodox and indigenous medicine: professional interests and attitudes among university-trained Nigerian physicians. *Soc. Sci. Med. 16*, 1611–17.

Pearson, M. 1982a: Social factors and leprosy in Lamjung, west central Nepal: implications for disease control. *Ecol. of Dis. 1*, 229–36.

_____ 1982b: Leprosy moves along the Nepalese valleys. *Geog. Mag. 54*, 504–9.

_____ 1984: Demographic and spatial distribution of leprosy in West Central Nepal: a case study of Lamjung Jilla. *Indian Geog. J. 59*, 46–54.

_____ 1985: Leprosy in west Nepal: social and spatial perspectives. University of Liverpool, Department of Geography, PhD thesis.

Pedgley, D.E. 1982: *Windborne Pests and Diseases: meteorology of airborne organisms*. Chichester: Ellis Horwood.

Peeters, E.-G. 1980: A propos de la répartition géographique des cancers. *Méd. Biol. Env. 8*, 26–36.

Pellett, P.L. 1983: Changing concepts on world malnutrition. *Ecol. Food and Nutr. 13*, 115–25.

Peltola, H. 1983: Meningococcal disease: still with us. *Reviews of Infect. Dis. 5*, 71–91.

———, Jónsdóttir, K., Lystad, A., Sievers, C.J. and Kallings, I. 1982: Meningococcal disease in Scandinavia. *British Med. J. 284* (29 May), 1618–21.

Pendleton, B. and Yang, Shu-O.W. 1985: Socioeconomic and health effects on mortality declines in developing countries. *Soc. Sci. Med. 20*, 453–60.

Pène, P., André, L.J., Rougemont, A., Bourgeade, A. and Barabé, P. (eds) 1980: *Health and Medicine in Tropical Africa*. Vol. 1. Paris: Doin Editeurs.

———, Bourgeade, A. and Delmont, J. 1982: *Tropical Medicine in Temperate Regions*. Paris: Doin Editeurs.

Pensaert, M., Ottis, K., Vandeputte, J., Kaplan, M.M. and Bachmann, P.A. 1981: Evidence for the natural transmission of influenza A virus from wild ducks to swine and its potential importance for man. *Bull. WHO 59*, 75–8.

Percy, C., Stanek, III. E., Gloeckler, L. 1981: Accuracy of cancer death certificates and its effect on cancer mortality statistics. *American J. Public Health 71*, 242–50.

Perdrizet, S. and Liard, R. 1981: Variations géographiques de la fréquences des maladies réspiratoires en France. In H. Picheral (ed.) 1981, pp. 109–28.

Perine, P.L., Hopkins, D.R., Niemel, P.L.A., St John, R.K., Causse, G. and Antal, G.M. 1984: *Handbook of Endemic Treponematoses*. Geneva: WHO.

Périsse, J. and Polacchi, W. 1980: Geographical distribution and recent changes in world supply of vitamin A. *Food and Nutr. 6/1*, 21–7.

Peterman, T.A., Drotman, D.P. and Curran, J.W. 1985: Epidemiology of the acquired immunodeficiency syndrome (AIDS). *Epidem. Reviews 7*, 1–21.

Peters, W. and Gilles, H.M. 1981: *Wolfe Medical Atlases 17. A colour atlas of tropical diseases and parasitology*. London: Wolfe Medical.

Peterson, W. and Newman, M. 1977: A selection of key documents on the Sahel: drought recovery and long-term development. *Sahel Bibliog. Bull. 1*, 5–20.

Petit, M.M. 1984: Les besoins de santé dans les régions rurale Africains: l'example de la région de Batoumé (Togo). In *Géosanté* Symposium 1984, pp. 273–88.

———, Houin, R., Mayroud, J., Dumas, J.M., Breuil, J., Randrianarison, J., Rajaona, T. and Coulanges, P. 1982: Geographical contribution to the study of an endemic tropical disease, intestinal bilharzia, the example of the Malagasy east coast. *Madagascar Rev. de Géog. 41*, 9–39.

Pettingale, K.W. 1985: Towards a psychobiological model of cancer: biological considerations. *Soc. Sci. Med. 20*, 779–87.

Philippe, P. 1985: Generation et évaluation des hypothèses étiologiques en épidemiologie. *Soc. Sci. Med. 20*, 681–9.

Picardat, C. 1982: *Le paludisme au Gujerat*. Mémoire de maîtrise, Université de Paris IV.

Picheral, H. 1976: *Espace et santé: géographie médicale du Midi de la France*.

Montpellier: Imprimerie du Paysan du Midi.

———— 1979: Une géocancerologie urbaine en France: première approche. *Méd. Biol. Env.* 7(2), 13–24.

———— 1981: Le déclin de la mortalité par maladies coronariennes dans les pays développés. In H. Picheral (ed.) 1981, pp. 91–108.

———— 1982: Medical geography, geography of diseases, geography of health. *France Géographique 11*, 161–75.

———— 1983: Complexes et systèmes pathogènes: approche géographique. In CEGET 1983, pp. 5–24.

———— (ed.) 1981: Etudes de géographie médicale. II Pays temperés et Sociétés développées. *Bull. de la Section de Géog., Comité des Travaux Hist. et Scient. Tome 83 (1978)*. Paris: Bibliothèque Nationale.

Pickles, W.N. 1948: Epidemiology in country practice. *New England J. Med. 239*, 419–27.

Picq, J.J. 1983: Onchocercose de savane et de forêt en Afrique de l'Ouest et complexe pathogène de l'onchocercose. In CEGET 1983, pp. 243–52.

———— and Albert, J.-P. 1979: Sudan-savannah and rain-forest onchocerciasis in West Africa: an epidemiological problem. *Rev.d' Epidem. et de Santé Publique 27*, 483–98.

Pinheiro, F.P., Travassos da Rosa, A.P.A. and Moraes, M.A.P. 1981. An epidemic of yellow fever in central Brazil, 1972–73. II Ecological studies. *American J. Trop. Med. and Hyg. 30*, 204–11.

Piot, P. and Meheus, A. 1983: Epidemiology of STD in developing countries. *Ann. de la Soc. Belge de Méd. Trop. 63*, 87–110.

Pisa, Z. and Uemura, K. 1982: Trends of mortality from ischaemic heart disease and other cardiovascular diseases in 27 countries, 1968–77. *World Health Stats Quart. 35*, 11–47.

Pisani, J.F., Angulo, J.J. and Takiguti, C.K. 1984: An objective reconstruction of the chain of contagion. *Soc. Sci. Med. 18*, 775–82.

Pitchford, J.T. 1981: Temperature and schistosome distribution in South Africa. *South African J. Sci. 77*, 252–61.

Polderman, A.M. 1984: Cost-effectiveness of different ways of controlling intestinal schistosomiasis: a case study. *Soc. Sci. Med. 19*, 1073–80.

———— and Manshande, J.P. 1981: Failure of targeted mass treatment to control schistosomiasis. *Lancet* i (3 Jan.), 27–8.

Popkin, B.M., Solon, F.S., Fernandez, T. and Latham, M.C. 1980: Benefit–cost analysis in the nutrition area: a project in the Philippines. *Soc. Sci. Med. 14C*, 207–16.

Popović, N. and Tadíc, I. 1979: Animal species living in freedom in the area of Belgrade, and their significance as active or potential carriers of causal agents of diseases common to humans and animals. *Vet. Glasnik 10*, 777–84.

Population Reports, 1986: AIDS: a public health crisis. Series L, no. 6, Population Information Program. Baltimore: Johns Hopkins University.

Posner, T. 1977: Magical elements in orthodox medicine. In R. Dingwall et al. (eds). *Health Care and Health Knowledge*. London: Croom Helm.

Potts, M., Janowitz, B.S. and Fortney, J.A. (eds) 1983: *Childbirth in Developing Countries*. Boston: MTP Press.

Prasad, S.R. 1984: Malaria in project areas: a study on Nagarjunasagar and Srisailam project areas. *Indian Geog. J.* 59, 18–21.

———, George, S. and Gupta, N.P. 1982: Studies on an outbreak of Japanese encephalitis in Kolar district, Karnataka state in 1977–78. *Indian J. Med. Res.* 75, 1–6.

Premier Ministre, Haut Comité d'Etude et d'Information sur l'Alcoolisme 1983: *L'Alcoolisme: morbidité, mortalité*. Paris: La Documentation Française.

Prentice, M.A. and Barnish, G. 1981: Snail infections following chemotherapy of *Schistosoma mansoni* in St Lucia, West Indies. *Trans. Roy. Soc. Trop. Med. and Hyg.* 75, 713–14.

Prescott, N.M. 1979: Schistosomiasis and development. *World Development 7*, 1–14.

Prescott, N. and Jancloes, M.F. 1984a: Selected issues in helminth control. *Soc. Sci. Med. 19*, 1057–60.

———, Prost, A. and Le Berre, R. 1984b: The economics of blindness prevention in Upper Volta under the onchocerciasis control program. *Soc. Sci. Med. 19*, 1051–5.

Preston, S.H. 1976: *Mortality Patterns in National Populations*. New York: Academic Press.

——— 1977: Mortality trends. *Annual Rev. Sociol. 3*, 163–78.

Preventive Medicine 1983: Proceedings of the international symposium on epidemiology and prevention of atherosclerotic disease. *12*, 1–234.

Price, E.W., McHardy, W.J. and Pooley, F.D. 1981: Endemic elephantiasis of the lower legs as a health hazard of barefooted agriculturists in Cameroon, West Africa. *Ann. Occup. Hyg. 24*, 1–8.

——— and Bailey, D. 1984: Environmental factors in the etiology of endemic elephantiasis of the lower legs in tropical Africa. *Trop. Geog. Med. 36*, 1–5.

Pringle, D. 1985: Regional variations in mortality in the Republic of Ireland. IBG/AAG symposium on medical geography, University of Nottingham, July.

Prost, A., Rougemont, A. and Omar, M.-S. 1980: Epidemiological, clinical and biological features of savannah and forest onchocerciasis in West Africa. Critical review and new data. *Ann. de Parasit. Humaine et Comparée 55*, 347–55.

Prothero, R.M. 1963: Population mobility and trypanosomiasis in Africa. *Bull. WHO 28*, 615–26.

——— 1965: *Migrants and Malaria*. London: Longmans.

——— 1977: Disease and mobility: a neglected factor in epidemiology. *International J. Epidem. 6*, 259–67.

——— 1983: Medical geography in tropical Africa. In N.D. McGlashan and J.R. Blunden (eds) 1983, pp. 137–53.

——— 1984: Population movement and health hazards in Africa. In R. Akhtar (ed.) 1987, pp. 83–9.

Pryer, J. 1986: Production and reproduction of malnutrition in an urban slum in Khulna, Bangladesh. IBG Conference University of Reading, January.

Pugh, R.N.H., Burrows, J.W. and Tayo, M.A. 1980a: Malumfashi Endemic Diseases Research Project XIV. Increasing schistosomiasis transmission. *Ann. Trop. Med. and Parasit. 74*, 569–70.

———, Bell, D.R. and Gilles, H.M. 1980b: Project as above XV. The potential medical importance of bilharzia in northern Nigeria: a suggested rapid, cheap and effective solution for control of *Schistosoma haematobium* infection. *Ann. Trop. Med. and Parasit. 74*, 597–613.

———, Burrows, J.W. and Bradley, A.K. 1981: Project as above XVI. The findings of a survey for *Schistosomiasis mansoni*. Hookworm, giardiasis and nutritional status. *Ann. Trop. Med. and Parasit. 75*, 281–92.

Pyle, G.F. 1969: The diffusion of cholera in the United States in the nineteenth century. *Geog. Analysis 1*, 59–75.

——— 1971: Heart disease, cancer and stroke in Chicago: a geographical analysis with facilities plans for 1980. *Research Paper no. 134* University of Chicago, Department of Geography.

——— 1979: *Applied Medical Geography*. Washington DC: V.H. Winston/New York: Wiley.

——— 1980: Geographical perspectives on influenza diffusion: the United States in the 1940s. In M.S. Meade (ed.) 1980, pp. 222–49.

——— and Cook, R.M. 1978: Environmental risk factors of California encephalitis in man. *Geog. Rev. 68*, 157–60.

——— and Patterson, K.D. 1983: Influenza diffusion in European history: patterns and paradigms. *Ecol. of Dis. 2*, 173–84.

Queguiner, F. 1981: Evaluation of the traditional Arab technique of couching in the treatment of cataract in Mali. *Méd. Trop. 41*, 535–40.

Quillévéré, D., Guillet, P. and Séchan, Y. 1981: Geographical distribution of the *Simulium damnosum* complex species in the Senegambia project zone. *ORSTOM Série Entom. Méd. et Parasit. 19*, 303–13.

Qureshi, N.A. and Kharbanda, V.P. 1980: A comparative study of the health systems of India and China. *Health and Popul. Perspect. and Issues 3*, 187–203.

Radford, J. 1984: Group home locational strategies in Toronto. In *Géosanté Symposium 1984*, pp. 636–65.

Radley, A.R. 1982: Theory and data in the study of coronary proneness (type A behaviour pattern). *Soc. Sci. Med. 16*, 107–14.

——— 1984: The embodiment of social relations in coronary heart disease. *Soc. Sci. Med. 19*, 1227–34.

Raghavan, N.G.S. 1955: National filaria control programme. *Bull. National Soc. India Malaria and Mosquito-borne Dis. 3*, 175–81.

——— 1957: Epidemiology of filariasis in India. *Bull. WHO 16*, 553–79.

Raghuramulu, N. and Reddy, V. 1982: Studies on vitamin D metabolism in malnourished children. *British J. Nutr. 47*, 231–4.

Rahu, M. 1986: The USSR. In G.M. Howe (ed.) 1986, pp. 223–37.

Ramachandra Rao, T. 1984: *The anophelines of India*. Delhi: Malaria Research Centre, Indian Council of Medical Research.

Ramalingaswami, V. 1984: Health without wealth. *World Health Forum 5*, 252–5.

Ramesh, A. 1983: Developments in medical geography in India. In N.D. McGlashan and J.R. Blunden (eds) 1983, pp. 19–36.

——— and Hyma, B. 1981a: Traditional Indian medicine in practice in an Indian metropolitan city. *Soc. Sci. Med. 15D*, 69–81.

——— 1981b: Traditional Indian medical systems as a field of study for medical geographers. *Geographia Medica 11*, 116–40.

———, Barai, D.C. and Hyma, B. 1984: The scope and limitations of insecticide spraying in rural vector control programmes in the states of Karnataka and Tamil Nadu. *Indian Geog. J. 59*, 89–97.

Ransford, O. 1983: *'Bid the Sickness Cease': disease in the history of black Africa.* London: John Murray.

Rashid, A., Mohammed, T., Stephens, W.P., Warrington, S. Berry, J.L. and Mawer, E.B. 1983: Vitamin D state of Asians living in Pakistan. *British Med. J. 286* (15 Jan.), 182–4.

Razi, Z. 1980: *Life, Marriage and Death in a Medieval Parish: economy, society and demography in Halesowen 1270–1400.* Cambridge: Cambridge University Press.

Rée, G.H. 1977: Schistosomiasis. In G.M. Howe (ed.) 1977, pp. 17–32.

——— 1982: Schistosomiasis and human behaviour. *Ecol. of Dis. 1*, 131–3.

Rees, R.J.W. and McDougall, A.C. 1977: Airborne infection with *Mycobacterium leprae* in mice. *J. Med. Microbiol. 10*, 63–8.

Reiss, P., Large, J.M. and Goudsmit, J. 1985: LAV/HTLV III infection after a single sexual contact with an AIDS patient. *Nederlands Tijdschr. v. Geneeskunde 129*, 1933–4.

Rémy, G. 1984: Un concept intégrateur: l'espace épidémiologique. In *Géosanté Symposium 1984*, pp. 508–18.

Rhodain, F. 1983: Mécanismes de diffusion et de persistence de la dengue. In CEGET 1983, pp. 65–71.

Richardson, S.A., Koller, H., Katz, M. and Albert, K. 1978: The contributions of differing degrees of acute and chronic malnutrition to the intellectual development of Jamaican boys. *Early Hum. Dev. 2*, 163–70.

Riley, M.W. 1982: Ageing and health in modern communities. *Ekistics 49*(296), 381–3.

Ringen, K. 1980: Norway's nutrition policy: directing the consumer's choice. *World Health Forum 1*, 184–5.

Ritson, E.B. 1973: Alcoholism as a reflection of environment. In G.M. Howe (ed.) 1973, pp. 208–18.

Roberts, A. 1982: Cervical cytology in England and Wales. *Health Trends 14*, 41–3.

Robertson, I., Ford, J.A., McIntosh, W.B. and Dunnigan, M.G. 1981: The role of cereals in the aetiology of nutritional rickets: the lessons of the Irish National Nutrition Survey 1943–48. *British J. Nutr. 45*, 17–22.

Robinson, S., Streetly, A., Farrant, M., MacSweeny, S. and McCracken, A. 1980: Famine relief in Karamoja, Uganda. *Lancet* ii (18 Oct.), 849–51.

Rodenwaldt, E. 1956: Die Geomedizinische Bedeutung menschlicher Einwirkungen auf die Oberflächengestalt der Erde. *International Geographical Union 18th Congress, Rio de Janeiro Medical Geography* 618–22, also *Z. Tropenmed. Parasit.* 1957 8, 227–33.

——— and Jusatz, H.J. 1956: Zür Methodik der Kartographische Darstellung von Seuchenkommen und Seuchenbewegungen. As above 623–9.

——— 1952–61: *World Atlas of Epidemic Diseases.* Hamburg: Falk.

Rodger, F.C. 1981: *Eye Disease in The Tropics: a practical textbook for developing countries*. Edinburgh: Churchill-Livingstone.

Rohan, T. and McMichael, A.J. 1981: Alimentary tract cancer mortality in Australia 1908–78 – an epidemiological appraisal. *Med. J. Australia 1*, 232–5.

Rose, E. 1976: Environmental influences on cancer incidence. *Méd. Biol. Env. 4*(1), 51–9.

———— 1979: A comparative analysis of two areas of differing oesophageal cancer incidence in the Transkei. *Méd. Biol. Env. 7*(2), 30–9.

———— and Fellingham, S.A. 1981: Cancer patterns in Transkei. *South African J. Sci. 77*, 555–61.

Rose, G. and Marmot, M.G. 1981: Social class and coronary heart disease. *British Heart J. 45*, 13–19.

Rose, G.A., Blackburn, H., Gillum, R.F. and Prineas, R.J. 1982: *Cardiovascular Survey Methods* 2nd edn. Geneva: WHO Monograph series no. 56.

Rosenfield, P.L. 1979: The management of schistosomiasis. *Resources for the Future, RFF Research Paper R-16* Washington.

————, Smith, R.A. and Wolman, M.G. 1977: Development and verification of a schistosomiasis transmission model. *American J. Trop. Med. and Hyg. 26*, 505–16.

————, Golladay, F. and Davidson, R.K. 1984: The economics of parasitic diseases: research priorities. *Soc. Sci. Med. 19*, 1117–26.

Rothenberg, R.B. 1983: The geography of gonorrhea: empirical demonstration of core group transmission. *American J. Epidem. 117*, 688–94.

Rotimi, V.O. and Duerden, B.I. 1981: The development of bacterial flora in normal neonates. *J. Med. Microbiol. 14*, 51–62.

Roundy, R.W. 1978a: Toilet facilities in peninsular Malaysia: hazards from faecal-borne diseases for the populace. In D.S.K. Tan (ed.) *Current concept in the diagnosis and treatment of parasitic and other tropical diseases in South East Asia.* SEAMED Regional Tropical Medicine and Public Health Project, pp. 183–97.

———— 1978b: A model for combining human behavior and disease ecology to assess disease hazard in a community: rural Ethiopia as a model. *Soc. Sci. Med. 12*, 121–30.

———— 1985: Clean water provision in rural areas of less developed countries. *Soc. Sci. Med. 20*, 293–300.

Roy, B.K. 1984: Causes of death statistics: a transformation approach in geographic pathology. *Indian Geog. J. 59*, 67–85.

Roy, D. 1982: Breast cancer in developing countries. *Med. Digest 8*, 5–14.

Russell, J. 1986: *Coronary Heart Disease and Asians in Britain.* London: Coronary Prevention Group.

Sabin, A.B. 1981: Paralytic poliomyelitis: old dogmas and new perspectives. *Reviews Infect. Dis. 3*, 543–64.

Sahel Bibliographic Bulletin 1977: Selected post-1970 publications of Sahelian interest at the Office de la Recherche Scientifique et Technique Outre-Mer (ORSTOM) *1*, 23–32.

Sakamoto-Momiyama, M. 1977: *Seasonality in Human Mortality.* Tokyo: University of Tokyo Press.

_____ 1978: Changes in the seasonality of human mortality: a medico-geographical study. *Soc. Sci. Med. 12D*, 29–42.

Sakya, G.M. 1981: Present status of malaria in Nepal. *J. Nepalese Med. Assoc. 19*, 21–8.

Samadi, A.R., Huq, M.I., Shahid, N., Khan, M.U., Eurof, A., Rahman, A.S.M.M., Yunus, M. and Faruque, A.S.G. 1983: Classical *Vibrio cholerae* biotype displaces El Tor in Bangladesh. *Lancet* i (9 Apr.), 805–7.

Sanderson, F.H. 1975: The great food fumble. *Science 188*(4188), 503–9.

Sarre, P. 1978: The diffusion of Dutch elm disease. *Area 10*, 81–8.

Sasaki, O., Karoji, Y., Kuroda, A., Karaki, T., Takenokuma, K. and Maeda, O. 1982: Protection of pigs against mosquito-borne Japanese encephalitis virus by vaccination with a live attenuated vaccine. *Antiviral Res. 2*, 355–60.

Sathe, B.D., Mukerji, S., Gaitonde, B.B. and Renapurkar, D.M. 1981: Reinvestigation of an old focus of schistosomiasis in Gimvi village, District Ratnagiri in Maharashtra State, India. *Bull. Haffkine Inst. 9*, 34–7.

Sauer, H.I. 1962: Epidemiology of cardiovascular mortality – geographic and ethnic. *American J. Public Health 52*, 94–105 and later papers.

Schad, G.A. and Anderson, R.M. 1985: Predisposition to hookworm infection in humans. *Science USA 228* (28 June), 1537–40.

Schaller, K.F. and Kuls, W. 1972: *Ethiopia*. Geomedical monograph series, Regional studies in geographical medicine 3. Berlin: Springer.

Schulpen, T.W.J. 1982: Rickets, back in the Netherlands. *Nederlands Tijdschr. v. Geneeskunde 126*, 610–13.

Schwartz, D.A. 1981: Helminths in the induction of cancer II. *Schistosoma haematobium* and bladder cancer. *Trop. and Geog. Med. 33*, 1–7.

Schwarz, E., Freese, U.K., Gissman, L., Mayer, W., Roggenbuck, B., Stremlau, A. and Hausen, H.Z. 1985: Structure and transcription of human papilloma virus sequences in cervical carcinoma cells. *Nature 314* (7 Mar.), 111–14.

Schwefel, D. 1986: Unemployment, health and health services in German-speaking countries. *Soc. Sci. Med. 22*, 409–30.

Schweinfurth, U. 1979: Regional studies – the importance of geoecological and geomedical analysis and synthesis: Ceylon (Sri Lanka). In H.J. Jusatz (ed.) *Geomedizin in Forschung und Lehre*. Wiesbaden: Franz Steiner, pp. 88–96.

_____ 1983: Filarial diseases in Ceylon: a geographic and historical analysis. *Ecol. of Dis. 2*, 309–19.

_____ 1984: Filariasis in Ceylon: its distribution and historical analysis. *Geog. Zeitschr. 72*, 113–28.

Scott, E.P. (ed.) 1984: *Life before the Drought*. London: George Allen and Unwin.

Selya, R.M. 1980: Deaths due to accidents in Taiwan: a possible indication of development. *Soc. Sci. Med. 14D*, 361–8.

Sembajwe, I.S.L. 1983: Socioeconomic factors affecting mortality in rural Tanzania. *J. Biosocial Sci. 15*, 487–500.

Sen, A.K. 1981: *Poverty and famines*. Geneva: International Labour Office (and see N. Black et al. (eds) 1984, pp. 83–8).

Serenius, F., Elidrissy, A. and Dandona, P. 1984: Vitamin D nutrition in pregnant women at term and in newly born babies in Saudi Arabia. *J. Clin. Path. 37*, 444–7.

Service, M.W. 1980: *A Guide to Medical Entomology*. London: Macmillan.

Serwadda, D., Mugerwa, R.D., Sewankambo, N.K., Lwegata, A., Carswell, J.W., Kirya, G.B., Bayley, A.C., Downing, R.G., Tedder, R.S., Claydon, S.A., Weiss, R.A. and Dalgleish, A.G. 1985: Slim disease: a new disease in Uganda and its association with HTLV-III infection. *Lancet* ii (19 Oct.), 849–52.

Serzhanov, O.S., Aubakirov, S.A., Fomushkin, V., Ageev, V.S. and Turkpenbaev, N. Zh. 1982: Typing of the Central Asian group of desert plague foci by levels of the hydrothermic coefficient. *Med. Parazit. i Parazitarnya Bol. 60/4,* 46–50.

Shabad, L.M., Khesina, A.Ya., Solenova, L.G., Dikun, P.P., Kalinina, I.A., Engst, R. and Fritz, V. 1982: Comparative studies of contamination of vegetable food with polycyclic aromatic hydrocarbons in the USSR and German Democratic Republic. *Voprosy Pitaniya* (1) 56–9.

Shah, F.H., Begum, N., Adil, R. and Sheikh, A.S. 1981: Aflatoxins in food and feedstuffs. *Pakistan J. Med. Res. 20*, 40–3.

Shannon, G.W. and Dever, G.E.A. 1974: *Health Care Delivery: spatial perspectives*. New York: McGraw Hill.

———— and Spurlock, C.W. 1976: Urban ecological containers, environmental risk cells and the use of medical services. *Econ. Geog. 52*, 171–80.

———— and Cromley, R.G. 1980: The great plague of London. *Urban Geog. 1*, 254–70.

Sharaf, A.T. 1968: A geographical assessment of health problems and disease incidence in the Sudan. *Geographia Medica 3*, 30–106.

Sharif, M. 1951: The spread of plague in Southern and Central Divisions of Bombay Province and plague endemic centres in the Indo-Pakistan subcontinent. *Bull. WHO 4*, 75–109.

Sharma, S.P., Biswas, H., Das, M. and Dwivedi, S.R. 1983: Present status of the filariasis problem in India. *J. Communicable Dis. 15*, 53–60.

Sharma, V.P., Uprety, H.C., Nanda, N., Raina, V.K., Parida, S.K. and Gupta, W.K. 1982a: Impact of DDT spraying on malaria transmission in villages with resistant *Anopheles culicifacies*. *Indian J. Malariol. 19*, 5–12.

———— and Mehrotra, K.N. 1982b: Return of malaria. *Nature 210* (8 July), 210 (correspondence).

Sherlock, S. (ed.) 1980: Virus hepatitis. *Clinics in gastroenterology 9*, 1–228.

Shigematsu, I. 1978 Vol. I; 1979 Vol. II: *Atlas of Cardiovascular Mortality for Cities, Towns and Villages in Japan 1969–74*. Tokyo: Daiwa Health Foundation.

Shortridge, K.F. and Stuart-Harris C.H. 1982: An influenza epicentre? *Lancet* ii (9 Oct.), 812–3.

Shoshin, A.A. 1962: *Principles of Medical Geography*. Moscow/Leningrad: Academy of Sciences of the USSR.

Shute, P.G. 1954: Indigenous *P. vivax* malaria in London believed to have been transmitted by *Anopheles plumbeus*. Monthly Bull. Ministry of Health and Public Health Lab. Service *13* (March), 48–51.

Sidney M. Cantor Associates Inc. Haverford, Penn.19041. 1973: *The Tamil Nadu Nutrition Survey Vols. I and II A, B, C, D, E*. Report to the US Agency for International Development Contract No. AID/ness-399 Mission to India.

Singh, B.P. and Singh, R.P.B. 1980: Spatial pattern of thyroid disorder – goitre – in eastern Uttar Pradesh, India: a geomedical analysis. *Geographia Medica* *10*, 61–85.

Singh, C.M. 1980: The problem of rabies in India. *Health and Popul. Perspect. and Issues 3*, 215–23.

Singh, S. and Dutta, H.M. 1981: Smallpox pattern and its correlates: a case study of an Indian city. *GeoJournal 5*, 77–82.

Singla, P.N., Agarwal, K.N., Singh, R.M., Reddy, E.C.G., Tripathi, A.M. and Aggarwal, D.K. 1980: Deficiency anaemias in schoolchildren: estimation of prevalence based on response to haematinic supplementation. *J. Trop. Pediatrics 26*, 239–42.

Slack, P. 1981: The disappearance of plague: an alternative view. *Econ. Hist. Rev. 34*, 469–76.

Smart, R.G., Natera, G. and Bonilla, J.A. 1980: A trial of a new method for studying drinking and drinking problems in three countries of the Americas. *Bull. Pan American Health Organ. 14*, 318–26.

Smith, C.J. 1978: Recidivism and community adjustment amongst former mental patients. *Soc. Sci. Med. 12*, 17–27.

——— 1985: The wrath of grapes: the health-related implications of changed American drinking habits. *Area 17*, 97–108.

Smith, R. 1982: Alcohol in the Third World: a chance to avoid a miserable trap. *British Med. J. 284* (16 Jan.), 183–5.

Snow, J. 1849, 1855, reprinted 1936: *Snow on Cholera* with a biographical note by B.W. Richardson and an introduction by W.H. Frost. New York: The Commonwealth Fund/London: Humphrey Milford, Oxford University Press.

Snow, W.F. 1983: Mosquito production and species succession from an area of irrigated rice fields in The Gambia, West Africa. *J. Trop. Med. and Hyg. 86*, 237–45.

Sobo, A.O. 1984: Comparative study of the age standardized cancer ratio (ASCAR) in Liberia, Cameroon and the Moshe district of Tanzania. *Public Health 98*, 216–24.

Social Science and Medicine 1980: Health problems in Australia and New Zealand. *140*, 81–269.

——— 1983a: Geomedical problems in Africa. *17*, 525–616.

——— 1983b: Ocular needs in Africa. *17*, 1683–1830.

——— 1983c: Health and development with special reference to Africa. *17*, 1945–2043.

——— 1985: Developments in France. *20*, 119–80.

——— 1986a: Medical sociology and the WHO's programme for Europe. *22*, 113–284.

——— 1986b: Health problems in southern Africa. *22*, 737–90.

——— 1986c: The resurgence and eradication of malaria. *22*, 835–86.

Sokolova, L.V. and Volegova, K.V. 1980: Changes in the population density of *Anopheles messeae* in the Moscow region after discontinuation of DDT treatment, as exemplified by the Solnechnogorsk district. *Med. Parazit. i. Parazitarnye Bol. 49/4*, 68–9.

Solon, F.S., Popkin, B.M., Fernandez, T.K. and Latham, M.C. 1980: Control of vitamin A deficiency in the Philippines – a pilot project. *Food and Nutr.* 6/2, 27–36, 43.

Sommer, A. 1982a: *Field guide to the detection and control of xerophthalmia.* Geneva: WHO.

———— 1982b: *Nutritional Blindness, Xerophthalmia and Keratomalacia.* New York: Oxford University Press.

————, Tarwotjo, I., Hussaini, G., Susanto, T. and Soegiharto, T. 1981: Incidence, prevalence and scale of blinding malnutrition. *Lancet* i (27 June), 1407–8.

Sondel, D.P. 1983: Road safety: putting people first. *World Health Forum 4,* 167–8.

Sorre, M. 1951: *Les fondements de la géographie humaine. Tome premier, Les fondements biologiques: essai d'une écologie de l'homme.* Ch.1, Livre VIII. Les complexes pathogènes. Paris: Armand Colin.

Southgate, B.A. 1984: Recent advances in the epidemiology and control of filarial infections including entomological aspects of transmission. *Trans. Roy. Soc. Trop. Med. and Hyg.* 78 (supplement), 19–28.

South Pacific Commission 1982: Regional workshop on hepatitis, Noumea 9–12 Jun 1981. Noumea, New Caledonia, pp. 1–70.

Souza, R.C. 1982: Forecasting the progress of epidemics by means of a Bayesian-entropy framework. *Env. and Planning A14,* 49–60.

Spruit, I.P. 1982: Unemployment and health in macrosocial analysis. *Soc. Sci. Med. 16,* 1903–17.

Srinivasan, H. 1984: Models for leprosy: an appraisal of graphic representation of the 'spectrum' concept as models and a suggestion for a catastrophe theory model for leprosy. *International J. Leprosy 52,* 402–13.

Staessen, J., Fagard, R., Lijnen, P., Amory, A., Bulpitt, C. and Joossens, J.V. 1981: Salt and blood pressure in Belgium. *J. Epidem. and Commun. Health 35,* 256–61.

Staluppi, G. 1983: Diffusione e caratteri geografici della malattie veneree in ambiente montano: il caso del Trentino. In IGU Working Group on the Geography of Health 1983, pp. 547–62.

Stampfer, H., Reymond, J., Burvill, P.W. and Carlson, J. 1984: The relationship between distance from inpatient facilities and the rate of psychiatric admissions in Western Australia. *Soc. Sci. Med. 19,* 879–84.

Stanfield, J. and Galazka, A. 1984: Neonatal tetanus in the world today. *Bull. WHO 62,* 647–90.

Stanley, N.F. and Joske, R.A. (eds) 1980: *Changing Disease Patterns and Human Behaviour.* London: Academic Press.

Stenkvist, B., Bergström, R., Eklund, G. and Fox, C.H. 1984: Papanicolaou smear screening and cervical cancer. What can you expect? *J. American Med. Assoc.* 252, 1423–6.

Stephens, W.P., Klimiuk, P.S., Warrington, S., Taylor, J.L., Berry, J.L. and Mawer, E.B. 1982: Observations on the natural history of vitamin D deficiency amongst Asian immigrants. *Quart. J. Med. 51,* 171–88.

Stephenson, L.S., Crompton, D.W.T., Latham, M.C., Schulpen, T.W.J., Nesheim, M.C. and Jansen, A.A.J. 1980: Relationships between *Ascaris* infection and growth of malnourished preschool children in Kenya. *American J. Clin. Nutr. 33*, 1165–72.

Steudler, F. 1986: The state and health in France. *Soc. Sci. Med. 22*, 211–21.

Stevens, R.G., Moolgavkar, S.H. and Lee, J.A.H. 1982: Temporal trends in breast cancer. *American J. Epidem. 115*, 759–77.

Stewart, G.J., Taylor, J.P.P., Cunningham, A.L., Barr, J.A., Driscoll, G.L., Gold, J. and Lamont, B.J., 1986: Transmission of human T-cell lymphotropic virus type III (HTLV III) by artificial insemination by donor. *Lancet* ii (14 Sep.) 581–5.

Stock, R.F. 1976: Cholera in Africa: diffusion of the disease 1970–75, with special reference to West Africa. *African Environment Special Report 3*, International African Institute.

_____ 1981: Traditional healers in rural Hausaland. *GeoJournal 5*, 363–8.

Stocks, P. 1936, 1937, 1939: Distribution in England and Wales of cancers of various organs. *Annual Reports, British Empire Cancer Campaign*, pp. 239–80, 198–223, 308–43.

Stott, H. and Gupta, S.P. 1930–31: The distribution and cause of endemic goitre in the United Provinces. *Indian J. Med. Res. 18*, 1059–85.

Strassburg, M. 1982: The global eradication of smallpox. *American J. Infect. Control 19*, 53–9.

Strode, G.K. 1951: *Yellow Fever*. New York: McGraw Hill.

Strong, J.A. and Blaxter, K. (chairmen) 1982: Travel, disease and other hazards. *Proc. Roy. Soc. Edinburgh 82B*, 1–144.

Sturrock, R.G. 1982a: Comment on J.F.M. Nguma et al. (1982). *Trop. Dis. Bull. 79*, no. 2543, 889.

_____ 1982b: Comment on P.T. White et al. (1982). *Trop. Dis. Bull. 79* no. 2768, 957–8.

_____ 1982c: Comment on K.C. Haddock (1982). *Trop. Dis. Bull. 79* no. 2774, 961.

_____ 1982d: Comment on F. DeWolfe Miller et al. (1981). *Trop. Dis. Bull. 79* no. 2769, pp. 958–9.

Sugiura, Y. 1977: Spatial diffusion of Spanish influenza in Japan 1916–26. *Geog. Rev. Japan 50*, 201–15.

Sukhatme, P.V. 1977: Incidence of undernutrition. *Indian J. Agr. Econs 32*, 1–7.

Susser, M. 1973: *Causal Thinking in the Health Sciences*. New York, London: Oxford University Press.

Swift, J. 1977: Desertification and man in the Sahel. *African Environment Special Report 5*, 171–8.

Takahashi, E. 1967: Geographic distribution of mortality rate from cerebrovascular disease in European countries. *Tohoku J. Exper. Med. 92*, 345–78.

_____ 1978: *Ecologic Human Biology*. Medical Information Service (Japan).

_____ 1981: Geographic distribution of cerebrovascular disease and environmental factors in Japan. *Soc. Sci. Med. 15D*, 163–72.

Tandon, B.N., Gupta, H., Irshad, M., Joshi, Y.K. and Chawla, T.C. 1984: Associated infection with non-A non-B virus as a possible cause of liver failure in Indian HBV carriers. *Lancet* ii (29 Sep.), 750–1 (correspondence).

Tarrant, J.R. 1980: The geography of food aid. *Trans. Inst. British Geogrs 5*, 125–40.

Taylor, P. and Pugh, A. 1982: Plague in Zimbabwe: a review of the situation in 1982. *Central African J. Med. 28*, 249–53.

Taylor, R., Parker, M., Ansford, A. and Davison, A. 1983: Cancer in Solomon Islands 1970–82. *Papua New Guinea Med. J. 26*, 102–10.

Tayo, M.A., Pugh, R.N.H. and Bradley, A.K. 1980: Malumfashi Endemic Diseases Research Project XI Water-contact activities in the schistosomiasis study area. *Ann. Trop. Med. and Parasit. 74*, 347–54.

Tedder, R.S. and O'Connor, T. 1987: HIV–2 in UK (correspondence). *The Lancet 1* (11 Apr.), 869.

Tedesco, L.R. 1980: Trachoma and environment in the Northern Territory of Australia. *Soc. Sci. Med. 14D*, 111–17.

Teilhard de Chardin 1960: *The Phenomenon of Man*. London: Collins.

Thambypillai, V. 1985: Smoking among urban Malaysian schoolchildren. *Soc. Sci. Med. 21*, 819–23.

The East Midland Geographer 1986: The geography of health and health care in the East Midlands. 9, iii and 1–60.

Thévenin, G.F. 1983: *L'evénement alcool dans le parcours migratoire*. Paris: La Documentation Française.

Thouez, J.-P. 1978: La dureté de l'eau potable et le mortalité cérébrale vasculaire dans l'Est du Québec. *Bull. Assoc. Géog. Français 451*, 115–23.

―――― 1979: Physicochemical characteristics of drinking water and death from ischaemic heart disease: application to the Eastern Townships, Quebec. *Canadian Geog. 23*, 308–21.

――――, Beauchamp, Y. and Simard, A. 1981a: Cancer and physicochemical quality of drinking water in Quebec. *Soc. Sci. Med. 15D*, 213–23.

―――― and Munan, L. 1981b: Obesity and regional space. *Geographica Medica 11*, 86–94.

Thouvenot, C. 1978: Studies in food geography in France. *Soc. Sci. Med. 12*, 43–54.

Tildon, J.T., Roeder, L.M. and Steinschneider, A. (eds) 1983: *Sudden Infant Death Syndrome*. London: Academic Press.

Timmer, C.P. 1977: Access to food: the ultimate determinant of hunger. *Ann. New York Acad. Sci. 300*, 59–68.

Tinline, R. 1982: The epizootiology and control of rabies in southern Ontario. *Geographia Medica 12*, 150 (abstract only).

―――― and Bond, P. 1981: The uses of a geographical information system: a mini-computer example. *Geoscope 12*, 13–19.

Tkacheva, M.N., Lobanova, E.A. and Atakian, R.V. 1981: Viral hepatitis as an actual world health problem. *Zhurnal Mikrobiol. Epidem. i Immunobiol. 9*, 6–13.

Todson, D.R. 1980: Spatial perspectives of infant health care: the distribution of infant health care facilities in Hillsborough County, Florida. *Soc. Sci. Med. 14D*, 379–87.

Tolley, H.D., Burdick, D., Manton, K.G. and Stallard, E. 1978: A compartment model approach to the estimation of tumor incidence and growth: investigation of a model of cancer latency. *Biometrics 34*, 377–89.

Toupet, C. 1977: The great drought in Mauretania. *African Environment Special Report* 6, 109–13.

Townsend, P., Phillimore, P. and Beattie, A. 1986: *Inequalities in health in the Northern Region.* Northern Regional Health Authority, Newcastle-upon-Tyne/ University of Bristol.

Tran Ba Loc, P. 1976: Transmission experimentale du virus oncogène VT4 par des larves d'*Aëdes aegypti* élevées en milieu de culture. *Méd. Biol. Env.* 4 (Jan.–Juin), 64–5.

_____ 1981: Pollution de l'eau et cancers. *Méd. Biol. Env.* 9 (Juill.–Déc.), 11–14.

Transactions of the Royal Society of Tropical Medicine and Hygiene. 1980: Symposium on schistosomiasis in the Sudan. *74*, 557–64.

Trivedi, C.R. 1981: Profile of dog bites, rabies and default in antirabic immunisation at V.S.G. Hospital, Ahmedabad. *J. Indian Med. Assoc. 76*, 134–6.

Tromp, S.W. 1973: The relationship of weather and climate to health and disease. In G.M. Howe and J.A. Loraine (eds) 1973, pp. 72–99.

_____ 1976: A review of possible effects of soil, water and meteorological factors on cancer. *Méd. Biol. Env.* 4 (Jan.–Juin), 66–74.

Trop. Dis. Bull. especially 1978, 75 onwards; a general source.

Trowell, H.C., Davies, J.N.P. and Dean, R.F.A. 1954: *Kwashiorkor.* London: Arnold.

_____ and Burkitt, D.P. 1981: *Western Diseases: their emergence and prevention.* London: Arnold.

Tulchinsky, D. and Modan, B. 1967: Epidemiological aspects of cancer of the stomach in Israel. *Cancer 20*, 1311–17.

Tuomilehto, J. and Wolf, E. (eds) 1984: Proceedings of the symposium on diet and primary prevention of hypertension. *Ann. Clin. Res. 16* (Suppl. 43), 1–183.

Tuyns, A.J. 1983: Oesophageal cancer in non-smoking drinkers and in non-drinking smokers. *International J. Cancer 32*, 443–4.

_____, Péquignot, G., Gignoux, G. and Valla, A. 1982: Cancers of the digestive tract, alcohol and tobacco. *International J. Cancer 30*, 9–11.

Tymowski, M. 1978: Famines and epidemics at Qualata and Tichit in the 19th century. *Africana Bull. 27*, 35–53.

Tyndall, R.M. 1983: *Patterns of cardiovascular disease mortality in Greater Glasgow.* University of Strathclyde, PhD Thesis.

United Nations Children's Fund 1984: *The State of the World's Children.* Oxford: Oxford University Press.

_____ Department of International Social and Economic Affairs 1982: *Levels and trends of mortality since 1950: a joint study by the UN and the WHO.* New York: United Nations.

Usmanov, M.K. and Glinyanova, L.M. 1982: Meningococcal infection in the Uzbek SSR. *Zhurnal Mikrobiol Epidem. i Immunobiol. 7*, 30–4.

van Heyningen, W.E. and Seal, J.R. 1983: *Cholera: the American Scientific Experience 1947–1980.* Essex UK: Bowker Publishing.

van Poppel, F.W.A. 1981: Regional mortality differences in western Europe: a review of the situation in the seventies. *Soc. Sci. Med. 15D*, 341–52.

van Rensburg, S.J. 1985: Recent studies on the etiology of oesophageal cancer. *South African Cancer Bull. 29*, 22–31.

———, Cook-Mozaffari, P., van Schalkwyk, D.J., van der Watt, J.J., Vincent, T.J. and Purchase, I.F. 1985: Hepatocellular cancer and dietary aflatoxin in Mozambique and Transkei. *British J. Cancer 51*, 713–26.

Vaskilampi, T. and MacCormack, C.P. (eds) 1982: *Folk medicine and health culture: role of folk medicine in modern health care.* Proceedings of Nordic Research Symposium 27–28 Aug. 1981. Kuopio, Finland: University of Kuopio, 1–261.

Velimirovic, B. 1984a: *Infectious diseases in Europe: a fresh look.* Copenhagen: WHO Regional Office for Europe.

——— 1984b: Traditional medicine is not primary health care: a polemic. *Courare 7*, 61–79, 85–93 and comments 95–102.

Vellar, O.D. 1964: Acute viral hepatitis in Norwegian track finders: an epidemiological study in Norway. *Acta Med. Scandinavia 176*, 651–5.

Verhasselt, Y. 1976: Some aspects of geocancerology. *Méd. Biol. Env. 4* (Jan.–Juin), 75–7.

——— 1981: Geography of stomach cancer in Belgium: an approach. *Geographia Medica 11*, 104–15.

——— 1985: Recent trends in cancer mortality in Belgium. IBG/AAG symposium on medical geography, University of Nottingham, July.

——— and Logie, F. 1984: Geography of nutrition in Belgium: a preliminary analysis. *Géosanté Symposium 1984*, 370–80.

Vérin, Ph. and Peyresblanques, J. 1983: Un modèle géographique médical: la pathologie ophthalmique au Viet Nam. In CEGET 1983, pp. 39–41.

Vijayaraghavan, K., Rameshwar Sarma, K.V., Pralhad Rao, N. and Reddy, V. 1984: Impact of massive doses of vitamin A on incidence of nutritional blindness. *Lancet* ii (21 July), 149–50.

Vincent, P., Dubois, G. and Leclerc, H. 1983: Nitrate in drinking water and cancer mortality: epidemiological study in the north of France. *Rev. d'Epidem. et de Santé Publique 31*, 199–207.

Vrijens, N. 1982: Trends in mortality from diseases of the circulatory system and cancer by site in Antwerp, Belgium 1900–75. *Soc. Sci. Med. 16*, 293–302.

Waaler, H.T. and Sterky, G. 1984: What is the best indicator of health care? *World Health Forum 5*, 276–9.

Waddington, J.I. 1983: The International Drinking Water Supply and Sanitation Decade in Europe. *J. Roy. Soc. Health 103*, 21–4.

Walker, A.R.P. 1980: The epidemiology of ischaemic heart disease in the different ethnic populations in Johannesburg. *South African Med. J. 57*, 748–52.

Walker, W.J. 1983: Changing US life style and declining vascular mortality – retrospective. *New England J. Med. 308*, 649–51 (editorial).

Wang Yaobin, Lan Lizun, Ye Benfa, Xu Yaochu, Liu Yunyuan and Li Wenguang 1983: Relation between geographical distribution of liver cancer and climate – aflatoxin B_1 in China. *Scientia Sinica* Series B 26, 1166–75.

Ward, R.H. 1980: Genetic epidemiology: promise or compromise? *Soc. Biol. 27*, 87–100.

Warren, H.V. 1972: Variations in the trace element contents of some vegetables. *J. Roy. Coll. General Practitioners 22*, 56–60.

———— 1973: Some trace element concentrations in various environments. In G.M. Howe and J.A. Loraine (eds) 1973, pp. 9–24.

Wasserstrom, R. and Chapin, G. 1982: Malaria resurgence. *Nature 299* (7 Oct.), 482 (correspondence).

Waterhouse, J.A.H. 1985: International epidemiology of cancer. *J. Roy. Coll. Phys. London 19*, 10–22.

Waterhouse, J., Muir, C., Shanmugaratnam, K. and Powell, J. (eds) 1982: Cancer incidence in five continents. Vol. IV. *IARC Scientific Pubn. no. 42*, 1–812.

Waterlow, J.C. 1982: Nutrient needs for man in different environments. In K. Blaxter and L. Fowden (eds), London: Applied Science Publishers, pp. 271–86.

———— 1984a: Kwashiorkor revisited: the pathogenesis of oedema in kwashiorkor and its significance. *Trans. Roy. Soc. Trop. Med. and Hyg. 78*, 436–41.

———— 1984b: Comment on Dixon et al. (1982). *Trop. Dis. Bull. 81* (922), 228–9.

————, Ashworth, A. and Griffiths, M. 1980: Faltering in infant growth in less developed countries. *Lancet* ii (29 Nov.), 1176–8.

Waterston, T. 1982: What causes kwashiorkor in the older child? *J. Trop. Pediatrics 28*, 132–4.

Watts, S.J. 1984: Population mobility, urban development and dracunculiasis in Kwara State, Nigeria. *Soc. Sci. Med. 19*, 471–3.

Weatherall, M. 1982: An end to the search for new drugs? *World Health Forum 3*, 409–13.

Webb, A. and Steven, M. 1985: Solar ultraviolet radiation and the production of vitamin D. IBG/AAG symposium on medical geography, University of Nottingham, July.

Webber, R.H. and Southgate, B.A. 1981: The maximum density of anopheline mosquitoes that can be permitted in the absence of continuing transmission of filariasis. *Trans. Roy. Soc. Trop. Med. and Hyg. 75*, 499–506.

Weil, C. and Kvale, K.M. 1985: Current research on geographical aspects of schistosomiasis. *Geog. Rev. 75*, 186–216.

Wellmer, H., in collaboration with H.J. Jusatz 1981: Geoecological analysis of the spread of tick-borne encephalitis in central Europe. *Soc. Sci. Med. 15D*, 159–62.

———— 1983: *Dengue haemorrhagic fever in Thailand: geomedical observations on developments over the period 1970–79*. Berlin: Springer/Heidelberger Akademie der Wissenschaften, pp. 1–40.

———— 1984: Dengue haemorrhagic fever in Thailand. *Indian Geog. J. 59*, 6–9.

WER (*Weekly Epidemiological Record*) 1980: Yellow Fever in 1979. *55*, 345–51, 355–60.

———— 1981a: Endemic treponematoses. *56*, 241–4.

———— 1981b: Surveillance of meningococcal meningitis. *56*, 225–6.

———— 1982a: Yaws and yellow fever surveillance. *57*, 142.

———— 1982b: Plague surveillance. *57*, 262–3.

———— 1983: Orthopox surveillance: post-smallpox eradication policy. *58*, 149–54.

420   References

_____ 1984a: Xerophthalmia surveillance: prevalence of xerophthalmia in Lombok. *59*, 129–30.

_____ 1984b: Nutritional surveillance: global trends in protein–energy malnutrition. *59*, 189–92.

_____ 1985a: Acquired immune deficiency syndrome (AIDS): report on the situation in Europe as of 30 June 1985. *60*, 305–12.

_____ 1985b: Dracunculiasis: global surveillance summary. *60*, 61–5.

Wheeler, E.F. 1981: Comment on Popkin et al. (1980), *Trop. Dis. Bull.* 78, no. 671, p. 300.

White, P.T., Coleman, M. and Jupp, B.P. 1982: Swamp rice development, schistosomiasis and onchocerciasis in southeast Sierra Leone. *American J. Trop. Med. and Hyg. 31*, 490–8.

Whitehead, M. 1987: *The Health Divide: Inequalities in health in the 1980s*. London, Health Education Council. A review commissioned by the HEC.

Whitelegg, J. 1982: *Inequalities in Health Care*. Retford, Nottinghamshire: Straw Barnes.

_____ 1985: A geography of road accidents. IBG/AAG symposium on medical geography, University of Nottingham, July.

Whitfield, D., Curtis, C.F., White, G.B., Targett, G.A.T., Warhurst, D.C. and Bradley, D.J. 1984: Two cases of falciparum malaria acquired in Britain. *British Med. J. 289* (8 Dec.), 1607–9.

Whittle, H.C., Mee, J., Werblinska, J., Yakuba, A., Onuora, C. and Gomwalk, N. 1980: Immunity to measles in malnourished children. *Clin. and Exper. Immunology 42*, 144–51.

_____, Brown, C.J., Marshall, K., Greenwood, B.M., Seidelen, P., Tighe, H. and Wedderburn, L. 1984: T-cell control of Epstein-Barr virus is lost during *Plasmodium falciparum* malaria. *Nature 312* (29 Nov.), 449–50.

WHO (World Health Organization) 1960: Endemic goitre. *WHO Monograph Series no. 44.* Geneva: WHO.

_____ 1979a: *Schizophrenia, an international follow-up study*. Geneva: WHO/New York: Wiley.

_____ 1979b: *Guidelines for programmes for the prevention of blindness*. Geneva: WHO.

_____ 1980: *Towards a better future: maternal and child health*. Geneva: WHO.

_____ 1981: *Health services in Europe 3rd edn. Vol. I Regional analysis, Vol. 2 Country review and statistics*. Copenhagen: WHO Regional Office for Europe.

_____ 1983: *Apartheid and Health*. Geneva: WHO.

_____ 1984a: Control of oral cancer in developing countries. *Bull. WHO 62*, 817–30.

_____ 1984b: *Strategies for the prevention of blindness in national programmes: a primary health care approach*. Geneva: WHO.

_____ 1984c: Recent progress in the development of malaria vaccines: memorandum from a WHO meeting. *Bull. WHO 62*, 715–27.

_____ 1984d: *Lymphatic filariasis*. Fourth report of the Expert Committee on Filariasis.

_____ 1985: *Informal consultation on the development of* Bacillus sphaericus *as a microbial larvicide*. UNDP/World Bank/WHO SPRT Trop. Dis. TDR/BCV/Sphaericus/85.3.

—— 1987 *Vaccination certificate requirements and health advice for international travel*. Geneva: WHO.

WHO Chronicle 1978: Malaria control – a reoriented strategy. *32*, 226–30.

—— 1980: The inequality of death: assessing socioeconomic influences on mortality. 34, 9–15.

WHO Environmental Health Criteria 1978: Nitrates, nitrites and N-nitroso compounds.

—— 1979: II. Mycotoxins.

WHO Malaria Action Programme 1986: World malaria situation 1984 *Wld Hlth Statist. Quart. 39*, 171–205.

WHO Scientific Working Group on Social and Economic Research 1983: *Community participation in tropical disease control*. TDR/SER-SWG(4) CP/83.3.

WHO Technical Report Series 1980: no. 643. Epidemiology and control of schistosomiasis pp. 1–63.

—— 1980: no. 650. Problems related to alcohol. Report of a WHO Expert Committee, pp. 1–72.

—— 1980: no. 654. Peripheral neuropathies. Report of a WHO study group, pp. 1–138.

—— 1980: no. 655. Resistance of vectors of disease to pesticides. Fifth report of the WHO expert committee on vector biology and control, pp. 1–82.

—— 1982: no. 671. Tuberculosis control. Report of a joint IUAT/WHO study group, Geneva 14–18 Sep. 1981, pp. 1–26.

—— 1982: no. 672. Control of vitamin A deficiency and xerophthalmia. Report of a joint WHO/UNICEF/USAID/Helen Keller International/IVACG meeting, pp. 1–70.

—— 1982: no. 674. Treponemal infections. Report of a WHO Scientific Group, pp. 1–75.

—— 1982: no. 678. Prevention of coronary heart disease. Report of a WHO expert committee, Geneva 30 Nov.–8 Dec. 1981, pp. 1–53.

—— 1982: no. 682. Bacterial and viral zoonoses, pp. 1–146.

WHO Working Group on Rickettsial Diseases 1982: Rickettsioses: a continuing disease problem. *Bull. WHO 60*, 157–64.

Whyte, K.F., Dunnigan, M.G. and McIntosh, W.B. 1982: Excessive beer consumption and beri-beri. *Scottish Med. J. 27*, 288–91.

Wickramasinghe, M.B. 1981: Malaria and its control in Sri Lanka. *Ceylon Med. J. 26*, 107–15.

Wilkins, H.A., Goll, P.G., Marshall, T.F. de C. and Moore, P.J. 1984: Dynamics of *Schistosoma haematobium* infection in a Gambian community. I The pattern of human infection in the study area. *Trans. Roy. Soc. Trop. Med. and Hyg. 78*, 216–21.

Willcox, R.R. 1977: Venereal diseases. In G.M. Howe (ed.) 1977, pp. 201–35.

—— 1980: Venereal diseases in the Pacific Islands, Papua New Guinea. *British J. Venereal Dis. 56*, 277–81.

—— 1981a: Sexual behaviour and sexually transmitted disease patterns in male homosexuals. *British J. Venereal Dis. 57*, 167–9.

—— 1981b: The rectum as viewed by the venereologist. *British J. Venereal Dis. 57*, 1–6.

Williams, A., O'Connor, G.T., de Thé, G.B. and Johnson, C.A. (eds) 1985:

Virus-associated Cancers in Africa. New York: Oxford University Press/IARC Scientific Pubn no. 63.

Wills, J.H. 1982: Nasal carcinoma in woodworkers: a review. *J. Occup. Med.* **24**, 526–30.

Wilson, A., Taylor, R., Nugumi, G., Cameron, I., Keke, L. and MacLennan, R. 1983: *Solomon Islands oral cancer study*. Noumea: South Pacific Commission, Technical Paper no. 183.

Wilson, M.G.A. 1978: The geographical analysis of small area/population death rates. *Australian Geog. Studies 16*, 149–60.

_____ 1979: Infant death in metropolitan Australia 1970–73. *Canadian Studies in Population 6*, 127–42.

Wilson, R.A. 1979: An Introduction to Parasitology. *Studies in biology no. 4*. London: Arnold.

Wingate, P. 1972: *The Penguin Medical Encyclopedia*. Harmondsworth: Penguin.

Winterstein, L. 1980: The correlation between the circulatory and cardiovascular diseases in the different communities in Israel and their countries of origin. *Geographia Medica 10*, 20–7.

Woodham-Smith, C. 1964: *The Great Hunger*. Harmondsworth: Penguin/New York: Signet.

Woodruff, A.W., Grant, J., El Bashir, E.A., Baya, E.I., Yugusuk, A.Z. and El Suni, A. 1984: Neonatal tetanus: mode of infection, prevalence, and prevention in southern Sudan. *Lancet* i (18 Feb.), 378–9.

Woodruff, G. 1957: Personal communication.

Woods, R. and Woodward, J. 1984: *Urban Disease and Mortality in Nineteenth Century England*. London: Batsford.

Working Group on Fortification of Salt with Iron 1982: Use of common salt fortified with iron in the control and prevention of anemia – a collaborative study. *American J. Clin. Nutr. 35*, 1442–51.

World Health Forum 1980: Mass screening in disease prevention (series). *1*, 87–116.

_____ 1981a: In Focus: The world's main health problems. *2*, 264–80.

_____ 1981b: Notes and news: an overview of health in New Zealand. *2*, 449–50.

_____ 1982a: Inequalities in health in the United Kingdom: report of a working group. *3*, 68–73.

_____ 1983: In Focus: Hepatitis. *4*, 135–41.

_____ 1984: Round table: coronary risk factors – should we not forget about mass control? (M. Oliver et al., *5*, 5–18; and see comment by J.T. Hart in *5*, 237–9).

_____ 1985: In Focus: Acquired immunodeficiency syndrome: the present situation. *6*, 30–4.

Worsley, P. 1982: Non-western medical systems. In *Annual Rev. of Anthrop.* vol. 11 (Annual Reviews Inc., Palo Alto), pp. 315–48.

Wretlind, A. 1982: Standards for nutritional adequacy of the diet: European and WHO/FAO viewponts. *American J. Clin. Nutr. 36*, 366–75.

Wrigley, E.A. and Schofield, R.S. 1981: *The Population of England 1541–1871: a reconstruction*. Cambridge: Cambridge University Press.

Wyke, J.A. 1981: Oncogenic viruses. *J. Path. 135*, 39–85.

Wyler, D.J. 1983: Malaria – resurgence, resistance and research. *New England J. Med.* *308*, 875–8, 934–40.

Xu, Z. and Su, D.L. 1984: *Schistosoma japonicum* and colorectal cancer: an epidemiological study in the People's Republic of China. *International J. Cancer 34*, 315–8.

Yamamoto, H. 1981: Arbovirus infections in the mosquitoes of Fukuoka area, Kyushu, Japan. 3 Natural infection of mosquitoes with Japanese encephalitis in the period from 1963 to 1972. *Japanese J. Sanitary Zool. 32*, 37–46.

Yanai, H., Inaba, Y., Takagi, H. and Yamamoto, S. 1979: Multivariate analysis of cancer mortality for selected sites in 24 countries. *Environmental Health Perspectives 32*, 83–101.

Yekutiel, P. 1980: Eradication of infectious diseases. A critical study. *Contributions to epidemiology and biostatistics vol. 2*. Basel: S. Karger, pp. 1–164.

_____ 1981: Lessons from the big eradication campaigns. *World Health Forum 2*, 465–8.

Ying, Y.Y., Yan, R.Q., Xu, B.D., Wang, L.X., Wang, Y.L. and Qian, Y.L. 1984: Relationship of hepatocellular carcinoma, liver cirrhosis, and hepatitis B virus: a pathologic study of 1069 autopsy cases in different areas of China. *Chinese Med. J. 97*, 758–64.

Yoshida, I., Takagi, M., Inokuma, E., Goda, H., Ono, K., Takaku, K. and Oku, J. 1981: Establishment of an attenuated ML-17 strain of Japanese encephalitis virus. *Biken J. 24*, 47–67.

Yu, M.C., Ho, J.H.C., Ross, R.K. and Henderson, B.E. 1981: Nasopharyngeal carcinoma in Chinese – salted fish or inhaled smoke? *Preventive Med. 10*, 15–24.

Yue, W., Lu, Z.Y. and Cai, C.Y. 1983: Longitudinal study of schistosomiasis in Nanzhang project area, Shanghai. *J. Parasit. and Parasitic Dis. 1*, 113–7.

Zakharova, N.F. 1983: A comparative evaluation of the influence of sterilization with bisavir and thiophosphamide on the sex activity of male mosquitoes. *Med. Parazit. i Parazitarnye Bol. 61*, 38–42.

Zaridze, D.G., Blettner, M., Trapeznikov, N.N., Kuvshinov, J.P., Matiakin, E.G., Poljakov, B.P., Poddubni, B.K., Parshikova, S.M., Rottenburg, V.I., Chamrakulov, F.S., Chodjaeva, M.C., Stich, H.F., Rosin, M.P., Thurnham, D.I., Hoffmann, D. and Brunnemann, K.D. 1985: Survey of a population with a high incidence of oral and oesophageal cancer. *International J. Cancer 36*, 153–8.

Zhang, S., Zhu, S. and Wu, J. 1980: Screening and prevention of colorectal cancer in Haining County. *Chinese Med. J. 93*, 843–8.

Zhao, E.-S, 1981: Cancer of the colon and schistosomiasis. *J. Roy. Soc. Med. 74*, 645.

Zhong, C. and Zheng, H. 1980: Studies on control of malayan filariasis in China. *Chinese Med. J. 93*, 537–44.

Zhong, H.L., He, L.Y. and Cao, W.J. 1981: Present situation of filariasis in China. *Chinese Med. J. 94*, 567–84.

Zhong, X.-L. 1982: Diabetes mellitus survey in China. *Chinese Med. J. 95*, 423–30.

Zhou, Z.J. 1981: The malaria situation in the People's Republic of China. *Bull.*

WHO 59, 931–6.

Zhuang, H., Coulepis, A.G., Zimmet, P., Taylor, R., Ram, P., Banuve, S. and Gust, I.D. 1982: Seroepidemiology of infection with hepatitis B virus in Fiji. *American J. Epidem. 116*, 608–16.

Ziegenfus, R.G. and Gesler, W.M. 1984: Geographical patterns of heart disease in the northeastern United States. *Soc. Sci. Med. 18*, 63–72.

Zinsser, H. 1935: *Rats Lice and History*. London: Routledge.

Zuckerman, A.J. 1982: Primary hepatocellular carcinoma and hepatitis B virus. *Trans. Roy. Soc. Trop. Med. and Hyg. 76*, 711–18.

_____ 1986a: AIDS in primates. *British Med. J. 292* (18 Jan.), 158.

_____ 1986b: AIDS and insects. *British Med. J. 292* (26 Apr.), 1094–5 (editorial).

Index of Authors

Only first authors are indexed. For second or subsequent authors please see list of references.

Index of Subjects

Figure numbers are in italics.

Acacia-Themeda plant association, 333
acarine mites, *see Leptotrombidium deliense*
accessibility, *see* health care
accidents, 19; alcohol and, 34, 35; alcohol
  and road a., 20, 33–4, 76, *4.6*;
  bystanders and, 34; children and
  cyclists, 34; distance from hospital, 34;
  home, 20; industrial 20; international
  comparisons 34 (Australia, USA,
  Kuwait); rural and urban 34
acquired immune deficiency syndrome, *see*
  AIDS
advertising, tobacco, 36
Aëdes aegypti, 132, 183, 220; *A.caspius*,
  132; *A.dorsalis* 132
aestivation, 208
aflatoxins, epidemics of 269; a. and
  kwashiorkor, 297; a. and liver cancer,
  104, 265, 269
Africa, cholera in, 176; East A., cancers,
  266, 274; food and famines, 293–4;
  goldminers in South A., cancers, 266;
  heart disease, black Africans in South
  A., 22; regional studies 326–8 (different
  scales, 326–8; Francophone, 328–9;
  Kenya, 326–34)
ageing, 11, 37–8; immune system and,
  277; "inverse interest law" and, 353;
  morbidity, compression of, in a., 38
age-structure, cohort risks, 48; groups at
  risk, 49
aggregate data, aggregative fallacy, 9, 124;
  see also ecology (ecological fallacy)

aggregation of administrative unit data,
  136
ague, marsh, 159, *8.11–14*
aid, food, *see* famine
AIDS (acquired immune deficiency
  syndrome), 4, 29–33; Africa, 32; anal
  intercourse, 31; behavioural change, 33;
  birth to infected mother, 32; central
  Africa, 32; diffusion, 4, 30, 32–3
  (Caribbean, Europe, 32; UK, USA, US
  cities); lymphomas, 275; milk,
  mother's, 32; monkeys 32–3; mucous
  membrane, vaginal 32; nomenclature of
  virus 30–1 (LAV II/HTLV III/HIV,
  HIV 1 and HIV 2?); oral intercourse,
  31; saliva, 32; social networks and, 33;
  Third World, 30, 32; transmission by
  arthropods (bed-bugs, mosquitoes)
  unlikely, 32; vaccine, 32; vaginal
  intercourse, 31
air, conditioning, 121; *see also* pollution
air travel, 115; airport malaria, 202
Akufo, Nigeria, 326
alcohol, 21, 35–6, 68, 163; cancers and,
  269, 271 (c. of the oesophagus, 271);
  France, general, ministerial report, 35
  (the Midi, and France, 340, the Midi
  341–4); malnutrition, 271, 300 ('specific
  overnutrition 300); Third World, 35;
  USA, Rand Report etc. 35; wine *cf*
  spirits 343
algae, 10; in water sources 316
American Geographical Society College